Perfectionism, Health, and Well-Being

Fuschia M. Sirois • Danielle S. Molnar
Editors

Perfectionism, Health, and Well-Being

Springer

Editors
Fuschia M. Sirois
Department of Psychology
University of Sheffield
Sheffield
United Kingdom

Danielle S. Molnar
Research Institute on Addictions
University at Buffalo, The State University of New York
Buffalo, NY
United States of America

Department of Psychology
Brock University
St. Catharines
Canada

ISBN 978-3-319-18581-1 ISBN 978-3-319-18582-8 (eBook)
DOI 10.1007/978-3-319-18582-8

Library of Congress Control Number: 2015944712

Springer Cham Heidelberg New York Dordrecht London

Printed on acid-free paper

Springer International Publishing AG Switzerland is part of Springer Science+Business Media (www.springer.com)

To my angels Domenic and Madeline,
for always believing in me; and to
Alice Cooper—I couldn't have done this
without you!

— Danielle Sirianni Molnar

To my husband, Mike,
for his never-ending support; and to my
girls, Cyan and Teala for reminding me to
take joy in the imperfections of life.

— Fuschia M. Sirois

Preface

The drive to improve oneself, to strive for the ideal, to seek better performance, and even higher standards, are in many ways the characteristics of the human condition. Indeed, this striving for betterment has served our species well and driven many great accomplishments throughout history. In today's performance-focused society, an unrelenting pursuit of ideal standards that leave no room for error, or perfectionism, is often revered with little consideration of its consequences. Understanding these consequences is becoming an increasingly important concern, especially in light of evidence that personality can confer risk or resilience for health-related outcomes. Whether we view perfectionism as a situationally bound quality induced by social or intra-psychic pressures for peak performance and flawless outcomes, or as an enduring tendency to have frequent cognitions about the attainment of ideal and often unrealistic standards, research has begun to highlight the ways in perfectionism may impact health and well-being.

The public health implications of perfectionism are evidenced by the growing body of research demonstrating that perfectionism, (i.e., the setting and striving for unrealistically high standards, often accompanied by harsh self-criticism) can have important consequences not only for mental health, but also for physical health and well-being. Yet, to date there are no books or edited volumes that provide a focused account of the different ways and domains in which perfectionism contributes to health and well-being, for better or worse. Our purpose for this edited volume was to address this surprising gap by presenting the latest theoretical and empirical perspectives from leading researchers in the perfectionism field on this important topic.

A significant limitation plaguing the perfectionism and health field is that aside from a few noteworthy exceptions, research on perfectionism and health has been largely atheoretical. To this end, a central goal in organizing this book was to include contributions that provide an overview of not only the most recent advances on this topic, but also those that present new conceptual models that may help further our understanding of when, how, and why perfectionism may be implicated in health and well-being. Collectively, these contributions provide in depth analyses and discussions of the specific mechanisms and processes that may render certain perfectionists particularly vulnerable to poor health and well-being, but leave other perfectionists less vulnerable to these same consequences.

Perfectionism is a topic that has relevance for not only scholars and researchers, but also for those who work therapeutically with people experiencing issues related to perfectionism, or who work in a setting in which perfectionism may be particularly rampant due to performance pressures and expectations. For these reasons, we have included contributions that focus on how perfectionism may relate to well-being, with a particular emphasis on, health-related and social contexts. For example, this volume includes chapters explicating the role of perfectionism in the context of general and specific chronic illness, psychopathology, and eating disorders, and in the relationship, academic, and work-life arenas. To further highlight the translational value and application of the book, we have also encouraged contributors to include a discussion of prevention and treatment issues surrounding perfectionism, where possible, which may be useful for clinicians and service providers. In doing so, we hope that this volume will be an important resource not only for researchers, but also for those who wish to use it in applied and clinical settings.

The chapters offer important and exciting new insights into the role of perfectionism in health and well-being written by authors who are well-respected international scholars. Each of these chapters presents the most up-to-date and cutting edge research on perfectionism, health, and well-being, and importantly, also highlights how these latest findings impact longstanding debates in these fields such as how perfectionism is best conceptualized and whether or not perfectionism can be healthy. As research on perfectionism has grown exponentially in the past 2 decades, these debates have also grown in their complexity. Accordingly, the contributors have weighed in on these controversial issues from a variety of different critical perspectives to provide the reader with an engaging, comprehensive, and up-to-date understanding of the current field of perfectionism with respect to health and well-being.

This book is structured to first provide an introductory overview of the fundamental conceptualization issues that need to be navigated for understanding the nuances that characterize the research on perfectionism, health, and well-being. Following this, the book is organized into three main sections, each concentrating on important and related topic areas. The first section examines the role of perfectionism in physical health—an area that has been relatively understudied by perfectionism researchers. In the second section, perfectionism as it relates to well-being and psychopathology is explored. The final section of the book focuses on specific social contexts and how they may contour the associations of perfectionism with health and well-being. We then conclude the book with a final chapter that highlights potentially fruitful and important avenues of research on perfectionism, health, and well-being yet to be explored that will hopefully contribute to the momentum of this fast growing field of research.

Given its focus and coverage, we believe that this volume will be useful to a number of different groups. It should serve as a useful reference book for researchers and scholars and also as a textbook suitable for advanced undergraduate and graduate courses dealing with personality and health, and/or personality and well-being. This book may also be of particular interest to those who work in applied settings where perfectionism is more common or more problematic, and where there is a pressing need to understand the processes linking perfectionism to health and well-being outcomes. As such, it may be a useful resource for those working in clinical, counselling, health, educational, and organizational areas, to name just a few. By presenting the latest theory and research on perfectionism, health, and well-being, we hope that this book makes a unique and useful new addition to the perfectionism literature that helps underscore the need to address the potential burden of perfectionism for health and well-being.

Contents

Chapter 1
Conceptualizations of Perfectionism, Health, and Well-Being: An Introductory Overview

Fuschia M. Sirois and Danielle S. Molnar

Perfectionism research has burgeoned over the past two decades. During this time, there have been a number of empirical and theoretical advances providing insight into the nature of perfectionism and its associated risks. Broadly, perfectionism can be described as setting and striving for excessively high and often unrealistic standards, accompanied by frequent thoughts focused on attainment of these standards and overly critical self-evaluation (Frost, Marten, Lahart, & Rosenblate, 1990). However, it is now recognized that the perfectionism construct is multidimensional, as shown simultaneously by the work of Frost and associates (1990) and by Hewitt and Flett (1990, 1991). This recognition has, nonetheless, complicated the field with respect to understanding the implications of different perfectionism dimensions for health and well-being. Yet, navigating the complexities of these issues has important theoretical and clinical repercussions. If we consider perfectionism as a relatively stable tendency, as many researchers do, then the potential benefits of understanding how, why, and when perfectionism may confer risk or resilience for health and well-being can be far-reaching. For example, personality is increasingly being recognized as an important epidemiological factor for understanding health-related trajectories and outcomes, including morbidity and mortality, in part through its associations with modifiable risk factors for the development of mental

As of July 1, 2015, Fuschia Sirois is with the Department of Psychology, the University of Sheffield, Western Bank, Sheffield, UK.

F. M. Sirois (✉)
Department of Psychology,
University of Sheffield, 309 Western Bank, Sheffield, S10 2TP, UK
e-mail: f.sirois@sheffield.ac.uk

Centre for Research on Aging, Sherbrooke, QC, Canada

D. S. Molnar
Research Institute on Addictions, University at Buffalo,
The State University of New York, Buffalo, NY, USA

Department of Psychology, Brock University, St. Catharines, ON, Canada

F. M. Sirois, D. S. Molnar (eds.), *Perfectionism, Health, and Well-Being,*
DOI 10.1007/978-3-319-18582-8_1

and physical health issues (Bogg & Roberts, 2013; Friedman, 2011; Hampson, Goldberg, Vogt, & Dubanoski, 2007).

This surge of interest in personality as risk or resilience for health in recent years has lent momentum to a burgeoning literature focused on the role of perfectionism in health. Two important themes have tended to capture the lion's share of researchers' attention in this rapidly growing literature. The first concerns perfectionism's role in psychological distress with an extensive body of work clearly implicating perfectionism in a vast array of adjustment problems including anxiety, depression, and eating disorders in both clinical and nonclinical samples (see Bardone-Cone et al., 2007; Flett & Hewitt, 2002; Frost & DiBartolo, 2002). Accordingly, it has been suggested that perfectionism be considered as a significant and unique form of personality dysfunction when revising diagnostic systems (see Ayearst, Flett, & Hewitt, 2012). From this perspective, perfectionism can confer risk for poor psychological well-being.

The other predominant theme in the perfectionism literature is whether perfectionism has adaptive or "healthy" components that may promote well-being. This theme has grown from the zeitgeist of positive psychology (Seligman & Csikszentmihalyi, 2000), in which some contemporary researchers have begun to question the traditional view of perfectionism as being entirely maladaptive and to demand a more inclusive model of perfectionism that considers the possibility that perfectionism can be both beneficial and detrimental to one's health, sense of well-being, and overall functioning. The logic here is that it may be plausible for individuals to display perfectionistic traits, but use them in ways that promote success rather than lead to dysfunction. Proponents and opponents of this notion have examined this issue at both the conceptual and empirical levels (see Bieling, Israeli, & Antony, 2004; Flett & Hewitt, 2006; Stoeber & Otto, 2006). However, as you will see throughout the chapters of this volume, it remains a topic ripe with controversy and complexity.

We suggest that there is a third theme that is of equal or even greater importance from a public health perspective, but it is a domain in the perfectionism field that has not thus far received the sustained attention it deserves—that is, the role of perfectionism in physical health. The notion that perfectionism might be linked to not only poor mental health, but also poor physical health outcomes is not new (see Wolff, 1937, 1948, and Flett, Hewitt, & Molnar, Chap. 2, this volume). Yet, perfectionism as it relates to physical health has only recently begun to be a primary focus for perfectionism researchers (e.g., this volume, Kempke, van Houdenhove, Claes, & Luyten, Chap. 5; Molnar, Sirois, & Methot-Jones, Chap. 4), perhaps because a focus on physical health in relation to perfectionism has been eclipsed by the preponderance of evidence indicating that certain forms of perfectionism pose a risk for mental health (see this volume Burgess & DiBartolo, Chap. 8; Dunkley, Solomon-Krakus, & Moroz, Chap. 7; Flett, Hewitt & Nepon, Chap. 6). From a biopsychosocial perspective, psychological states and social factors play an integral role in the development and exacerbation of physical health issues and are therefore essential factors to consider for understanding how perfectionism may confer risk or resilience for physical health outcomes. Accordingly, we propose that widening the scope of perfectionism and mental health research to include a more specific and routine emphasis on physical health is a natural next step in the evolution of this important research literature and one that can have significant implications for understanding a range of health-related outcomes.

After introducing and summarizing the different ways that the perfectionism construct has been conceptualized and measured, we then present a brief introduction to how the terms "health and well-being" have been defined in the literature, highlighting areas that may be particularly relevant for understanding the potential linkages to perfectionism dimensions. We then conclude with an overview of the structure and organization of this book, which provides the latest perspectives and research on perfectionism, health, and well-being organized into three sections: Perfectionism and Health; Perfectionism, Psychopathology, and Well-Being; and Perfectionism, Health, and Well-Being in Context.

Conceptualization and Measurement of Perfectionism

It is important to recognize up front that there are striking differences among researchers with respect to how they define, conceptualize, and assess perfectionism. These discrepancies are important to acknowledge because the way in which perfectionism is conceptualized and measured has a considerable impact on the results that emerge from empirical research. Typically, research conducted on perfectionism and health does not incorporate multiple measures of perfectionism representing different theoretical "camps," and it should not be presumed that measures that seem substantially related to each other are indeed equivalent, especially in terms of their implications for health outcomes. Fry and Debats (2011), for example, examined the link between perfectionism and mortality risk in a sample of older adults with diabetes. Contrary to their hypotheses, they found that trait perfectionism was associated with greater longevity. However, when they focused on the role of perfectionistic dysfunctional attitudes in mortality risk in the same sample, they found that perfectionism was associated with greater mortality risk. These conflicting findings that have divergent and potentially critical implications attest to the importance of considering measurement issues when assessing links between perfectionism and health. Consequently, the first section of the book will introduce the reader to the different ways that the perfectionism construct has been conceptualized and measured.

A Unitary or a Multifarious Construct?

A careful reading of the literature on perfectionism reveals that most of the discussion concerning the conceptualization and measurement of perfectionism can be boiled down to three central issues. The first issue concerns whether perfectionism should be considered as a unidimensional or as a multidimensional construct. Originally, there was a general consensus regarding the essence of perfectionism, as early theorists from different theoretical orientations, such as Sigmund Freud (1926/1959), Karen Horney (1950), Aaron Beck (1976), Albert Ellis (1962), and W. H. Missildine (1963), were quite explicit in treating perfectionism as a unitary construct that was pathological in nature. Indeed, they characterized perfectionists as individuals who set and strive compulsively toward excessively high standards, not because of a drive toward excellence, but because of a punishing fear of failure resulting from poor self-esteem. Horney's (1950) seminal writings speak directly to this point as she stated,

> He holds before his soul his image of perfection and unconsciously tells himself: Forget about the disgraceful creature you actually are; this is how you should be; and to be this idealized self is all that matters. You should be able to endure everything, to understand everything, to like everybody, to always be productive. (p. 65)

These classic theorists further observed that perfectionists scrutinize themselves and others harshly and approach life with a cognitive style characterized by rigidity and all or none thinking. This was best illustrated by Ellis (2002) when he stated in a rather terse manner that "perfectionists are more rigid and persistent in their irrational beliefs than what I call the 'nice neurotics'" (p. 228) and further emphasized by Asher Pacht (1984) when during his awards address to the American Psychological Association he spoke of perfectionists as having the "God/scum complex," in which perfectionists think that they must either be perfect or be a total failure. Finally, the early writings on perfectionism stressed that perfectionists lack the ability to experience joy and satisfaction even when they do reach their standards. This point was made glaringly clear when Weisinger and Lobsenz (1981) wrote, "The need to be perfect places a person in a self-destructive double bind. If one fails to meet the unrealistic expectation, one has failed; but if one does meet it, one feels no glow of achievement for one has only done what was expected" (p. 237).

Hamachek (1978) was the first to diverge from this unidimensional conceptualization of perfectionism and to suggest that perfectionism is multidimensional and that the different dimensions have distinct functional effects, allowing for both positive and negative outcomes. Specifically, he postulated that there are two distinct types of perfectionism: normal and neurotic. He delineated "normal perfectionists" as "those who derive a very real sense of pleasure from the labors of a painstaking effort and who feel free to be less precise as the situation permits" (p. 27). Conversely, he described neurotic perfectionists as "the sort of people whose efforts—even their best ones—never seem quite good enough, at least in their own eyes. It always seems to these persons that they could—and should—do better … they are unable to feel satisfaction because in their own eyes they never seem to do things good enough to warrant the feeling" (p. 27).

Early investigations tended to employ various unidimensional perfectionism measures such as the Burns Perfectionism Scale or the perfectionism subscales of the Eating Disorder Inventory (e.g., Burns, 1980; Garner, Olmstead, & Polivy, 1983). However, with the exception of a few researchers who favor a unitary construct that focuses on the clinical aspects of perfectionism (e.g., Shafran, Cooper, & Fairburn, 2002), most contemporary researchers have followed from the work of Hamachek (1978) and adopted a multidimensional conceptualization of perfectionism in light of convincing evidence demonstrating the construct validity of multidimensional measures of perfectionism and strong support for the contention that different dimensions of perfectionism often have distinct functional consequences (Hewitt & Flett, 1991; Stoeber & Otto, 2006). However, accepting that perfectionism is a multifarious construct has only fueled the debate concerning the nature of perfectionism, as there is currently a general lack of agreement concerning what dimensions best define the core facets of perfectionism.

What are the Central Components of Perfectionism?

This leads us to the next layer of complexity in the conceptualization of perfectionism: What are the central components of perfectionism? Perfectionism is best understood at different levels, depending on one's theoretical orientation and research question. A typical approach is to treat perfectionism as a fairly stable personality trait. However, other potentially relevant aspects of perfectionism come to light when understood from other theoretical perspectives. For instance, the frequency with which individuals experience automatic perfectionistic thoughts concerning the need to be perfect (e.g., Perfectionistic Cognitions Inventory (PCI); Flett, Hewitt, Blankstein, & Gray, 1998; The Multidimensional Perfectionism Cognitions Inventory-English; Kobori, 2006; Stoeber, Kobori, & Tanno, 2010) are a source of interest when studying perfectionism through the lens of cognitive psychology, whereas the tendency to engage in perfectionistic self-presentation, such as perfectionistic self-promotion and defensive self-concealment (e.g., Perfectionistic Self-Presentation Scale (PSPS); Hewitt et al., 2003), is emphasized when examining perfectionism from the perspective of social psychology.

Also, some researchers have stressed the importance of the distinction between "general perfectionism," which assesses broad tendencies toward having unrealistically high standards and harsh self-scrutiny, and "domain-specific" perfectionism, which assesses perfectionism in particular areas of life. An example is "romantic perfectionism," which assesses perfectionistic beliefs and standards specifically about romantic relationships (Matte & Lafontaine, 2012). Indeed, research has supported that "romantic perfectionism" has incremental predictive utility beyond general perfectionism with regard to relationship adjustment (Matte & Lafontaine, 2012; Shea, Slaney, & Rice, 2006). The addition of these measures has surely enriched our understanding of perfectionism by allowing a more nuanced approach to its study. For instance, findings from several studies now provide compelling evidence to support the notion that experiencing automatic perfectionistic thoughts uniquely predicts several important and diverse outcomes such as athletic burnout (Hill & Appleton, 2011), depression (Flett et al., 2012), and eating disturbance (Downey, Reinking, Gibson, Cloud, & Chang, 2014) after accounting for trait measures of perfectionism. However, they also complicate the field such that contemporary researchers are now faced with choosing between a seemingly endless assortment of possibly relevant perfectionism measures with divergent findings often resulting from different conceptualizations and measures of perfectionism being employed.

Perfectionism as a Trait

This issue is perhaps best illustrated when examining perfectionism at the trait level. Several measures that assess perfectionism at the trait level are currently available for use (Enns & Cox, 2002). However, it is clear that there are three primary models of trait perfectionism that dominate the field. Frost et al. (1990) developed the Multidimensional Perfectionism Scale (MPS-F) to assess their conceptualization of perfectionism which posits that perfectionism consists of six key dimensions tapping high standards, organization, concern over mistakes, doubts about actions, parental criticism, and high parental expectations. Although the MPS-F has been shown to have good psychometric properties and continues to be widely used in both clinical and nonclinical samples (Frost & DiBartolo, 2002), it has also drawn criticism on both empirical and conceptual grounds. For instance, the stability of Frost et al.'s (1990) factor structure has come into question with some arguing in favor of a three-factor structure (Purdon, Antony, & Swinson, 1999) and others demonstrating evidence to support a four-factor structure (Stöber, 1998).

On conceptual grounds, the MPS-F has received two primary criticisms. First, some have questioned the validity of the MPS-F on the basis that some of the subscales tap measures of psychopathology that are seen as correlates or outcomes of perfectionism rather than perfectionism per se. For instance, Shafran and Mansell (2001) claimed that the doubt about actions subscale of the MPS-F assesses checking symptoms of obsessive-compulsive disorder (OCD), rather than perfectionism itself, a criticism that may have validity, as this subscale consists primarily of items taken from the Maudsley Obsessive Compulsive Inventory (MOCI; Hodgson & Rachman, 1977) which measures OCD symptoms. Second, the MPS-F has been challenged on the basis that the parental expectations and parental criticism subscales confound etiological factors with the core components of perfectionism. For instance, Rheaume et al. (2000) pointed out that "the inclusion of developmental aspects of perfectionism makes it difficult to interpret results and understand perfectionism itself" (p. 120). This criticism has merit, given that parental factors have been given the greatest emphasis regarding the etiology of perfectionism.

Based on their review of the literature and clinical observations, Hewitt and Flett (1991) concluded that perfectionism includes intrapersonal as well as interpersonal aspects and asserted that perfectionism should be conceptualized as three dimensions centered on interpersonal source and direction: self-oriented perfectionism (i.e., the setting of excessively high personal standards, accompanied by strict guidelines and evaluations of personal behavior); other-oriented perfectionism (i.e., the tendency to hold exceedingly high standards for other people); and socially prescribed perfectionism (i.e., the need to attain standards perceived to be imposed by significant others) (Flett & Hewitt, 2002). They further developed their own Multidimensional Perfectionism Scale (MPS-HF; Hewitt & Flett, 1991) to assess each of these components, and the reliability and validity of the MPS-HF have been shown to be quite impressive (Hewitt, Flett, Turnbull-Donovan, & Mikail, 1991). Hence, whereas Frost et al.'s (1990) model treats perfectionism primarily as a self-focused construct, Hewitt and Flett's (1991) conceptual framework places equal emphasis on both the personal and social aspects of perfectionism.

A large body of literature supports that self-oriented perfectionism, other-oriented perfectionism, and socially prescribed perfectionism are differentially related to myriad important outcomes such as psychopathology, relationship functioning, and health (Hewitt & Flett, 1991; Hewitt, Flett, & Mikail, 1995; Molnar, Reker, Culp, Sadava, & DeCourville, 2006). However, the MPS-HF is not without its critics. Shafran et al. (2002), for example, argue that consistent with historical definitions, only self-oriented perfectionism assesses the construct of perfectionism and that the other two dimensions (i.e., other-oriented perfectionism and socially prescribed perfectionism) are only tangential to the construct. They then go on to blame the widespread acceptance and use of the Frost et al.'s (1990) and the Hewitt and Flett's (1991) Multidimensional Perfectionism Scales as bolstering the view that perfectionism is multidimensional rather than remain a clinically based construct. However, Hewitt, Flett, Besser, Sherry, and McGee (2003) maintain that perfectionism is multidimensional by drawing attention to evidence indicating that each of the MPS-HF dimensions is differentially related to numerous outcomes, such as psychopathology, and by highlighting that both socially prescribed and other-oriented perfectionism disrupt the therapeutic alliance, thus showing that the interpersonal dimensions of perfectionism also have important clinical implications.

Finally, Slaney and colleagues (see Slaney, Rice, & Ashby, 2002; Slaney, Rice, Mobley, Trippi, & Ashby, 2001) developed the Almost Perfect Scale-Revised (APS-R) in an effort to assess both positive and negative features of perfectionism, especially with regard to their implications for therapy. According to their model, perfectionism consists of three dimensions: high standards, order, and discrepancy. Standards assess individuals' self-performance expectations and incorporate some elements of personal standards, as measured by the MPS-F, and some features of self-oriented perfectionism, as measured by the MPS-HF, whereas the unique dimension of discrepancy measures the degree of self-critical evaluation in an individual's perceived capability to achieve expected standards (e.g., doing my best never seems to be enough). Order assesses preferences for order and organization, but it appears to be less pivotal in gauging the central aspects of perfectionism (Stoeber & Otto, 2006). Research has supported the psychometric properties of the APS-R, demonstrating adequate reliability and that the standards and the order factors are positively and moderately associated, whereas the association between the standards and discrepancy scales is generally inconsequential (Ashby & Rice, 2002; Slaney et al., 2001). This last finding is worth noting as it indicates that the APS-R is likely measuring two very well-defined forms of perfectionism.

However, as seen with the previous two trait measures of perfectionism, there are also criticisms of the APS-R as well. First, it can be argued that some of the dimensions assessed in the APS-R do not seem to conceptually map onto other measures of perfectionism (e.g., the MPS-F and the MPS-HF) very well, thus making comparison of studies difficult. Some researchers have also called the construct validity of the APS-R into question. Flett and Hewitt (2002), for instance, have argued that discrepancy is not a fundamental element of perfectionism, but is a related and independent construct. Specifically, they contend that there are important temporal differences between trait perfectionism and self-evaluation, such that perfectionism is relatively stable, whereas self-evaluation varies based on one's experiences and feedback (Flett & Hewitt, 2002). In support of their argument, they drew attention to research on perfectionism and self-efficacy, which demonstrates that the two constructs are separable.

Perfectionistic Strivings and Perfectionistic Concerns

Although each of these models and accompanying measures of trait perfectionism continue to be widely used in the field, contemporary research has indicated that two underlying higher order dimensions of trait perfectionism can be extrapolated from the most widely used perfectionism measures (e.g., the MPS-HF, Hewitt & Flett, 1991; the MPS-F, Frost et al., 1990; and the APS-R, Slaney et al., 2001). Although they have been cast with different labels, most researchers tend to refer to these underlying factors as perfectionistic strivings (PS) and perfectionistic concerns (PC). *PS* refers to the propensity to set excessively high personal standards that are often unrealistic in nature and to demand nothing less than perfection from the self. Indicators of PS include the personal standards subscale of the MPS-F along with the self-oriented perfectionism subscale from the MPS-HF and the standards subscale from the APS-R. *PC* includes extraordinarily critical appraisals of one's own behavior, chronic harsh self-scrutiny, excessive preoccupations with others' evaluations, expectations, and criticism, and an inability to gain satisfaction even when one is successful in an endeavor. Subscales tapping this dimension include concern over mistakes, parental expectations, parental criticism, and doubt about actions from the MPS-F, socially prescribed perfectionism from the MPS-HF, and discrepancy from the APS-R.

Not only do factor analytic studies support these two high-order factors of perfectionism using a variety of samples and measures of perfectionism (Bieling et al., 2004; Slade & Owens, 1998; Terry-Short, Owens, Slade, & Dewey, 1995), but researchers have also documented that these factors are differentially related to health and well-being. PC is consistently related to poorer health (Molnar, Sadava, Flett, & Colautti, 2012), greater psychopathology (see Shafran & Mansell, 2001), and poorer well-being (Chang, 2000, Chang, Watkins, & Banks, 2004; Dunkley et al., 2003). PS, on the other hand, is associated with both better and worse health and well-being. On the one hand, PS is associated with higher levels of positive affect

(Bieling, Israeli, Smith, & Antony, 2003), greater life satisfaction (Bergman, Nyland, & Burns, 2007; Chang et al., 2004), and better physical health (Molnar et al., 2006). Yet, on the other hand, it is also a risk factor for eating disorders (Bardone-Cone et al., 2007) and poorer physical health (Fry & Debats, 2011; Molnar et al., 2012) and is related to experiencing greater psychopathology after a performance failure (Besser, Flett, & Hewitt, 2004).

Finally, consistent with Hewitt and Flett's (1991) model of perfectionism, some researchers are beginning to argue in favor of a three-factor model, suggesting that other-oriented perfectionism (OOP) should be included along with PS and PC. OOP measures the extent to which individuals rigidly demand perfection from others in an exacting and entitled way and are being highly critical of others. Indeed, research has demonstrated that OOP is most relevant in the domain of interpersonal functioning as it has been related to maladaptive relational outcomes, such as higher levels of negative affect, higher levels of marital conflict, and lower levels of sexual satisfaction (Blatt, 1974; Habke, Hewitt, & Flett, 1999). Further, it has been established that OOP is uniquely related to other markers of poor relationship functioning, such as the dark triad traits of narcissism, Machiavellianism, and psychopathy (Sherry, Gralnick, Hewitt, Sherry, & Flett, in press; Stoeber, 2014). However, our understanding of OOP is rather limited since this dimension of perfectionism has received far less attention in the research literature in comparison with PS and PC.

Health and Well-Being: An Introductory Primer

The terms "health and well-being" are common conceptual companions in the contemporary vernacular that refer to related but distinct concepts. A frequent underlying assumption in pairing these concepts is that in experiencing good health, one may also expect to experience well-being. However, this also implies the converse; that without good health, well-being may be elusive. The assumed directionality of these statements aside, theory and research indicates that health and well-being are inextricably linked.

Unpacking the Dynamics of Health

One of the most widely recognized and used conceptualizations of health is from the World Health Organization (WHO) which in 1948 defined health as "a complete state of physical, mental, and social well-being and not merely the absence of disease or infirmity."

Current conceptualizations of health have emerged largely from this positive and inclusive view of health which acknowledges the importance of assessing health not just in physical terms, but also with respect to psychological and social well-being. Extending this view, public health promotion perspectives conceptualize health as "the capacity of people to adapt to, respond to, or control life's challenges and changes" (Frankish, Green, Ratner, Chomik, & Larsen, 1996, p. 6). This definition moves from a primarily descriptive view of health to one that highlights the key roles of factors such as coping and health behaviors for maximizing, promoting, and maintaining health. Characteristic coping responses can up- or down-regulate the physiological stress response, through differences in how potential stressors are appraised and perceptions of the availability of coping resources (Lazarus & Folkman, 1984). The magnitude and length of activation of the stress response (and the hypothalamic–pituitary–cortical–adrenal (HPCA) system in particular) in turn, can have important implications for the regulation of the immune system and inflammatory processes which are known precursors of a variety of acute and chronic illnesses (Cohen et al., 2012; Juster, McEwen, & Lupien, 2010; McEwen, 2007). Similarly, maximizing health-promoting behaviors and minimizing health risk behaviors are key for maintaining health and reducing risk of disease (Bogg & Roberts, 2013; Hampson et al., 2007).

Consistent with this view and relevant for our focus on perfectionism, models linking personality to health include coping and health behaviors as routes through which personality may influence health and well-being outcomes (Smith, 2006). Not surprisingly, current research confirms that perfectionism is linked to both coping and health behaviors (see this volume, Dunkley et al., Chap. 7; Sirois, Chap. 3, this volume). Moreover, in the context of chronic illness which poses an ongoing challenge, perfectionism may confer particular risk for poor adjustment and disease management because of its links to poor coping and health behaviors (Sirois & Molnar, 2014; see also Kempke et al., Chap. 5; Molnar et al. Chap. 4, this volume).

No discussion of how we understand health would be complete without the mention of the biopsychosocial model of health and illness. Implicit within the name of this model is the notion that health and illness are based on multifactorial processes. Specifically, health is viewed as the intersection of biological, psychological, and social systems, and the interaction of micro- and macroprocesses across these systems. For example, microlevel processes, including cellular and immune system changes, are viewed as being nested within macrolevel processes, including availability of social support and levels of depressive affect, with changes in one level affecting the other and vice versa (Taylor & Sirois, 2014). Thus, the biopsychosocial model presents a dynamic and comprehensive framework for understanding the multiplicity of factors that can create risk or resilience for health.

With respect to perfectionism and physical health, the complexity of the biopsychosocial factors involved is only just beginning to be fully explored. For example, research is now providing compelling evidence that perfectionism may play a predisposing, precipitating, or perpetuating role in certain chronic health conditions (see Kempke et al., Chap. 5; Molnar et al., Chap. 4, this volume). Moreover, the mood disturbances associated with certain forms of perfectionism can create risk for the development of psychopathologies, such as eating disorders which are known to have a direct effect on physical health (see Wade, O'Shea, & Shafran, Chap. 9, this volume). The influence of perfectionism on stress and coping can also contribute to poor health outcomes in general (see Dunkley et al., Chap. 7, this volume) and especially for those living with a chronic health condition (see Molnar et al., Chap. 4, this volume). Given the key role of social factors and social support for health in the biopsychosocial model, the social disconnection associated with perfectionism may also confer further risk for health (see Sherry, Mackinnon, & Gautreau, Chap. 10, this volume).

Well-Being: A Convergence of Competing Perspectives

Whether conceived of as a transitory state of positive feelings and satisfaction, or as a continuing process of growth and adaptation to changing life circumstances, well-being is an increasingly popular topic for researchers and clinicians alike (Sirois, 2011). In the past 5 years alone, the term "well-being" has more than 475,000 citations indexed within the scholarly research literature. Yet, despite this proliferation of interest, consensus regarding a single definition of well-being is lacking (Dodge, Daly, Huyton, & Sander, 2012). Instead, the term "well-being" is often viewed as being synonymous with related terms such as happiness, wellness, mental health, and quality of life. Indeed, the World Health Organization (2005, p. 2) defines mental health as "a state of well-being in which the individual realizes his or her own abilities, can cope with the normal stresses of life, can work productively and fruitfully, and is able to make a contribution to his or her community." This and similar views of well-being are in sharp contrast to early conceptualizations which focused on the absence of distress as the key defining quality of well-being (McDowell, 2010). In this respect, the evolution of our understanding of well-being has paralleled the trajectory for how we view health, moving towards definitions of inclusion rather than exclusion, but without one clear, universally agreed upon conceptualization.

This lack of agreement aside, a commonality among modern conceptualizations of well-being is that their roots come from one of two ancient Greek traditions. The first is aligned with the ancient Greek Epicurean conceptions of the nature of living the "Good Life" (Waterman, 1993, 2008) and emphasizes maximizing pleasure—"hedonia"—and minimizing pain. From this hedonic perspective, well-being is comprised of two broad components: an emotional component that includes high levels of positive emotions (e.g., happiness, contentment) and low levels of negative emotions (e.g., anxiety, depression) and an evaluative component that includes overall satisfaction with life and satisfaction with specific, important life domains such as family life, work, and personal life (Ryan & Deci, 2001). Given the subjective evaluation involved in both of these components, researchers often adopt the term "subjective well-being" to describe this particular hedonic view of well-being (Diener, 1984; Diener, Suh, Lucas, & Smith, 1999). In short, well-being in the hedonic tradition is feeling good and evaluating one's life as satisfying.

The alternative and rivalling view of well-being is rooted in the classical Greek teachings of Aristotle and his Nicomachean ethics (1985). The eudaimonic view proposes that well-being arises, not from the pursuit of pleasure, but from the pursuit of goals that are aligned with the authentic self or *daimon*. To Aristotle, eudaimonia was not a subjective, but an objective state that arose from contemplating the best within oneself and personal excellence (Waterman, 2008). Modern scholars who subscribe to this particular view of well-being have extended this to acting upon personal contemplations of authenticity (Ryff, 1989; Ryff & Keyes, 1995), with well-being as an emergent property of engaging in growth-promoting pursuits that help develop one's potential (Sirois, 2011). Consistent with this view, Ryff and colleagues (1989; Ryff & Keyes, 1995) have proposed a model of *psychological well-being* comprised of multiple dynamic dimensions which reflect optimal psychological functioning. Three core dimensions—personal growth, purpose in life, and positive relations with others—are proposed to capture the essence of eudaimonic well-being and its dynamic, action-oriented focus on purposefully pursuing meaningful goals and cultivating rewarding relationships. Thus, well-being from the eudaimonic tradition is focused more on the process of flourishing rather than the outcome of simply feeling good (Sirois, 2011).

Despite the distinctions in how well-being is conceptualized in each of these models, researchers have nonetheless acknowledged that considerable overlap does exist. For example, knowing that one is engaged in the pursuit of meaningful goals that reflect fulfilling one's potential may increase feelings of happiness and life satisfaction. Researchers have therefore suggested that from a practical standpoint, it makes sense to think of each type of well-being as running in tandem with each other (Biswas-Diener, Kashdan, & King, 2009; Kashdan, Biswas-Diener, & King, 2008), rather than being separate and distinct.

Elements from each of these conceptualizations have relevance for understanding how perfectionism dimensions may relate to different levels of well-being. From the lens of hedonic models of well-being, the high levels of negative affect such as worry, anxiety, and distress associated with PC perfectionism would be an indicator of poor well-being (see Burgess & DiBartolo, Chap. 8; Dunkley et al., Chap. 7; Flett et al., Chap. 6, this volume). In terms of the evaluative component of well-being, not being easily satisfied with one's performance is arguably one of the defining features of perfectionism, and especially PC perfectionism, which is linked to burnout and dissatisfaction with work (see Stoeber & Damian, Chap. 12, this volume) and lower academic satisfaction (see Rice, Richardson, & Ray, Chap. 11, this volume). However, there is some evidence that PS perfectionists also experience little satisfaction from their achievements (Hewitt & Flett, 1991; Mor, Day, Flett, & Hewitt, 1995) and may be more inclined to dissatisfaction with their performance after failure than PC perfectionists (Besser et al. 2004). Regarding general life satisfaction, several studies have now shown clear links between PC perfectionism and lower life satisfaction. (Ashby, Noble, & Gnilka, 2012; Chang, 2000; Williams & Cropley, 2014).

If we map perfectionism onto the eudaemonic landscape of well-being, the prospects are not as encouraging as what might be expected. Ostensibly, the setting and striving for high standards that is the hallmark of PS perfectionism should contribute to increased eudaemonic well-being, insomuch that this striving reflects pursuing one's purpose in life and/or promotes personal growth. However, when this striving becomes excessive, unrelenting, and based on the standards of others rather than one's own, or on the standards that are inherently unrealistic rather than authentic, well-being may be at risk (see this volume, Rice et al., Chap. 11; Stoeber & Damian, Chap. 12). In addition, there is mounting evidence that many perfectionists are interpersonally distressed and find having positive relations with others a challenge (see Sherry et al., Chap. 10, this volume). Collectively, this constellation of findings suggests that perfectionism, and PC perfectionism in particular, creates risk for well-being.

Overview of the Book

Following this introductory chapter, the latest perspectives on perfectionism, health, and well-being will be presented in three main sections. Each chapter will not only present the most up-to-date and cutting-edge research on perfectionism, health, and well-being, but will also highlight how the latest findings impact long-standing debates in the field such as whether perfectionism has an adaptive component or not. The first section will cover both historical and emerging research perspectives on the linkages between perfectionism and physical health. The second section will examine the dynamic interrelations of affect and cognition that underlie how perfectionism relates to well-being and associated psychopathologies. The third section puts perfectionism, health, and well-being in context by discussing the latest findings on the implications of excessive striving for high standards in life domains that often demand excellence (work life and academics), or where having excessively high standards may be particularly problematic for both the perfectionist and those around the perfectionist (relationships).

Part I: Perfectionism and Health

Physical health is arguably a fundamental factor in the experience of well-being. Yet, until recently, understanding how perfectionism may be implicated in physical health has been an understudied area of the perfectionism literature. This initial set of chapters addresses this gap from historical, empirical, and theoretical perspectives.

Flett et al. (Chap. 2) take us on a historical journey of the theoretical, methodological, and ideological issues in the literature on perfectionism and health. Using case studies and early empirical research, their summary of the "hidden literature" highlights the value of a rich, but often overlooked source of information for both understanding and conceptualizing the linkages among perfectionism, physical health, and illness. They conclude that perfectionism is more of a liability than a benefit for physical health and call for a more person-centered rather than variable-centered approach to understanding when and why perfectionism may pose health risks.

The contribution by Sirois (Chap. 3) focuses on positive health behaviors as an important route through which perfectionism may influence health. Sirois argues that taking a self-regulation approach is necessary for understanding how and why perfectionism dimensions may promote or prevent the practice of health-promoting behaviors and reviews the theory and research on perfectionism and self-regulation. Combining this limited literature with preliminary supportive evidence, Sirois proposes a new self-regulation resource model that highlights the reciprocal and dynamic roles of affective and temporal self-regulation resources and liabilities for conceptualizing how perfectionism relates to the practice of important health behaviors.

Next, Molnar et al. (Chap. 4) present a contemporary view of perfectionism in the context of chronic illness. Throughout this chapter, they propose that perfectionism should not only be considered when examining the etiological factors involved in illness, but also when examining adjustment to illness. After critically reviewing the literature relating perfectionism to chronic illness, they present their new Stress and Coping Cyclical Amplification Model of Perfectionism in Illness (SCCAMPI) that underscores the importance of the intrapsychic and interpersonal processes that link perfectionism to important health outcomes through the amplification of stress and maladaptive coping.

Moving from a broad to a more focused perspective of perfectionism and chronic illness, Kempke et al. (Chap. 5) review and discuss the involvement of perfectionism in the development and maintenance of chronic fatigue syndrome (CFS). Their research and review of this topic supports a working model of self-critical perfectionism and CFS that places chronic stress in a central role for understanding the deleterious effects of perfectionism in this context. They conclude that a greater emphasis on, and therapeutic attention to, the dysfunctional cognitive and affective patterns associated with self-critical perfectionism may be beneficial for treatment of CFS patients with high levels of self-critical perfectionism.

Part II: Perfectionism, Psychopathology, and Well-Being

As noted earlier in this chapter, well-being and health are inextricably linked. But like health, well-being is often defined as being more than just the absence of distress or psychopathology. This more inclusive conceptualization aside, when distress and/or psychopathology is present, it is usually an indicator of poor well-being. The chapters in this section tackle the issue of how perfectionism may relate to both global and more specific indicators of poor well-being and provide unique perspectives on the latest research and theory to help guide both researchers and clinicians.

Flett et al. (Chap. 6) open this section with a review and discussion of the central roles of rumination and worry in poor health and well-being outcomes. Noting that tendencies to excessively worry and overthink are key features of both self-oriented and socially prescribed perfectionists, they introduce a perfectionism cognition theory that explains how "perseverating perfectionists" may be vulnerable to both emotional distress and physical health problems. Their comprehensive review argues for the need to consider how issues concerning self and identity underlie a tendency toward perfectionistic rumination.

Dunkley et al. (Chap. 7) address the important issue of how perfectionism dimensions may differentially relate to stress and coping processes and associated well-being outcomes. Reviewing the literature with a focus on mediators and moderators of perfectionism and stress, they highlight the central roles of coping strategies and social support for understanding how and why self-critical and personal standards perfectionism may be related to different well-being outcomes. They further highlight several methodological limitations in the current perfectionism and stress research that should be addressed, including the predominance of self-report rather than physiological measures of stress and a lack of experimental and sophisticated event-sampling methodologies.

Burgess and DiBartolo (Chap. 8) continue and extend the theme of perfectionism and psychological distress by focusing more specifically on how the perfectionism–anxiety relationship is qualified by the multidimensional nature of perfectionism. In reviewing how perfectionism dimensions relate to a broad spectrum of anxiety symptomology, they note potential mediating and moderating roles for stress regulation, social factors, and cognitions. They conclude with recommendations for advancing the field that focus on theory-driven and methodological appropriate research to better elucidate the often complex nature of the perfectionism–anxiety relationship.

In their chapter, Wade et al. (Chap. 9) provide a comprehensive overview of the literature linking perfectionism to eating disorders. Their review of the prominent theories on this topic, along with the extant research suggesting a causal role for different perfectionism dimensions, highlights the complexities of mechanisms that may link perfectionism to both the development and maintenance of eating disorders. They argue for the importance of and need for interventions that target perfectionism not only in the treatment of, but also in the prevention of eating disorders.

Part III: Perfectionism, Health, and Well-Being in Context

The associations among perfectionism, health, and well-being do not manifest themselves in a social vacuum. It is therefore important that these linkages be studied within the context of the interpersonal worlds in which they occur. The chapters in this final section place perfectionism, health, and well-being in context by examining three key social arenas—interpersonal relationships, academic settings, and work life—where striving for perfection may have some expected as well as unexpected consequences.

Sherry et al. (Chap. 10) present their expanded social disconnection model (SDM) of perfectionism and psychopathology and argue that distinguishing between personality-dependent and personality-independent moderators is important for gaining insights into the interpersonal ramifications of perfectionism. The expanded SDM provides an inclusive view of how different perfectionism dimensions create vulnerabilities for poor interpersonal relationships and elucidates the mechanisms that explain the link between perfectionism and psychopathology. Using two case studies of well-known public figures to illustrate the utility of the expanded SDM, they provide compelling evidence for their assertion that perfectionists do not play well with others.

Rice et al. (Chap. 11) navigate the important issue of how perfectionism may affect students across the academic setting continuum and present evidence supporting a multivalenced view of perfectionism in this context. They note that although perfectionism is fundamentally a performance-based construct, issues in the conceptualization and analysis of perfectionism can often make understanding the implications of perfectionism in academic settings difficult. Nonetheless, their review suggests that unhealthy forms of perfectionism put students at an overall disadvantage in terms of academic performance and well-being, due in part to the self-critical aspects of perfectionism.

Next, Stoeber and Damian (Chap. 12) provide an overview of how perfectionism relates to key well-being indicators in the context of working life. Their review of the limited research on how perfectionism dimensions relate to burnout, work engagement, and workaholism among employees reveals important distinctions between perfectionistic strivings and perfectionistic concerns. They propose two hypothetical models to explain these differential results and guide future research and note the importance of conducting more methodologically rigorous research to better understand the implications of perfectionism for well-being in the workplace.

In the concluding chapter of this volume, Molnar and Sirois (Chap. 13) highlight prominent themes that arise when studying the interface of perfectionism, health, and well-being. They then offer suggestions for future research to help guide the next generation of perfectionism researchers.

Conclusions

Empirical and theoretical advances into the nature of perfectionism and its associated outcomes have heightened awareness and understanding of the effects of setting and striving for excessively high, and often unrealistic, standards. Although striving for perfection may be viewed as desirable and even may be rewarded in certain contexts, the evidence to date is often equivocal regarding the nature of the linkages of perfectionism to health and well-being, and especially in light of more sophisticated and interrelated views of these concepts. Consistent with biopsychosocial and public health promotion views of health, understanding the implications of perfectionism for health and well-being requires integrating rather than separating research on these related outcomes as well as studying them in the contexts in which they occur. What becomes clear from these issues is that whether perfectionism is healthy or unhealthy may not be the best question to ask. Rather, asking when, why, and how perfectionism can pose risk or resilience for health and well-being may provide richer and more accurate insights into these important issues. We believe that navigating the complexities of these often controversial issues and questions is a worthwhile endeavor as the answers can have significant public health implications. By taking different perspectives, the contributions in this book illustrate that there is strength in diversity when examining the mechanisms and processes that may render certain perfectionists particularly vulnerable to poor health and well-being. As editors, we hope that bringing these contributions fields together into one volume will provide a unique and useful resource for readers that will stimulate further research, theory, and debate.

References

Albert Ellis, A. (1962). *Reason and emotion in psychotherapy*. New York: Lyle Stuart.

Aldea, M. A., & Rice, K. G. (2006). The role of emotional dysregulation in perfectionism and psychological distress. *Journal of Counseling Psychology, 53,* 498–510.

Aristotle. (1985). *Nicomachean ethos* (T. Irwin, Trans.). Indianapolis: Hackett. (Original work published 4th Century BC).

Ashby, J. S., & Rice, K. G. (2002). Perfectionism, dysfunctional attitudes, and self-esteem: A structural equations analysis. *Journal of Counseling & Development, 80*(2), 197–203.

Ashby, J. S., Noble, C. L., & Gnilka, P. B. (2012). Multidimensional perfectionism, depression, and satisfaction with life: Differences among perfectionists and tests of a stress-mediation model. *Journal of College Counseling, 15*(2), 130–143.

Ayearst, L., Flett, G., & Hewitt, P. (2012). Where is multidimensional perfectionism in DSM-5? A question posed to the DSM-5 personality and personality disorders work group. *Personality Disorders-Theory Research and Treatment, 3,* 458–469. doi:10.1037/a0026354.

Bardone-Cone, A. M., Wonderlich, S. A., Frost, R. O., Bulik, C. M., Mitchell, J. E., Uppala, S., et al (2007). Perfectionism and eating disorders. Current status and future directions. *Clinical Psychology Review, 27,* 384–405. doi:10.1016/j.cpr.2006.12.005.

Beck, A. T. (1976). *Cognitive therapy and the emotional disorders*. New York: International Universities Press.

Bergman, A. J., Nyland, J. E., & Burns, L. R. (2007). Correlates with perfectionism and the utility of a dual process model. *Personality and Individual Differences, 43,* 389–399. doi:10.1016/j.paid.2006.12.007.

Besser, A., Flett, G., & Hewitt, P. L. (2004). Perfectionism, cognition, and affect in response to performance failure vs. success. *Journal of Rational-Emotive & Cognitive Behaviour Therapy, 22*(4), 297–324.

Bieling, P. J., Israeli, A. L., Smith, J., & Antony, M. M. (2003). Making the grade: The behavioural consequences of perfectionism in the classroom. *Personality and Individual Differences, 35,* 163–178.

Bieling, P. J., Israeli, A. L., & Anthony, M. M. (2004). Is perfectionism good, bad, or both? Examining models of the perfectionism construct. *Personality and Individual Differences, 36,* 1373–1385. doi:10.1016/S0191-8869(03)00235-6.

Biswas-Diener, R., Kashdan, T. B., & King, L. A. (2009). Two traditions of happiness research, not two distinct types of happiness. *The Journal of Positive Psychology, 4*(3), 208–211.

Blatt, S. (1974). Levels of object representation in anaclitic and introjective depression. *Psychoanalytic Study of the Child, 29,* 107–157.

Bogg, T., & Roberts, B. W. (2013). The case for conscientiousness: Evidence and implications for a personality trait marker of health and longevity. *Annals of Behavioral Medicine, 45*(3), 278–288.

Burns, D. (1980, November). The perfectionist's script for self-defeat. Psychology Today, 34–51.
Chang, E. C. (2000). Perfectionism as a predictor of positive and negative psychological outcomes: Examining a mediation model in younger and older adults. *Journal of Counseling Psychology, 47*(1), 18–26.
Chang, E. C., Watkins, A., & Banks, K. H. (2004). How adaptive and maladaptive perfectionism relate to positive and negative psychological functioning: Testing a stress-mediation model in black and white female college students. *Journal of Counseling Psychology, 51,* 93–102.
Cohen, S., Janicki-Deverts, D., Doyle, W. J., Miller, G. E., Frank, E., Rabin, B. S., & Turner, R. B. (2012). Chronic stress, glucocorticoid receptor resistance, inflammation, and disease risk. *Proceedings of the National Academy of Sciences, 109*(16), 5995–5999.
Diener, E. (1984). Subjective well-being. *Psychological Bulletin, 95,* 524–575.
Diener, E., Suh, E. M., Lucas, R. E., & Smith, H. L. (1999). Subjective well-being: Three decades of progress. *Psychological Bulletin, 125*(2), 276–302.
Dodge, R., Daly, A. P., Huyton, J., & Sander, L. D. (2012). The challenge of defining wellbeing. *International Journal of Wellbeing, 2,* 222–235.
Downey, C. A., Reinking, K. R., Gibson, J. M., Cloud, J. A., & Chang, E. C. (2014). Perfectionistic cognitions and eating disturbance: Distinct mediational models for males and females. *Eating Behaviors, 15,* 419–426. doi:10.1016/j.eatbeh.2014.04.020.
Dunkley, D. M., Zuroff, D. C., & Blankstein, K. R. (2003). Self-critical perfectionism and daily affect: Dispositional and situational influences on stress and coping. *Journal of Personality and Social Psychology, 84*(1), 234–252.
Ellis, A. (2002). The role of irrational beliefs in perfectionism. In G. L. Flett, & P. L. Hewitt (Eds.), *Perfectionism: Theory, research, and treatment* (pp. 217–229). Washington, DC: American Psychological Association.
Enns, M. W., & Cox, B. J. (2002). The nature and assessment of perfectionism: A critical analysis. In G. L. Flett, P. L. Hewitt, G. L. Flett, & P. L. Hewitt (Eds.), *Perfectionism: Theory, research, and treatment* (pp. 33–62). Washington, DC: American Psychological Association. doi:10.1037/10458-002.
Flett, G. L., & Hewitt, P. L. (2002). *Perfectionism: Theory, research, and treatment*. Washington, DC: American Psychological Association.
Flett, G. L., & Hewitt, P. L. (2006). Positive versus negative aspects of perfectionism in psychopathology: A comment on Slade and Owen's dual process model. *Behavior Modification, 30,* 11–24. doi:10.1177/0145445506288026.
Flett, G. L., Hewitt, P. L., Blankstein, K. R., & Gray, L. (1998). Psychological distress and the frequency of perfectionistic thinking. *Journal of Personality and Social Psychology, 75,* 1363–1381.
Flett, G. L., Hewitt, P. L., Demerjian, A., Sturman, E. D., Sherry, S. B., & Cheng, W. (2012). Perfectionistic automatic thoughts and psychological distress in adolescents: An analysis of the Perfectionism Cognitions Inventory. *Journal of Rational-Emotive and Cognitive-Behavior Therapy, 30,* 91–104. doi:10.1007/s10942-011-0131-7.
Frankish, C. J., Green, L. W., Ratner, P. A., Chomik, T., & Larsen, C. (1996). Health impact assessment as a tool for population health promotion and health policy. http://www.phac-asp.gc.ca/ph-sp/phdd/impact. Accessed 26 Jan 2008.
Freud, S. (1926/1959). Inhibitions, symptoms, and anxiety. In J. Strachey (Ed. and Trans.), *The standard edition of the complete psychological works of Sigmund Freud, 20,* (Vol. 20, pp. 77–175). London: Hogarth.
Freud, S. (1959). Inhibitions, symptoms, and anxiety. In J. Strachey (Ed. and Trans.), *The standard edition of the complete psychological works of Sigmund Freud* (Vol. 20, pp. 77–172). London: Hogarth Press. (Original work published 1926).
Friedman, H. S. (2011). Personality, disease and self-healing. In H. S. Friedman (Ed.), *The Oxford handbook of health psychology* (pp. 215–240). New York: Oxford University Press.
Frost, R. O., & DiBartolo, P. (2002). Perfectionism, anxiety and obsessive compulsive disorder. In G. Flett & P. Hewitt (Eds.), *Perfectionism: Theory, research, and treatment*. Washington, DC: American Psychological Association Press.

Frost, R. O., Marten, P., Lahart, C., & Rosenblate, R. (1990). The dimensions of perfectionism. *Cognitive Therapy and Research, 14,* 449–468.
Fry, P. S., & Debats, D. L. (2011). Perfectionism and other related trait measures as predictors of mortality in diabetic older adults: A six-and-a-half-year longitudinal study. *Journal of Health Psychology, 16,* 1058–1070. doi:10.1177/1359105311398684.
Garner, D. M., Olmstead, M. P., & Polivy, J. (1983). Development and validation of a multidimensional eating disorder inventory for anorexia and bulimia. *International Journal of Eating Disorders, 2,* 15–34.
Habke, A. M., Hewitt, P. L., & Flett, G. L. (1999). Perfectionism and sexual satisfaction in intimate relationships. *Journal of Psychopathology and Behavior Assessment, 21,* 307–322.
Hamachek, D. E. (1978). *Encounters with the self.* New York: Holt, Rinehart and Winston.
Hampson, S. E., Goldberg, L. R., Vogt, T. M., & Dubanoski, J. P. (2007). Mechanisms by which childhood personality traits influence adult health status: Educational attainment and healthy behaviors. *Health Psychology, 26*(1), 121–125.
Hewitt, P. L., & Flett, G. L. (1990). Perfectionism and depression: A multidimensional analysis. *Journal of Social Behavior and Personality, 5,* 423–438.
Hewitt, P. L., & Flett, G. L. (1991). Perfectionism in the self and social contexts: Conceptualization, assessment, and association with psychopathology. *Journal of Personality and Social Psychology, 60,* 456–470.
Hewitt, P. L., Flett, G. L., Turnbull-Donovan, W., & Mikail, S. F. (1991). The multidimensional perfectionism scale: Reliability, validity, and psychometric properties in psychiatric samples. *Psychological Assessment, A Journal of Consulting and Clinical Psychology, 3,* 464–468. doi:10.1037/1040-3590.3.3.464.
Hewitt, P. L., Flett, G. L., & Mikail, S. F. (1995). Perfectionism and relationship maladjustment in chronic pain patients and their spouses. *Journal of Family Psychology, 9,* 335–347.
Hewitt, P. L., Flett, G. L., Besser, A., Sherry, S. B., & McGee, B. (2003). Perfectionism is multidimensional: A reply to Shafran, Cooper, and Fairburn (2002). *Behaviour Research and Therapy, 41,* 1221–1236.
Hewitt, P. L., Flett, G. L., Sherry, S. B., Habke, M., Parkin, M., Lam, R. W., & Stein, M. B. (2003). The interpersonal expression of perfection: Perfectionistic self-presentation and psychological distress. *Journal of Personality & Social Psychology, 84,* 1303–1315. doi:10.1037/0022-3514.84.6.1303.
Hill, A. P., & Appleton, P. R. (2011). The predictive ability of the frequency of perfectionistic cognitions, self-oriented perfectionism, and socially prescribed perfectionism in relation to symptoms of burnout in youth rugby players. *Journal of Sports Sciences, 29*(7), 695–703. doi:10.1080/02640414.2010.551216.
Hodgson, R. J., & Rachman, S. (1977). Obsessional-compulsive complaints. *Behaviour Research and Therapy, 15,* 389–395. doi:10.1016/0005-7967(77)90042-0.
Horney, K. (1950). Neurosis and human growth: the struggle toward self-realization. Norton.
Juster, R.-P., McEwen, B. S., & Lupien, S. J. (2010). Allostatic load biomarkers of chronic stress and impact on health and cognition. *Neuroscience & Biobehavioral Reviews, 35*(1), 2–16.
Kashdan, T. B., Biswas-Diener, R., & King, L. A. (2008). Reconsidering happiness: The costs of distinguishing between hedonics and eudaimonia. *The Journal of Positive Psychology, 3*(4), 219–233.
Kobori, O. (2006). *A cognitive model of perfectionism: The relationship of perfectionism personality to psychological adaptation and maladaptation.* Unpublished doctoral dissertation, University of Tokyo, Tokyo.
Lazarus, R. S., & Folkman, S. (1984). *Stress, appraisal, and coping.* New York: Springer.
Lynam, D. R., Hoyle, R. H., & Newman, J. P. (2006). The perils of partialling: Cautionary tales from aggression and psychopathy. *Assessment, 13,* 328–341.
Matte, M., & Lafontaine, M.-F. (2012). Assessment of romantic perfectionism: Psychometric properties of the romantic relationship perfectionism scale. *Measurement and Evaluation in Counseling and Development, 45,* 113–132. doi:10.1177/0748175611429303.
Missildine, W. H. (1963). *Your inner child of the past.* New York: Simon and Schuster.

McDowell, I. (2010). Measures of self-perceived well-being. *Journal of Psychosomatic Research, 69*(1), 69–79.
McEwen, B. S. (2007). Physiology and neurobiology of stress and adaptation: Central role of the brain. *Physiological Reviews, 87*(3), 873–904.
Molnar, D. S., Reker, D. L., Culp, N. A., Sadava, S. W., & DeCourville, N. H. (2006). A mediated model of perfectionism, affect, and physical health. *Journal of Research in Personality, 40,* 482–500. doi:10.1016/j.jrp.2005.04.002.
Molnar, D. S., Sadava, S. W., Flett, G. L., & Colautti, J. (2012). Perfectionism and health-related quality of life in women with fibromyalgia. *Journal of Psychosomatic Research, 73,* 295–300.
Mor, S., Day, H. I., Flett, G. L., & Hewitt, P. L. (1995). Perfectionism, control, and components of performance anxiety in professional artists. *Cognitive Therapy and Research, 19*(2), 207–225.
Organization, W. H. (2005). *Promoting mental health: Concepts, emerging evidence, practice.* Geneva: WHO.
Pacht, A. R. (1984). Reflections on perfection. *American Psychologist, 39*(4), 386–390. doi:10.1037/0003-066X.39.4.386.
Purdon, C., Antony, M., & Swinson, R. (1999). Psychometric properties of the Frost Multidimensional perfectionism scale in a clinical anxiety disorders sample. *Journal of Clinical Psychology, 55,* 1271–1286.
Rhéaume, J., Ladouceur, R., & Freeston, M. H. (2000). The prediction of obsessive–compulsive tendencies: Does perfectionism play a significant role? *Personality and Individual Differences, 28,* 583–592. doi:10.1016/S0191-8869(99)00121-X.
Ryan, R. M., & Deci, E. L. (2001). To be happy or to be self-fulfilled: A review of research on hedonic and eudaimonic well-being. In S. Fiske (Ed.), *Annual review of psychology* (Vol. 52, pp. 141–166). Palo Alto: Annual Reviews.
Ryff, C. D. (1989). Happiness is everything, or is it? Explorations on the meaning of psychological well-being. *Journal of Personality and Social Psychology, 6,* 1069–1081.
Ryff, C. D., & Keyes, C. L. M. (1995). The structure of psychological well-being revisited. *Journal of Personality and Social Psychology, 69,* 719–727.
Seligman, M., & Csikszentmihalyi, M. (2000). Positive psychology: An introduction. *American Psychologist, 55,* 5–14. doi:10.1037/0003-066X.55.1.5.
Shafran, R., & Mansell, W. (2001). Perfectionism and psychopathology: A review of research and treatment. *Clinical Psychology Review, 21,* 879–906. doi:10.1016/S0272-7358(00)00072-6.
Shafran, R., Cooper, Z., & Fairburn, C. G. (2002). Clinical perfectionism: A cognitive-behavioural analysis. *Behaviour Research and Therapy, 40,* 773–791. doi:10.1016/S0005-7967(01)00059-6.
Shea, A. J., Slaney, R. B., & Rice, K. G. (2006). Perfectionism in intimate relationships: The dyadic almost perfect scale. *Measurement and Evaluation in Counseling and Development, 39,* 107–125.
Sherry, S. B., Gralnick, T. M., Hewitt, P. L., Sherry, D. L., & Flett, G. L. (in press). Perfectionism and narcissism: Testing unique relationships and gender differences. *Personality and Individual Differences.*
Sirois, F. M. (2011). Psychological health and well-being: A research agenda for the Eastern Townships. *Journal of the Eastern Townships Studies, 37,* 77–94.
Sirois, F. M., & Molnar, D. S. (2014). Perfectionism and maladaptive coping styles in patients with chronic fatigue syndrome, irritable bowel syndrome and fibromyalgia/arthritis and in healthy controls. *Psychotherapy and Psychosomatics, 83*(6), 384–385.
Slade, P. D., & Owens, R. G. (1998). A dual process model of perfectionism based on reinforcement theory. *Behavior Modification, 22,* 372–390.
Slaney, R. B., Rice, K. G., Mobley, M., Trippi, J., & Ashby, J. (2001). The revised almost perfect scale. *Measurement and Evaluation in Counseling and Development, 34,* 130–145.
Slaney, R. B., Rice, K. G., & Ashby, J. S. (2002). A programmatic approach to measuring perfectionism: The almost perfect scales. In G. L. Flett, P. L. Hewitt, G. L. Flett, & P. L. Hewitt (Eds.), *Perfectionism: Theory, research, and treatment* (pp. 63–88). Washington, DC: American Psychological Association. doi:10.1037/10458-003.

Smith, T. W. (2006). Personality as risk and resilience in physical health. *Current Directions in Psychological Science, 15*(5), 227–231.

Stober, J. (1998). The frost multidimensional perfectionism scale revisited: More perfect with four (instead of six) dimensions. *Personality and Individual Differences, 24,* 481–491.

Stoeber, J. (2014). How other-oriented perfectionism differs from self-oriented and socially prescribed perfecitonism. *Journal of Psychopathology and Behavioral Assessment, 36,* 329–338. doi:10.1007/s10862-013-9397-7.

Stoeber, J., & Otto, K. (2006). Positive conceptions of perfectionism: Approaches, evidence, challenges. *Personality and Social Psychology Review, 10,* 295–319. doi:10.1207/s15327957pspr1004_2.

Stoeber, J., Kobori, O., & Tanno, Y. (2010). The Multidimensional Perfectionism Cognitions Inventory–English (MPCI-E): Reliability, validity, and relationships with positive and negative affect. *Journal of Personality Assessment, 92*(1), 16–25.

Taylor, S. E., & Sirois, F. M. (2014). *Health psychology (3rd Canadian ed.).* Toronto: McGraw-Hill Ryerson.

Terry-Short, L. A., Owens, R. G., Slade, P. D., & Dewey, M. E. (1995). Positive and negative perfectionism. *Personality and Individual Differences, 18,* 663–666.

Waterman, A. S. (1993). Two conceptions of happiness: Contrasts of personal expressiveness (eudaimonia) and hedonic enjoyment. *Journal of Personality and Social Psychology, 64*(4), 678–691.

Waterman, A. S. (2008). Reconsidering happiness: A eudaimonist's perspective. *The Journal of Positive Psychology: Dedicated to furthering research and promoting good practice, 3*(4), 234–252.

Weisinger, H., & Lobsenz, N. M. (1981). *Nobody s perfect: How to give criticism and get results.* New York: Warne.

Williams, C. J., & Cropley, M. (2014). The relationship between perfectionism and engagement in preventive health behaviours: The mediating role of self concealment. *Journal of Health Psychology, 19,* 1211–1221.

Wolff, H. G. (1937). Personality features and reactions of subjects with migraine. *Archives of Neurology & Psychiatry, 37,* 985–921

Wolff, H. G. (1948). *Headache and other head pain.* New York: Oxford University Press.

Part I
Perfectionism and Physical Health

Chapter 2
Perfectionism in Health and Illness from a Person-Focused, Historical Perspective

Gordon L. Flett, Paul L. Hewitt and Danielle S. Molnar

This chapter examines the role of perfectionism in health problems from a historical perspective. Our chapter qualifies what is known about the link between perfectionism and illness because most scholars and readers who are familiar with the perfectionism field would likely point to the last two decades of the previous century as the time period when the role of perfectionism in health and illness first became a significant topic. Indeed, this is the time period when several relevant papers and studies emerged. Initial investigations during this period tended to be based on the use of the various unidimensional perfectionism measures such as the Burns Perfectionism Scale, and the perfectionism subscales of the Eating Disorder Inventory and the Workaholism Inventory (e.g., Brewerton & George, 1993; Forman, Tosi, & Rudy, 1987; Kanai, Wakabayashi, & Fling, 1996). The eventual appearance of multidimensional perfectionism measures by Frost, Marten, Lahart, and Rosenblate (1990) and Hewitt and Flett (1990, 1991) made it possible to examine perfectionism using a more complex approach involving multiple trait dimensions.

Collective understanding of people with perfectionistic personalities has been substantially advanced over the past decade as a result of overall developments in the field. While the emphasis is now on multidimensional perfectionism and recent advances, the conceptual contributions and clinical observations of luminaries such as Alfred Adler, Karen Horney, and Hilde Bruch can never be discounted.

Adler suggested that all people have a need to be perfect and this stems from feelings of inferiority. These feelings are compensated for by striving for superior-

G. L. Flett (✉)
Department of Psychology, York University, Toronto, ON, Canada
e-mail: gflett@yorku.ca

P. L. Hewitt
University of British Columbia, Vancouver, Canada

D. S. Molnar
Research Institute on Addictions, University at Buffalo, The State University of New York, Buffalo, NY, USA

Department of Psychology, Brock University, St. Catharines, ON, Canada

F. M. Sirois, D. S. Molnar (eds.), *Perfectionism, Health, and Well-Being*,
DOI 10.1007/978-3-319-18582-8_2

ity and perfection. Adler left room for individual differences by noting variability in this tendency. Specifically, Adler (1938/1998) described certain people who strive for a godlike perfection as "…. perpetually comparing themselves with the unattainable ideal of perfection, are always possessed and spurred on by a sense of inferiority" (p. 35–36). This sense of striving for perfection as a way of trying to lessen feelings of inferiority can be viewed as a constant source of pressure that causes physiological dysregulation. This was illustrated in a case account in the very first issue of *Psychosomatic Medicine*. Alexander (1939) described a hypertensive, submissive man with an inferiority complex and a chronic need to be perfect and outperform others in order to establish his worth.

Adler's views linking perfectionism with the inferiority complex resulted in perhaps the first empirical attempts to assess perfectionism. Heidbreder (1927) included item content that tapped self-reported perfectionism when creating a self-report measure of the inferiority complex. Perfectionists with an inferiority complex were identified in this study, but Heidbreder (1927) found via statistical analyses that the component tapping perfectionism did not effectively distinguish people with or without the inferiority complex because many people lacking a sense of inferiority complex also seemed perfectionistic. It is interesting to note that Heidbreder (1927) suggested long ago that, after further inspection, the results were limited by how perfectionism was assessed; that is, the measure had elements of conscientiousness rather than perfectionism *per se*.

Karen Horney focused on perfectionism and its roots in the basic anxiety and basic hostility that children experience as a result of frustrating and disquieting early experiences with parents. The child who feels hostility that cannot be expressed for fear of punishment is characterized by a strong neurotic conflict. Horney (1945/1972), in her classic book *Our Inner Conflicts*, suggested that one way of addressing a neurotic conflict is to create an idealized image of the perfect self that the individual perceives can be attained at some point. She also posited ten neurotic needs that were prime motivators, and one of these ten needs was the neurotic need for perfection and unassailability (Horney, 1950). These neurotic tendencies reflect a simultaneous desire to move toward people, but also move away from and against these people. This observation suggests that the neurotic need for perfection is underscored by a complex array of motives.

The views and observations of Hilde Bruch are especially relevant given that she focused on perfectionism within the context of a potentially life-threatening disorder—anorexia nervosa—that combines complex physical and psychological processes and functioning. Bruch is known for her seminal books on anorexia nervosa (Bruch, 1973, 1978, 1988), but her insights about perfectionism first emerged in her analysis of how children and their families responded after the child was diagnosed with diabetes. She noted that this response is rooted in the family's tendency to have "… a repressive, perfectionistic attitude toward the child" (Bruch & Hewlett, 1947, p. 205). Her subsequent work on the nature and etiology of anorexia (e.g., Bruch, 1962) described how girls suffering from anorexia were driven to achieve perfect grades in school and this was traced back to the unresolved psychological needs of the girls' mothers and fathers. These views about the perfectionistic demands of parents were later reflected by specific test items on the

Eating Disorder Inventory perfectionism subscale reflecting parental expectations and parental criticism (see Garner, Olmstead, & Polivy, 1983). Bruch's views about the role of perfectionism were elaborated upon in a series of books that documented Bruch's remarkable clinical insights after having spent years treating young people with anorexia nervosa (see Bruch, 1973, 1978, 1988). Her work foreshadowed the contemporary emphasis on socially prescribed perfectionism (i.e., the pressure to be perfect imposed on the self by other people) because she discussed the pressures to conform that faced adolescent girls and the problems that ensue when they cannot live up to these very high expectations. The most detailed analysis can be found in the book *Conversations With Anorexics* that Bruch worked on just prior to her death, and it was published posthumously (see Bruch, 1988). It is here that Bruch outlines her views that perfectionism is largely a façade that covers up a highly inadequate self. She observed:

> "Deep down, every anorexic is convinced that basically she is inadequate, low, mediocre, inferior, and despised by others. She lives in an imaginary world with an assumed reality where she feels that people around her—her family, her friends, and the world at large—look down on her with disapproving eyes, ready to pounce on her with criticism. The image of human behavior and interaction that an anorexic constructs in her apparently well-functioning home is one of surprising cynicism, pessimism, and bitterness. All her efforts, her striving for perfection and excessive thinness, are directed toward hiding the fatal flaw of her fundamental inadequacy" (Bruch, 1988, p. 6).

Bruch's sage observations were acknowledged by Hewitt, Flett, and Ediger (1995) in our conceptualization of perfectionistic self-presentation and its role in eating disorders.

Unfortunately, scientific advances in research on perfectionism were hindered for several decades by the lack of available measures tapping perfectionism. The Irrational Beliefs Test (IBT) by Jones (1968) has a 10-item perfectionism subscale that taps the belief in perfect solutions to world problems. It fails to tap the core drive for achievement that is central to an understanding of perfectionism; this aspect of perfectionism is better captured by another IBT subscale tapping high self-expectations. Earlier we mentioned the Burns Perfectionism Scale (BPS), which was the first widely known measure constructed solely and specifically to assess perfectionism (see Burns, 1980). The BPS is a 10-item unidimensional measure that consists of attitude statements reflecting the importance of perfectionism and the catastrophes that await the person who is imperfect (e.g., If I don't set the highest standards for myself, I am likely to end up a second-rate person). Scale content is a reflection of the work that David Burns conducted with Aaron Beck on perfectionism within the context of the cognitive model of depression.

This measure was followed by the emergence of the six-item unidimensional perfectionism subscale of the Eating Disorder Inventory (EDI; Garner et al., 1983). It is more than symbolic that this subscale is one component of a measure designed to assess a form of psychopathology with clear health consequences. While perfectionism is often regarded as synonymous with eating disorders, people with an eating disorder vary in their levels of perfectionism. Clearly, perfectionism can have important consequences in the context of eating disorders, as illustrated by one of the initial studies with the EDI showing that more perfectionistic adolescents with anorexia were less likely to complete treatment and, as such, they have greater risk (see Steiner, Mazer, & Litt, 1990).

The "Hidden Literature" on Perfectionism in Health and Illness

We stated at the outset of this chapter that most analyses of the link between perfectionism and health would likely focus on the 1980s and 1990s. However, when a detailed historical analysis is conducted as we did for the purposes of the current chapter, it becomes apparent that the notion that perfectionism contributes to illness is not new; in fact, there is a substantial "hidden literature" comprised of case accounts and some intriguing empirical studies that are highly informative and that stretch back several decades. We refer to this work as "hidden" because to our knowledge, much of this work has never been cited or documented by contemporary authors despite the exponential increase in research and theory on perfectionism over the past 25 years.

In light of these observations, this chapter contains a description of this early research and theory on perfectionism and health in keeping with our primary goal of heightening awareness of these earlier contributions. Early papers on perfectionism and health represent a vital source of hypotheses that deserve to be considered and tested by contemporary researchers. Indeed, this work points to several key themes.

As will be illustrated in the material presented below, the clear picture that emerges from this earlier literature is that perfectionists have "a pressure personality" that involves continuous exposure to stress from external and internal demands. There are also clear indications of the tendency for perfectionists to make themselves vulnerable to health problems as a result of striving to the point of exhaustion. We found it particularly useful to consider perfectionism from a person-focused perspective that emphasizes the factors and processes that can contribute to health and illness in the individual person.

Our historical overview of previous theory and research is provided below. While our search yielded some empirical investigations of perfectionism and health, there was also an abundance of descriptive case accounts. While such cases have limited value from a strict scientific perspective, we nevertheless found these descriptive accounts to be highly informative in at least two key respects. First, these reports point to key factors that need to be considered by researchers who are seeking to identify the specific mechanisms and processes that link perfectionism with illness. For instance, stress is one process that has been emphasized continuously by early authors. We have sometimes been frustrated by contemporary research that is designed to test whether perfectionism is adaptive versus maladaptive because it is often the case that no attempt was made to examine the role of stress, despite clear statements about how perfectionism can be regarded as a vulnerability factor that is activated when the perfectionist encounters ego-involving and personally threatening stressors (see Hewitt & Flett, 1991, 1993, 2002).

Second, as alluded to earlier, the descriptive case accounts from the previous century serve as a reminder of the need to remain cognizant of the link between perfectionism and health problems from a person-centered perspective; most perfectionism research thus far has used a variable-centered perspective. At the level of the individual person, and in keeping with a clinical and counseling focus, it is essential to consider the pattern of perfectionism across various perfectionism dimensions and how it relates to other personality features and the situational contexts that have an impact on the individual person. A clear example of the potential complexities involved for the individual perfectionist is a remarkable psychoanalytic account of a highly perfectionistic woman with a severe case of colitis (see Karush & Daniels, 1953). This case clearly illustrates the interpersonal aspects of perfectionism and how interpersonal stressors and strains can fuel health problems long before perfectionism took on an interpersonal focus. Most notably, the woman described by these authors had tried to compensate for her unmet interpersonal needs by working hard to maintain the façade that her marriage with her husband was perfect (i.e., perfectionistic self-presentation), but life became far from perfect when her husband had an affair with her friend; the betrayed woman, in turn, became sexually involved with her friend's husband. In this case example, perfectionism represented a way of coping with circumstances that were far from ideal. Karush and Daniels (1953) also described how this woman experienced much hostility because her husband fell far short of her wish to have an ideal, perfect partner. Perfectionism was a theme throughout this case analysis, including the component focused on the therapy process. For instance, at one point, the client tried to project her older brother's demanding perfection onto the therapist, and she also noted that she had come to see the therapist as expecting her to be perfect (i.e., socially prescribed perfectionism).

The link between perfectionism and stress-related health symptoms has been described by several other authors. For instance, Rodger (1948) described Mrs. H., who was characterized as "… a young bride with an over-conscientious, perfectionist, meticulous personality" (p. 155) who continued to manage her parents' business after being married. She suffered symptoms following periods of emotional tension and stress.

Perhaps the clearest illustration of the need for a complex, person-centered focus that allows for complex blends of various perfectionism dimensions was provided by Lundh, Saboonchi, and Wangby (2008) who examined how patterns of perfectionism, as assessed by the Frost Multidimensional Perfectionism Scale (FMPS), are related to various forms of clinical disorder. They conducted a cluster analysis that yielded a ten-cluster solution with several combinations deemed to reflect clinically significant perfectionism. Three patterns involving extreme perfectionism across most of the FMPS subscales were overrepresented among the patients with social phobia but underrepresented among the nonclinical participants. Lundh et al. (2008) cautioned that it is inappropriate to characterize high scores on the personal standards factor as adaptive because when the focus is on the individual person, some patterns involving high perfectionism often reflect combinations that also include high concern over mistakes and high doubts about actions. These data have clear implications for variable-centered research that isolates perfectionism dimensions (e.g., personal strivings versus evaluative concerns perfectionism), and there is little attempt to think about the extreme perfectionist who is highly vulnerable due to elevations on both dimensions.

Themes Emerging from the Historical Work on Perfectionism and Health

Our historical overview is provided below. When this material is being considered, we found it helpful to remain cognizant of three key themes. First, it became evident early on that perfectionism is primarily maladaptive and there is little suggestion in these initial accounts that it is adaptive; by and large, perfectionism was implicated in various forms of illness by authors in ways that are not in keeping with the notion that perfectionism yields benefits to the individual. One way to frame this issue is that the costs of perfectionism, especially health costs, seem to far outweigh the benefits.

Our second theme is that the mind and body connection is clearly relevant in seeking to understand those people who are driven by a need to be perfect. This is particularly well illustrated by complex case studies of the various individuals who have also suffered from comorbid psychological and medical problems. These complexities continue to be evident in contemporary case accounts of perfectionists. For instance, a recently published case study of a young woman who died by suicide noted that she had diagnosed depression and psychotic features, but also a long-standing history of significant health issues, including migraine headaches, fibromyalgia, and Wolff–Parkinson–White syndrome (see Hassan, Flett, Ganguli, & Hewitt, 2014).

Finally, as mentioned earlier, a third theme that is highly salient is the notion of "the stressed perfectionist" who does not respond well to stress and pressure, but who nevertheless takes on too much responsibility and responds to challenge and threat by striving even harder and even longer to be perfect. A clear sense emerges of depleted and exhausted perfectionists who lack the resources and resilience to withstand further stresses and challenges to their well-being. Surprisingly, in this regard, one of the most cogent and insightful analyses of the role of stress in perfectionism was provided by the infamous Ewen Cameron, the psychiatrist who was later to be disgraced for his unethical treatment of his research participants in Montreal. Regarding perfectionism, Cameron (1944) described the "tensional breakdowns" of a cohort of workers who responded poorly to wartime pressures and job stress because they had to work under time pressures that did not allow for them to be as exacting, deliberate, and precise as they would like to be, yet they were not permitted to make mistakes. Cameron (1944) observed that "… there is a range of personalities running from those who are exceedingly meticulous and perfectionistic in their work and in their social relations, through those who are considered reliable and conscientious members of society …" (p. 117). Cameron

(1944) described the perfectionists as people who are painstaking, meticulous, and seldom satisfied and who are "… a little lacking in self-confidence unless they feel quite strongly that they are doing the right thing" (p. 117). He then suggested that there is a subset of particularly stress prone perfectionists "… who tend to be rather anxious-minded; who worry unduly about things that most of us take in stride; who may not be quite as careful to do the right thing as those whom I have just described, but who, when they fail to do so, worry quite excessively about it" (p. 117). Some insights from Cameron have yet to be tested empirically, but they fit with our notion that some perfectionists are overly anxious ruminators who are at risk for stress-related illnesses and associated difficulties.

The three themes outlined above are reflected throughout the remainder of this chapter. The summary overview we provide below is organized into various sections according to distinguishable health problems. Specifically, we describe the role of perfectionism in the following: (1) ulcers and other gastrointestinal illnesses; (2) migraine headaches; and (3) cardiovascular illnesses. We also provide a section that summarizes the early empirical research linking perfectionism with illness.

Initial Historical Links Between Perfectionism and Health Problems

Perfectionism in Ulcers and Other Gastrointestinal Illnesses

Initial links between perfectionism and health problems began to emerge in the 1930s when perfectionism was conceptualized as a monolithic construct focused on personal perfection. One of the earliest case studies was provided by Fremont-Smith (1932) who described a 39-year-old single man suffering from an ulcer. He was described as a perfectionist who had unrealistic relationship ideals and a tendency to take his responsibilities and mistakes far too seriously. His perfectionism reflected being raised by a domineering aunt and he learned to react to disappointment by developing exaggerated ambition and fear of failure. There was also a stated history of phobias and feelings of panic and guilt. As an adult, ulcer symptoms emerged when his work schedule became too heavy during the winter months. This man had a tendency to suffer symptoms when he felt that he was being pressured by more work than he could possibly accomplish in the period allowed; ulcer symptoms could be triggered simply by thinking about not getting all of his work done. This case study is one of the first illustrations of the potential relevance of perfectionism to workplace health. It also shows how long-standing stressors (i.e., a domineering aunt) can combine with current stressors and strains to elicit symptoms such as pain in perfectionistic people. Freemont-Smith (1932) emphasized that this type of case shows a clear link between states of mind and ulcer-related pain.

Mittelmann and Wolff (1942) also pointed to a link between perfectionism and ulcers by identifying perfectionism as a maladaptive response exhibited by their adult patients suffering from ulcers in response to feelings of low self-esteem. The family histories of these individuals often involved family discord and conflict and this elicited a common response according to reports of the patients' childhoods. Specifically, Mittelmann and Wolff (1942) noted that "in several instances, children threatened with fear of abandonment and rejection because of expressed conflict between parents attempted to gain approval through perfect performance, usually linked with repression or resentment. The development of such compensatory measures began in early childhood" (p. 6). To our knowledge, this emphasis on striving not just for perfection but also for approval is one of the earliest accounts of the self-worth contingencies that are arguably central to an understanding of perfectionism.

Mittelmann and Wolff (1942) also provided an exceedingly detailed case account that includes analyses of physiological reactions with objective data of an ulcer patient who dealt with feelings of abandonment, resentment, and submissiveness by trying to live up to high ideals and expectations by having flawless performance. This patient then condemned himself for inevitably failing to be perfect. This is one of the earliest documented cases of the self-critical perfectionism described by Blatt (1995). A clear conclusion that can be drawn from this case study is that the path to recovery must involve developing a sense of self-compassion and self-acceptance. Negative self-views can play a vital role in exacerbating the link between perfectionism and illness.

Further support for the role of perfectionism in ulcer came from an analysis of the first 50 cases of men with ulcer who were treated in a hospital in London, Ontario (see Ross, Geddes, Hauch, & Scratch, 1950). Detailed personality information was not gathered, but it was concluded that emotional tension was present in 35 of the 50 cases. Most of the patients were described as hard-driving perfectionists who found it difficult to leave work behind when it was time to go home for the day. Several were assembly-line foremen. It was noted that they showed less spontaneity in their responses than other patients. A similar description was provided by Bingham (1960) in his description of his 50 patients with an ulcer and how they were distinguished from 50 ulcer patients who were also suffering from alcoholism. Bingham (1960) noted that the perfectionism was often an overcompensation response that emerged during times of stress and challenge.

Parenthetically, it should be noted that in keeping with the case study noted above, perfectionism has also been implicated in non-ulcerative colitis. We will focus on two of the most detailed analyses. First, Mahoney, Bockus, Ingram, Hundley, and Yaskin (1949) provided a detailed description of 20 patients with non-ulcerative colitis based on psychiatric interviews and personality tests. The psychiatric interviews identified that 12 patients were characterized by perfectionism and aggression. Other associated features included nervous tension and anxiety, hostility, and immaturity. Comparative conclusions were limited, unfortunately, by the lack of a comparison group.

Second, White, Cobb, and Jones (1939) described the personality features of 60 patients with colitis as part of their detailed monograph. Their summary description sounds very much like depictions of neurotic perfectionists who need social approval. They described overconscientious, meticulous individuals with restricted emotional expression despite being filled with anxiety, guilt, and resentment. These people were highly focused on being mistreated by others, even when, according to the investigators, it involved forms of mistreatment that less sensitive people would probably not notice. They also linked this style with a rigid and obsessive form of rumination that involved a cognitive preoccupation with their problems. They observed that "This constant preoccupation is presumably responsible for the prolongation of tension and hence for the prolonged action of the parasympathetic system upon the colon" (p. 95). The role of rumination and other forms of cognitive perseveration in perfectionism are discussed at length by Flett et al., 2016 in Chap. 6.

Perfectionism in Migraine Headache

The 1930s decade also is the period when there was a great emphasis on the role of perfectionism in migraine headache. This really began with a detailed description of "the migrainous patient" by Touraine and Draper (1934). Their article in the *Journal of Nervous and Mental Disease* appeared in two separate parts of approximately 23 pages each. The second segment has brief descriptions of each one of 50 patients. These accounts focused on having an insecure attachment to one's mother, with the mother being someone who is difficult to please and who is capable of being quite critical. Touraine and Draper (1934) observed that people afflicted with migraine headaches often were people who seemed healthy, useful and of high intelligence. These people were described as reserved individuals who did not easily make social contacts. Perfectionism was first highlighted in the work context. Specifically, it was noted that:

> "In his (sic) occupation he is a detailed perfectionist, and the urge to check and re-check his work is a characteristic common to his sort. This is particularly the result of an extremely sensitive response to criticism, for it is his nature to seek the cause within himself. Unnecessary burdens and responsibilities are assumed…whether or not they are found in the reality or phantasy worlds. He is anxious, anticipates catastrophe, and is discouraged. He does not lose himself in the art of living. His emotions are deep, but the expression of them appears to be frustrated, and there is a tendency to revert to self-pity." (Touraine & Draper, 1934, p. 2).

Several associated attributes in this description ring true in terms of more recent accounts of perfectionists; key themes include being sensitive to criticism, being overly responsible, and an unwillingness or inability to express negative emotions.

Harold Wolff (1937) was also highly instrumental in highlighting the role of perfectionism in illness beginning with his observations that also pointed to the role of perfectionism in migraine headache. Wolff was a pioneer in the early study of head pain and was former president of the American Neurological Association. It was primarily his observations that led to perfectionism receiving very early consideration as one of the leading psychological causes of migraine headache (see Wolff, 1937, Wolff, 1948). Marcussen and Wolff (1949) concluded that people with these personality attributes are "not necessarily 'neurotic' in the usual sense"

(p. 251). Rather, they are tense, driven people who are rigid, ambitious, and perfectionistic. As a result, they tend to strive relentlessly and ignore bodily needs for rest and relaxation to the extent that they put themselves at risk. Marcussen and Wolff (1949) then outlined four case studies of migraine sufferers who had considerable stress and tension in their lives. Central themes emerging from these case studies portrayed these individuals as interpersonally sensitive and highly reactive to failure and feedback highlighting their lack of accomplishment.

A descriptive analysis of 500 people with "the migrainous personality" provided by a Mayo Clinic physician named Walter Alvarez (1947) also emphasized the role of perfectionism. Alvarez (1947) focused on women because women comprised the vast majority of his patients. He concluded that "The outstanding characteristics of the migrainous woman are her hypersensitiveness, her quickness of thought and movement and her tendency to get tense, to worry, to tire easily, to tire suddenly and to sleep poorly. Usually, she is a perfectionist who works fast and accurately and likes to push other persons along to work fast with her" (p. 3). Alvarez (1947) also noted that these women are also quite prone to marital problems because these women are prone to dissatisfaction because even a good husband does not approximate her ideal of the perfect husband.

The relevance of perfectionism as part of migraine personality involving perfectionism was also highlighted by Donahue (1949) as part of his comprehensive analysis of the link between migraine and ocular functioning. Donahue (1949) concluded his analysis with detailed case excerpts of five people who suffered from migraines that impacted their visual capacities. Three of the five people showed clear indications of perfectionism, while a fourth person was described as having a striving and ambitious temperament but her interest in graduate studies was discouraged by her husband. The most perfectionistic person was a 44-year-old male office worker referred to as "Case 2." He was described as someone who was an "… extremely hard-working, driving, perfectionistic and ambitious type of man who was interested in and able to keep a number of different activities in operation at the same time. In order to accomplish this, he was required to make quick decisions and to be constantly alert and attentive; if he encountered any delay, or if for some reason he was unable to maintain his high standard of efficiency, he became extremely tense and resentful. It was during these periods that his migraine attacks took place." Observation of Case 2 over a 6-month period showed that he would permit no compromises in terms of needing to be excellent and efficient at all times, but he was also prone to periods of great tension, irritability, and dejection. What is clear from this case analysis is that as was suggested initially by Hewitt and Flett (1991, 1993), it is essential to consider stressors and factors in the situational context that trigger the vulnerabilities of extreme perfectionists.

Perfectionism was also seen as highly relevant in cluster headaches (see Friedman, 1958). Some support for the existence of "the migraine personality" (i.e., meticulousness, preoccupation with achievement, and relentless striving for perfection) was found by Burns (1965) who determined that 57 of the 92 migraine patients in his rural practice were perfectionistic and had "the migraine personality" versus 20 of the 92 patients in the control group. Unfortunately, the methods and criteria used to establish the presence of this personality style were not outlined.

Some particularly useful insights about perfectionism and migraine headache were provided by Graham (1953), who conducted a descriptive study of 46 adults (36 women, 10 men) who had suffered for years from "normal" migraine headaches. Graham (1953) indicated that "the large majority" were perfectionists. In general, the patients were described succinctly as people, "who, by virtue of their personality, tend to seek stress but who, by virtue of their physiology, are ill-equipped to meet it. The advent of stress of various sorts tends to precipitate their attacks" (p. 73). Graham (1953) went on to note that his sample consisted largely of "thin, tense, intelligent housewives or white collar workers, who are perfectionists in their outlook and are chronically fatigued" (p. 62). They also have "conscientious drive," little rest, and irregular or disturbed sleep. Graham's (1953) work is particularly representative in that it emphasizes the association that perfectionism has with stress as well as the propensity for perfectionists to over-strive to the point of mental and physical exhaustion. An appended commentary on Graham's (1953) paper further highlighted the anger of perfectionists and "… chronic resentment resulting from inability to satisfy perfectionistic demands and compulsively assumed responsibilities" (p. 74).

More recently, perfectionism was featured in a descriptive analysis of 20 patients with migraine headaches and allergies to food (see Wilson, Kirker, Warnes, & O'Malley, 1980). This study involved a psychiatric interview, and it was deemed that 17 of the 20 patients had an obsessional personality, while all 20 were characterized by perfectionism. While intriguing, it should be noted that a detailed description of how perfectionism was conceptualized and assessed was not provided other than to note that the patients "… had traits of perfectionism, meticulosity, orderliness and high standards of behavior"(p. 618). However, a measure of "hysteroid-obsessional" style was used and "… it was noted that the whole group rated high on conscientiousness, stability, fear of change, tension, and a desire to live up to high standards and ideals"(Wilson et al., 1980, p. 618).

Perfectionism in Hypertension and Cardiovascular Illnesses

Contemporary research on how perfectionists cope with cardiac illness is now emerging (Dunkley et al., 2012; Shanmugasegaram et al., 2014), and this research has its roots in work conducted over 60 years ago on hypertension and cardiovascular illness. Alexander's (1939) case account of a man with hypertension was noted earlier. Simon's (1948) article on the role of the psychiatrist in cardiovascular illness supported previous observations by Binger, Ackerman, Cohn, Schroeder, and Steele (1945) who implicated perfectionism in hypertension. Simon observed that these people are described as individuals who "… worry over their jobs, everything must be just right, and in this way they display their compulsive drive to perfectionism which may be so intense as to interfere in the achievement of their goal… They dislike and resent criticism. However, they do not overtly express their anger, but tend to repress their feelings. Outwardly they act as though they want to please people and gain their approval, and inwardly they may be 'mad as hell'. As a result they are in a psychological turmoil because of the conflict between their need for approval and their need to express the anger they repress" (Simon, 1948, p. 187-188). Simon (1948) discussed at length the turmoil that characterizes perfectionistic people because their abiding need for approval does not mesh well with their unexpressed anger and resentment that sometimes cannot be controlled and creates interpersonal problems for the vulnerable perfectionist.

Other investigations focused on apparent links between perfectionism and cardiac difficulties and contributing conditions such as hypertension. Duncan, Stevenson, and Ripley (1950) provided another insightful account of the perfectionism–illness link following their thorough analysis of 14 patients with cardiac arrhythmias. All 14 patients showed signs of driven, compulsive tendencies, and they were all found to be perfectionistic in the standards they set both for themselves and for others. Emotional factors were seen as quite important in general in these cardiac patients. Overall, 11 of the 14 patients had long-standing problems with anxiety and observed difficulties with expressing hostility and resentment.

Finally, several authors considered perfectionism as part of the great initial interest in the Type A coronary-prone style. The initial descriptions of the Type A personality by Friedman and Rosenhan mentioned several characteristics that are often found among perfectionists, but the role of perfectionistic standards was not emphasized explicitly by these groundbreaking researchers (see Friedman & Rosenhan, 1974; Friedman & Ulmer, 1984). However, other clinical accounts made frequent references to perfectionism. For instance, a qualitative analysis of 12 people suffering from chest pains and migraines led to the observation that "all patients exhibited the aggressive, obsessive and perfectionistic make-up of Type A personality" (Leon-Sotomayor, 1974).

Perhaps the most insightful observations here were provided by Henry Russek (1959), a physician based in New York, who compared risk factors for 100 young patients under 40 years of age with coronary heart disease and 100 patients with other diseases. In general, Russek (1959) highlighted the role of emotional stress and strain in coronary heart disease, but key for our purposes is that Russek concluded that the Type A personality pattern "… presents a caricature rather than a portrait of the average coronary patient under the age of 40 in our series" (p. 505). Why? Russek (1959) noted that these people had seemingly high levels of self-control, reserve, and an outward complacency, but they were actually driven perfectionists who were victims of overwork and taking on too many responsibilities while feeling guilty and being unable to relax during those times when they were on vacation. Russek (1959) deserved particular credit for noting that these overmeticulous perfectionists were "stress-blind" (p. 505) with any attempt at self-care; instead, they "… minimized their symptoms, and neglected prudent rules of health." (p. 505). It is our experience that perfectionists are exceptionally low in self-care, especially those who are workaholics with heavy role demands (e.g., physicians, lawyers), and this lack of focus on self-protective behaviors likely contributes substantially to their susceptibility to illness. Contemporary research has yet to document the diminished self-care of those perfectionists who seemingly live in a world of stress.

Given the overlapping features of perfectionism and the Type A style, we find it surprising that with but few exceptions (e.g., Flett, Hewitt, Blankstein, & Dynin, 1994; Flett, Panico, & Hewitt, 2011), contemporary research has also failed to extensively evaluate the degree to which perfectionism and the Type A style are interrelated yet distinguishable. A very plausible hypothesis that merits future research from a person-centered perspective is that it is the highly perfectionistic Type A people who are particularly at risk for health problems, especially if their sense of being stressed and driven is accompanied by chronic feelings of resentment and hostility.

Early Empirical Research on Perfectionism and Health

We will conclude our chapter with a broader overview of some of the earliest empirical research on individual differences in perfectionism in the context of health. As noted earlier, a major difficulty that impeded early research on perfectionism was its focus on description rather than empirical assessment (e.g., Graham, 1953). And, of course, when perfectionism was actually measured, the results were constrained by significant limitations due to their less than optimal assessments of perfectionism. For instance, Moos and Solomon (1965) conducted their own investigation on perfectionism and arthritis to extend clinical accounts (e.g., Robinson, 1957). Their results were based on the identification of a subset of Minnesota Multiphasic Personality Inventory (MMPI) items that tapped perfectionism and compulsivity. A group of women with arthritis, when compared to their non-arthritic sisters, had significantly higher levels of perfectionism, compliance, nervousness, depression, and sensitivity to anger. Yet, related analyses established that perfectionism was among the factors associated with slower disease progress among those with arthritis (Moos & Solomon, 1964). This research, however, should be interpreted with substantial caution given that the degree to which the MMPI items provide an accurate assessment of perfectionism remains to be determined.

Heightened stress reactivity was implicated in perhaps the first detailed empirical investigation of perfectionism and chronic disease. This study by Prichard, Schwab, and Tillmann (1951) examined different personality styles associated with Parkinson's disease. To our knowledge, this study has never been cited by perfectionism researchers until now. Prichard et al. used a variety of pieces of information to group patients into one of four categories: (1) Group A had people with normal, placid personalities; (2) Group B had patients with dependent, submissive, and somewhat neurotic personalities; (3) Group C had patients described as having perfectionistic personalities; and (4) Group D had patients with more extreme forms of psychopathology and dysfunction. A total of 100 patients were classified into one of these four groups based jointly on the impressions that were reached when the patients came for appointments, but also based on informant feedback from the family doctor as well as from friends and families. In addition, each patient was asked to assign him or herself to one of the four groups. Prichard et al. (1951) reported close agreement between informant and self-classifications, and this yielded 48 patients in Group A, 33 patients in Group B, and 19 perfectionistic patients in Group C. Only two patients had Group D attributes, so they were not considered further. Those with the perfectionistic style were described as "… obsessive and perfectionistic and they all demand from life, their family, and their physician far more than is obtainable" (p. 106). Group comparisons established that these three groups differed significantly in two key respects. First, analyses of responses to drug treatment showed that much lower success rates were found with the Group C perfectionists relative to the other two groups. In all likelihood, this is the first empirical demonstration of perfectionism impeding treatment success. In addition, whereas Group A and Group B participants showed little evidence of being "stress affected," 58 % of the perfectionistic patients were deemed to be stress affected in terms of overt stressors, both minor and major, reported to the investigators. This impressive study by Prichard et al. (1951) clearly deserves to be cited because it shows with multiple forms of assessment that perfectionism can be linked with disease and stress, as well as with response to treatment. This paper was published over 60 years ago. It stands as an illustration of the usefulness of going back to examine the historical literature. This research is also remarkable because it incorporated informant feedback; going beyond self-reports seldom occurs in today's perfectionism research!

Another study evaluated patients with rheumatoid arthritis from clinics affiliated with McGill University (see Cormier & Whittkower, 1957). It was based on 18 patients who were interviewed by a psychologist and a psychiatrist on at least three occasions. One sibling of each patient who did not have rheumatoid arthritis was also interviewed for comparison purposes. Detailed family histories were gathered and personality judgments from a psychoanalytic perspective were made by the interviewers. Participants also completed projective personality tests. Accounts of family histories typically identified one or both parents as excessively demanding, suggesting a role for high parental expectations and parental criticism. One of the clearest differences was a tendency for the patients, relative to their siblings, to "… be punctual, tidy, and perfectionistic… Obsessional doubts and brooding are common manifestations of their inability to face a situation demanding immediate action" (p. 536), suggesting that the perfectionists with arthritis had difficulties in responding to challenging situations.

Earlier data were provided by Gressel, Shobe, Saslow, Dubois, and Schroeder (1949). They rated personality factors in three groups of participants: 50 people with essential hypertension, 50 people with normal blood pressure who had some form of psychiatric illness, and 50 people with chronic medical problems in which "psychologic factors are considered to have low etiologic relevance" (p. 267). Ratings tapped perfectionism as part of obsessive-compulsive style. Other personality ratings included impulsiveness, subnormal assertiveness (i.e., not showing overt assertiveness), anxiety, hysteria, and depressive behavior. Degree of hypertension was indeed associated significantly with obsessive-compulsive personality features ($r=.44$) and with subnormal assertiveness ($r=.38$), and it was not associated significantly with hysteria, anxiety, depression, and impulsiveness. These findings were generally in keeping with later research on obsessional perfectionism. Analyses of the personality component obsessionality subscale of the Crown–Crisp Experiential Index showed that the patients with myocardial infarction, relative to those who had not experienced an infarction, had higher mean scores on perfectionism, conscientiousness, and cleanliness (Crisp, Queenan, & D'Souza, 1984).

Adler, MacRitchie, and Engel (1971) conducted a retrospective study of "32 men with 35 strokes." No comparison group was included. A common pattern that emerged was a personality style described as "pressured" that involved satisfying elevated self-set goals, a sense of personal responsibility, and chronic problems controlling anger. This description has many elements in common with the Type A coronary-prone style. Most noteworthy were the conditions deemed to precede the onset of the stroke itself. The authors concluded that "The typical setting in which the stroke occurred was one in which the patient was reacting with a feeling of anger, hopelessness and sometimes shame when he (sic) felt he was not performing up to his standards, no longer was in control of his or her environment, or no longer was meeting the needs of others" (p. 1). This emphasis on the loss of key attributes and skills and diminished performance points to the potential role of temporal self-comparisons and a sense of a loss of self that leaves the vulnerable person with the sense of an emerging discrepancy between standards that are central to one's sense of self and identity and a self that may no longer be up to the challenge. The "pressured pattern" has five attributes: (1) pressure to keep busy; (2) a self-image focused on being an active and hard worker; (3) high standards and sense of responsibility; (4) urgency, time pressure, need to fulfill goals; and (5) sense of determination and strong will. High standards and responsibility were found in 84 % of the men who had strokes. Overall, 14 of the men (43 %) had all five attributes. Adler and associates (1971) described how they took steps to reduce interview bias as part of their observation that they unearthed many features of the Type A style despite not setting out to do so. Another feature that pointed to perfectionism was the tendency to have fleeting feelings of satisfaction experienced when goals were met. Work activity did not provide much pleasure; instead, it seemed to be a defensive form of distraction. Indeed, one participant noted that "being busy keeps me from thinking" (p. 22).

Another study contrasted 10 men with completed cerebral infarctions (strokes), 16 men with transient cerebral ischemic attacks (TIA), and 14 control participants who were hospitalized with various problems such as hernias or lumbar problems (see Gianturco, Breslin, Heyman, Gentry, Jenkins, & Kaplan, 1974). Group comparisons of the presence of "the pressured personality pattern" based on interview data found a marginally significant group difference ($p<.10$), with the pattern found in 7 (70 %) of the men in the stroke group, 5 of the 16 (31 %) men in the TIA comparison group, and 5 of the 14 (36 %) men in the control group. The high standards component indicative of perfectionism was found in 9 of the 10 men who had strokes, but was also found in at least 75 % of the men in the other two groups.

Most noteworthy for our purposes was the authors' observation that the men who had combined cerebral and coronary vascular disease were clearly perfectionistic. These men were described as having "… an intense striving toward self-imposed goals, a keen sense of responsibility and a determination to discharge responsibilities 'even if it kills me'. The need to maintain an image of a hard, active worker was frequently cited by these men as a motivation for their life styles" (p. 459). It was also noted that these men sought out work situations that afforded a sense of control.

The relevance of perfectionism in the "pressured pattern" was illustrated by the list of seven life stressors that preceded the illness. Several of these stressors are precisely the kinds of stressors deemed highly relevant in diathesis–stress accounts of perfectionism (see Hewitt & Flett, 2002). They were (1) personal inadequacies, (2) environmental demands, (3) loss of control over objects, (4) specific personal failure, (5) object loss, (6) loss of status of being useful and needed, and (7) failure to meet standards.

Subsequently, Adler was part of a team that examined personality features related to a high need for control among women who had a stroke (Goetz, Adler, Weber, & Siegrist, 1992). This study contrasted 19 women who had a stroke, 19 women with non-arteriovascular disease, and 19 healthy women. Participants completed a six-factor scale created for this study that included a "perfectionism/need for making plans" subscale. Participants were also evaluated with the Bortner Type A measure that was completed by themselves and a family member. Group comparisons of the six scale factors found that the women with a history of stroke were significantly higher than women in the other two groups on three subscales including the "perfectionism/need for making plans" subscale, and this difference was evident in terms of both self-ratings and informant ratings.

Summary

We have seen in this chapter that evidence of the association between perfectionism and illness goes back several decades and that there is an extensive "hidden literature" that includes some well-designed, controlled studies that were conducted despite the widespread ability of suitable perfectionism measures. In some respects, this chapter illustrates a growing problem in psychology, that is, the need to somehow come to grips with the previously published literature and use available past information to full advantage by building on it. In this particular instance, foreknowledge of the existing literature on the role of perfectionism in illness would likely have resulted in the early development of an extended diathesis–stress model of perfectionism and illness. We located several clear and detailed descriptions of the stress experienced by perfectionists and how this stress combined with dispositional characteristics to create or exacerbate health problems. Specific stressors were highlighted as well as the constant pressure to be perfect experienced by hyperconscientious, driven perfectionists.

It was also evident from the early literature on perfectionism and illness that there was little sense that perfectionism should be regarded as adaptive or beneficial. Moreover, perfectionists do not typically engage in protective health behaviors and self-care. A picture emerged of people who are excessively striving in ways that reflect their sense of responsibility and obligation, and their efforts get taken too far in ways that exact significant health costs. That is, people are holding themselves up to exceptionally high standards and paying a physiological price for it as if self-oriented perfectionism should be regarded as self-imposed or self-inflicted perfectionism.

Hopefully, the perfectionism and health field will advance in the future by focusing to a greater degree on specific illnesses rather than on health problems in general. The current chapter shows that this would simply be a return to earlier days when perfectionism was implicated in specific illnesses and health problems such as migraine headache and rheumatoid arthritis. We are not yet at the point of being able to ascertain whether certain perfectionism dimensions are more or less relevant in specific illnesses, and we also need much more evidence of the potential causal role of perfectionism in illness. In the meantime, we will remain hopeful and optimistic that future developments will be informative and will meaningfully extend previous work and detailed accounts of the link between perfectionism and illness.

References

Adler, A. (1938/1998). *Social interest: Adler's key to the meaning of life*. Oxford: Oneworld Publications.

Adler, R., MacRitchie, K., & Engel, G. L. (1971). Psychological processes and ischemic stroke (occlusive cerebrovascular disease): I. Observations on 32 men with 35 strokes. *Psychosomatic Medicine, 33,* 1–29.

Alexander, F. (1939). Psychoanalytic study of a case of essential hypertension. *Psychosomatic Medicine, 1,* 139–152.

Alvarez, W. C. (1947). The migrainous personality and constitution: The essential features of the disease: A study of 500 cases. *The American Journal of the Medical Sciences, 213,* 1–8.

Binger, C. A. L., Ackerman, N. W., Cohn, A. E., Schroeder, H. A., & Steele, J. M. (1945). *Personality in arterial hypertension*. New York, American Society for Research in Psychosomatic Problems (Psychosomatic Medicine Monograph No. 8).

Bingham, J. R. (1960). Precipitating factors in peptic ulcer. *Canadian Medical Association Journal*, 83, 205–210.

Blatt, S. J. (1995). The destructiveness of perfectionism. *American Psychologist, 50,* 1003–1020.

Brewerton, T. D., & George, M. S. (1993). Is migraine related to eating disorder? *International Journal of Eating Disorders, 14,* 75–79.

Bruch, H. (1962). Perceptual and conceptual disturbance in anorexia nervosa. *Psychosomatic Medicine*, 24, 187–194.

Bruch, H. (1973). *Eating disorders: Anorexia nervosa, obesity, and the person within*. New York: Basic Books.

Bruch, H. (1978). *The golden cage: The enigma of anorexia nervosa*. Cambridge: Harvard University Press.

Bruch, H. (1988). *Conversations with anorexics*. New York: Basic Books.

Bruch, H., & Hewlett, I. (1947). Psychological aspects of the medical management of diabetes in children. *Psychosomatic Medicine, 9,* 205–209.
Burns, C. (1965). Migraine in a rural practice (1958–1963): A five year study of a controlled clinical trial. *Journal of the College of General Practitioners, 10,* 230–238.
Burns, D. (1980). The perfectionist's script for self-defeat. P*sychology Today*, 34–51.
Cameron, D. E. (1944). Wartime pressures. *Canadian Medical Association Journal, 51,* 114–120
Cormier, B. M., & Wittkower, E. D. (1957). Psychological aspects of rheumatoid arthritis. *The Canadian Medical Association Journal, 77,* 533–541.
Crisp, A. H., Queenan, M., & D'Souza, M. F. (1984). Myocardial infarction and the emotional climate. *The Lancet, 323,* 616–619.
Donahue, H. C. (1949). Migraine and its ocular manifestations. *Transactions of the American Opthalmological Society, 47,* 554–605.
Duncan, C. H., Stevenson, I. P., & Ripley, H. S. (1950). Life situations, emotions, and paroxysmal auricular arrhythmias. *Psychosomatic Medicine, 12,* 23–37.
Dunkley, D. M., Schwartzman, D., Looper, K. J., Sigal, J. J., Pierre, A., & Kotowycz, M. A. (2012). Perfectionism dimensions and dependency in relation to personality vulnerability and psychosocial adjustment in patients with coronary artery disease. *Journal of Clinical Psychology in Medical Settings, 19,* 211–223.
Flett, G. L., Hewitt, P. L., Blankstein, K. R., & Dynin, C. (1994). Dimensions of perfectionism and Type A behaviour. *Personality and Individual Differences, 16,* 477–485.
Flett, G. L., Panico, T., & Hewitt, P. L. (2011). Perfectionism, Type A behaviour, and self-efficacy in depression and health symptoms among adolescents. *Current Psychology, 30,* 105–116.
Flett, G. L., Hewitt, P. L., & Nepon, T. (2016). Perfectionism, worry, and rumination in health and mental health: A review and a conceptual framework for a cognitive theory of perfectionism. In F. Sirois & D. M. Molnar (Eds). *Perfectionism, health, and well-being*. Berlin: Springer.
Forman, M. A., Tosi, D. J., & Rudy, D. R. (1987). Common irrational beliefs associated with the psychophysiological conditions of low back pain, peptic ulcers and migraine headache: A multivariate study. *Journal of Rational-Emotive Therapy, 5,* 255–265.
Fremont-Smith, M. (1932). Relationships between emotional states and organic disease. *Transactions of the American Clinical and Climatological Association, 48,* 62–72.
Friedman, A. P. (1958). Cluster headaches. *Neurology, 8,* 653–663.
Friedman, M., & Rosenman, R. H. (1974). *Type A behavior and your heart*. New York: Wildwood House.
Friedman, M., & Ulmer, D. (1984). Treating Type A behavior—and your heart. New York: Fawcett Crest.
Frost, R. O., Marten, P., Lahart, C., & Rosenblate, R. (1990). The dimensions of perfectionism. *Cognitive Therapy and Research, 14,* 449–468.
Garner, D., Olmstead, M., & Polivy, J. (1983). Development and validation of a multidimensional eating disorder inventory for anorexia nervosa and bulimia. *International Journal of Eating Disorders, 2,* 15–34.
Gianturco, D. T., Breslin, M. S., Heyman, A., Gentry, W. D., Jenkins, C. D., & Kaplan, B. (1974). Personality patterns and life stress in ischemic cerebrovascular disease. 1. Psychiatric findings. *Stroke, 5,* 453–460.
Goetz, S., Adler, R. H., Weber, R., & Siegrist, J. (1992). High "need for control" as a psychological risk factor in women suffering from ischemic stroke: A controlled retrospective exploratory study. *The International Journal of Psychiatry in Medicine, 22,* 119–129.
Graham, J. R. (1953). The natural history of migraine: Some observations and a hypothesis. *Transactions of the American Clinical and Climatological Association, 64,* 61–74.
Gressel, G. C., Shobe, F. O., Saslow, G., Dubois, P. H., & Schroeder, H. A. (1949). Personality factors in arterial hypertension. *Journal of the American Medical Association, 140,* 265–272.
Hassan, S., Flett, G. L., Ganguli, R., & Hewitt, P. L. (2014). Perfectionistic self-presentation and suicide in a young woman with major depression and psychotic features. *Case Reports in Psychiatry, 2014,* 1–6. (http://dx.doi.org/10.1155/2014/901981).

Heidbreder, E. F. (1927). The normal inferiority complex. *Journal of Abnormal and Social Psychology, 22,* 243–258.
Hewitt, P. L., & Flett, G. L. (1990). Perfectionism and depression: A multidimensional analysis. *Journal of Social Behavior and Personality*, 5, 423–438.
Hewitt, P. L., & Flett, G. L. (1991). Perfectionism in the self and social contexts: Conceptualization, assessment, and association with psychopathology. *Journal of Personality and Social Psychology, 60,* 456–470.
Hewitt, P. L., & Flett, G. L. (1993). Dimensions of perfectionism, daily stress, and depression: A test of the specific vulnerability hypothesis. *Journal of Abnormal Psychology, 102,* 58–65.
Hewitt, P. L., & Flett, G. L. (2002). Perfectionism and stress in psychopathology. In G. L. Flett & P. L. Hewitt (Eds.), *Perfectionism: Theory, research, and treatment* (pp. 255–284). Washington, DC: American Psychological Association Press.
Hewitt, P. L., Flett, G. L., & Ediger, E. (1995). Perfectionism traits and perfectionistic self-presentation in eating disorder attitudes, characteristics, and symptoms. *International Journal of Eating Disorders, 18,* 327–336.
Horney, K. (1945/1972). *Our inner conflicts: A constructive theory of neurosis*. New York: Norton.
Horney, K. (1950). *Neurosis and human growth*. New York: Norton
Jones, R. G. (1968). *A factored measure of Ellis' irrational belief system with personality and maladjustment correlates*. Unpublished doctoral dissertation. Texas; Technical College.
Kanai, A., Wakabayashi, M., & Fling, S. (1996). Workaholism among employees in Japanese corporations: An examination based on the Japanese version of the Workaholism Scales. *Japanese Psychological Research, 38,* 192–203.
Karush, A., & Daniels, G. (1953). Ulcerative colitis: The psychoanalyses of two cases. *Psychosomatic Medicine, 15,* 140–167.
Leon-Sotomayor, L. (1974). Cardiac migraine-report of twelve cases. *Angiology-the Journal of Vascular Disease, 25,* 161–172.
Lundh, L-G., Saboonchi, F., & Wangby, M. (2008). The role of personal standards in clinically significant perfectionism: A person-oriented approach to the study of patterns of perfectionism. *Cognitive Therapy and Research, 32,* 333–350.
Mahoney, V. P., Bockus, H. L., Ingram, M., Hundley, J. W., & Yaskin, J. C. (1949). Studies in ulcerative colitis. I. A study of the personality in relation to ulcerative colitis. *Gastroenterology, 13,* 547–563.
Marcussen, R. M. & Wolff, H. G. (1949). A formulation of the dynamics of the migraine attack. *Psychosomatic Medicine, 11,* 251–256.
Mittelman, B., & Wolff, H. G. (1942). Emotions and gastroduodenal function: Experimental studies on patients with gastritis, duodenitis, and peptic ulcer. *Psychosomatic Medicine, 4,* 5–61.
Moos, R. H., & Solomon, G. F. (1964). Minnesota Multiphasic Personality Inventory response patterns in patients with rheumatoid arthritis. *Journal of Psychosomatic Research, 8,* 17–27. doi:10.1016/0022-3999(64)90018-2
Moos, R. H., & Solomon, G. F. (1965). Psychologic comparisons between women with rheumatoid arthritis and their nonarthritic sisters: I. Personality test and interview rating data. *Psychosomatic Medicine, 27,* 135–149.
Prichard, J. S., Schwab, R. S., & Tillman, W. A. (1951). The effects of stress and the results of medication in different personalities with Parkinson's disease. *Psychosomatic Medicine, 13,* 106–111.
Robinson, C. E. G. (1957). Emotional factors and rheumatoid arthritis. *Canadian Medical Association Journal, 77,* 344–345.
Rodger, D. E. (1948). The challenge of colitis. *Canadian Medical Association Journal, 58,* 153–156.
Ross, C. C., Geddes, J. H., Hauch, P. P., & Scratch, N. W. (1950). Vagotomy and duodenal ulcer (An analysis of fifty cases at Westminster D.V.A. Hospital). *Canadian Medical Association Journal, 63,* 347–355.

Russek, H. I. (1959). Role of heredity, diet, and emotional stress in coronary heart disease. *Journal of the American Medical Association, 171,* 503–508.

Shanmugasegaram, S., Flett, G.L., Madan, M., Oh, P., Marzolini, S., Reitav, J., Hewitt, P. L., & Sturman, E.C. (2014). Perfectionism, Type D personality, and illness-related coping styles in cardiac rehabilitation patients. *Journal of Health Psychology, 19,* 417–426.

Simon, A. (1948). The role of the psychiatrist in cardiovascular disease. *California Medicine, 69,* 185–189.

Steiner, H., Mazer, C., & Litt, I. F. (1990). Compliance and outcome in anorexia nervosa. *Western Journal of Medicine, 153,* 133–139.

Touraine, G. A., & Draper, G. (1934). The migrainous personality: A constitutional study. *The Journal of Nervous and Mental Disease, 80*(1–23), 183–204.

White, B. V., Cobb, S., & Jones, C. M. (1939). *Mucous colitis: A psychological medical study of 60 cases*. *Psychosomatic Medicine Monograph, 1*. Washington, DC: National Research Council.

Wilson, C. M. W., Kirker, J. G., Warnes, H., & O'Malley, M. (1980). The clinical features of migraine as a manifestation of allergic disease. *Postgraduate Medical Journal, 56,* 617–621.

Wolff, H. G. (1937). Personality features and reactions of subjects with migraine. *Archives of Neurology & Psychiatry, 37,* 985–921.

Wolff, H. G. (1948). *Headache and other head pain*. New York: Oxford University Press.

Chapter 3
Perfectionism and Health Behaviors: A Self-Regulation Resource Perspective

Fuschia M. Sirois

Introduction

Perfect health and harmony, is the normal state of all life.

Hippocrates

Striving for a state of perfect health has been a highly valued goal for both ancient and modern societies. To the ancient Greeks, achieving and maintaining perfect health was considered a natural state that relied upon building the body's resistance to disease through proper diet and regular exercise. For modern Western society, public health promotion campaigns emphasizing the importance of maximizing healthy behaviors and minimizing health risk behaviors similarly reflect a striving for health perfection (Fugelli, 2006). Given this perspective, it is not surprising that personality is increasingly being recognized as an important epidemiological factor for understanding health outcomes through its associations with health behaviors (Bogg & Roberts, 2013; Hampson, Goldberg, Vogt & Dubanoski, 2007; Smith, 2006). Ostensibly, as a personality trait, perfectionism should be implicated in the practice of important health behaviors as a reflection of this quest for perfect health. Rather than confirming this common sense assertion, the research to date has instead yielded limited and equivocal results and therefore highlighted the complexities surrounding how different perfectionism dimensions may relate to health-promoting behaviors. In this chapter, I argue that self-regulation capacity is a critical consideration for bringing clarity to the issue of how different conceptualizations of

---

Preparation of this paper was supported by a Canada Research Chair in Health and Well-Being awarded to Fuschia M. Sirois.

F. M. Sirois (✉)
Department of Psychology, University of Sheffield,
309 Western Bank, Sheffield, S10 2TP, UK
e-mail: f.sirois@sheffield.ac.uk

Centre for Research on Aging, Sherbrooke, QC, Canada

F. M. Sirois, D. S. Molnar (eds.), *Perfectionism, Health, and Well-Being*,
DOI 10.1007/978-3-319-18582-8_3

perfectionism may or may not relate to health behaviors. As will be discussed, self-regulation approaches to health behaviors are particularly appropriate for addressing this issue as they provide a comprehensive framework for understanding the processes involved in committing to long-term goals while controlling immediate needs (de Ridder & de Wit, 2008). Although striving for perfection as a general life orientation may provide the necessary motivation for engaging in health-perfecting behaviors, when this striving becomes excessive and unrealistic, it may actually undermine the very resources needed to successfully follow through with and maintain a regimen of health-promoting behaviors. After briefly outlining the importance of health behaviors for health outcomes, and why self-regulation plays a central role, I critically review current research on perfectionism and health-promoting behaviors, underscoring the conceptual and methodological issues that characterize this understudied area of perfectionism and health research. I then present theory and research on self-regulation as it relates to perfectionism, and highlight the potential value of a self-regulation framework for understanding when and why perfectionism may be a liability for health behavior regulation. Next, I outline a self-regulation resource model (SRRM) as a new and potentially useful guiding conceptual lens for understanding how perfectionism dimensions may promote or prevent the practice of health-promoting behaviors. After presenting preliminary and illustrative empirical evidence that suggests the self-regulation processes and factors that may be involved in how perfectionism relates to health behaviors, I conclude with a provisional blueprint of how the SRRM may be applied to better understand the role of perfectionism in health behaviors across different settings and populations to guide future research in this area.

Health Behaviors and Health: The Central Role of Self-Regulation

Health behaviors are widely recognized as critical factors in understanding health trajectories and outcomes such as morbidity and mortality (Bogg & Roberts, 2013; Hampson et al., 2007). Healthy eating, regular physical activity, stress management, and good sleep hygiene are known precursors of health promotion and maintenance. In contrast, poor eating habits (Schulze & Hu, 2002), a sedentary lifestyle (Lee et al., 2012), excessive stress (Cohen et al., 2012), and poor sleep (Buxton & Marcelli, 2010) are the common pathways to the development of a host of lifestyle-based or noncommunicable diseases such as diabetes, hypertension, cardiovascular disease, and even cancer. Moreover, engaging in other health behaviors such as following medical regimens, seeking appropriate and timely care for important symptoms, and maintaining current health status are the corner stones of disease management for individuals diagnosed and living with chronic illness (Daskalopoulou et al., 2012; Gulliksson et al., 2011).

Aside from the obvious links to health outcomes, what all of these behaviors have in common is that they rely in part on the individual's ability to successfully regulate their immediate behavior to reach a long-term goal. That is, the ability to follow through with healthy actions while resisting unhealthy actions or inaction. This capacity of being able to control and regulate one's actions is commonly referred to as self-regulation (Forgas, Baumeister, & Tice, 2009). Although the control of behavior is the observable end result or goal of self-regulation, self-regulation also encompasses a broader spectrum of capabilities that are intertwined with, and contribute to, behavior. In addition to setting reasonable goals, self-regulation involves exerting self-control over the thoughts, feelings, and impulses necessary for adaptively monitoring behavior (Tice & Bratslavsky, 2000). Optimal self-regulation can therefore be viewed as a process of garnering the necessary cognitive and emotional resources to successfully regulate behavior in the service of long-term goals (Tice, Bratslavsky, & Baumeister, 2001).

If we consider that many health-promoting behaviors require focusing on the distal rather than immediate rewards and therefore can be challenging to initiate and maintain, it becomes clear that self-regulation is a key process to nurture for successful health behavior management and life-long health. For example, eating healthier foods requires foregoing immediate urges to eat more desirable, but less healthy food choices to reach long-term diet goals. Similarly, engaging in regular physical activity requires overcoming the inertia from more sedentary, passive activities such as television, gaming, and computer time and opting instead to be more physically active. Theory and research indicates that emotion regulation, in particular, may be important in such instances. Self-regulation tends to break down when people experience unpleasant negative emotional states, as the focus shifts to repairing short-term mood rather than controlling impulses and focusing on long-term gains (Sirois & Pychyl, 2013; Tice & Bratslavsky, 2000; Tice et al., 2001). Thus, when negative emotional states are high, people are more prone to give in to these more immediately pleasurable choices such as eating delicious, but unhealthy food and enjoying passive technology-based activities to feel good, at least temporarily (Tice & Bratslavsky, 2000; Tice et al., 2001). Moreover, the inevitable failures that can occur on the path toward trying to make health behavior changes can, for some individuals, trigger feelings of guilt and shame, which may increase susceptibility to goal-derailing temptations and further disrupt effective self-regulation of health behaviors (e.g., Sirois & Giguère, 2013).

Although the links between self-regulation and health behaviors outlined above can be applied to most health behaviors, for the purposes of this chapter only positive or health-promoting behaviors will be examined. This choice is informed by the empirically derived framework proposed by Vickers, Conway, and Hervig (1990), which suggests that there are two broad classifications of health behaviors: preventive health behaviors and risk-taking behaviors. Preventive behaviors include wellness maintenance behaviors such as engaging in healthy eating, regular physical activity, stress management, and healthy sleep behaviors. In contrast, risk-taking behaviors include exposure to hazardous substances such as excessive drinking, smoking, and drugs. These behaviors include an addictive component that can further complicate efforts at self-regulation. For these reasons, perfectionism will be examined only with respect to health-promoting behaviors.

Perfectionism and Health Behaviors: Limited but Promising Evidence

Before reviewing the current research on perfectionism and health behaviors, it is important to note the distinctions made by researchers in how perfectionism is conceptualized and measured. As noted in Chap. 1, perfectionism is a multidimensional construct that can be broadly described as the tendency to experience frequent cognitions about the attainment of ideal standards (Flett, Hewitt, Blankstein, & Gray, 1998). The two higher order dimensions of perfectionism are commonly referred to as perfectionistic concerns (PC) and perfectionistic strivings (PS), with the latter viewed by some researchers as a more adaptive or "healthy" form of perfectionism, and the former viewed as a maladaptive or "unhealthy" form of perfectionism (Bieling, Israeli, & Antony, 2004; Dunkley & Blankstein, 2000; Stoeber & Otto, 2006). These monikers derive from the empirical evidence which demonstrates that, on average, the two broad perfectionism dimensions are differentially related to mental (Ashby, Noble, & Gnilka, 2012; Bieling et al., 2004; Hewitt & Flett, 1991) and physical (Molnar, Reker, Culp, Sadava, & DeCourville, 2006) health outcomes, with PC linked to poorer outcomes. However, there is mounting evidence that calls into question whether the so-called "healthy" perfectionism is healthy at all, as several studies have noted either non-significant or negative associations with important health-related outcomes (Chang & Rand, 2000; Dunkley & Blankstein, 2000; Molnar, Sadava, Flett, & Colautti, 2012).

PC perfectionism is characterized by several important features, such as perceptions that others demand perfection from the self (socially prescribed perfectionism; Hewitt & Flett, 1991), a perceived discrepancy between unrealistically high standards and the progress toward meeting these standards (Slaney, Rice, Mobley, Trippi, & Ashby, 2001), and responding with strong negative reactions and self-doubt to perceived failure and mistakes (Frost, Marten, Lahart, & Rosenblate, 1990). PS perfectionism is characterized by the setting and striving for high standards for oneself (Frost et al., 1990; Slaney et al., 2001), but often with limited satisfaction for one's achievements (Hewitt & Flett, 1991). A key distinction between these two broad dimensions of perfectionism is reflected in their characteristic affective and cognitive responses to poor performance and failure, with PC perfectionism associated with an array of more dysfunctional responses including self-blame (Dunkley, Zuroff, & Blankstein, 2003), self-criticism (Stoeber, Hutchfield, & Wood, 2008), and rumination (Flett, Madorsky, Hewitt, & Heisel, 2002; Hewitt & Flett, 2002; Sirois, Monforton, & Simpson, 2010), in comparison with PS perfectionism.

To date, there is little research examining how perfectionism dimensions relate to health-promoting behaviors. The majority of research with respect to health behaviors has focused instead on behaviors linked to psychopathology such as disordered eating behaviors (Aruguete, Edman, & Yates, 2012; Bardone-Cone et al., 2007) and extreme exercise behavior (Goodwin, Haycraft, Willis, & Meyer, 2011; McLaren, Gauvin, & White, 2001). At the time of this writing, there were only four published studies investigating how perfectionism relates to the practice of health-promoting behaviors. Although there is some consistency in the findings, this is overshadowed by several methodological and conceptual issues which limit the conclusions that can be drawn.

Across the four studies available, the most consistent finding is that PC perfectionism tends to be associated with fewer health-promoting behaviors. Chang and colleagues (2008) examined the associations of several measures of PC perfectionism with a composite measure of different health behaviors that included items related to addictive behaviors (e.g., smoking). Despite this potential issue, three of the five scales used to measure PC perfectionism (i.e., concern over mistakes and doubts about actions subscales from the Multidimensional Perfectionism Scale (MPS-F; Frost et al., 1990), and socially prescribed perfectionism from the Multidimensional Perfectionism Scale (MPS-HF; Hewitt & Flett, 1991) were negatively correlated with the health behavior measure, and only socially prescribed perfectionism remained a unique predictor when all other perfectionism measures were included in the model tested. Similarly, Williams and Cropley (2014) used a general preventive behaviors checklist that included a wide variety of health-related behaviors. The behaviors spanned several of the health behavior categories proposed by Vickers and colleagues (1990), including accident control, avoidance of harmful substances, and health-promoting behaviors such as healthy eating and exercise. Again, PC perfectionism as measured by subscales from the MPS-F (Frost et al., 1990) was associated with the practice of fewer general health behaviors. In another study examining a single health-promoting behavior, PC perfectionism was similarly found to be negatively related to a measure of exercise commitment (Andrews, Burns, & Dueling, 2014). Although it would appear from these findings that PC perfectionism is associated with fewer health-promoting behaviors, the heterogeneity in the health behaviors assessed makes it difficult to determine the extent to which this is the case, or if the results jointly reflect the associations of PC perfectionism with a greater number of health risk behaviors.

The only published study to date which has distinguished between health-promoting behaviors and health-risk behaviors, in line with the suggestions by Vickers and colleagues (1990), was conducted by Molnar and colleagues (2012). This is important to note as their findings provide valuable insights into the potential differential relations between perfectionism dimensions and distinct classes of health behaviors. The results from the bivariate analyses confirmed the findings from the studies described previously: PC perfectionism, measured as socially prescribed perfectionism, was modestly and negatively associated with the measure of health-promoting behaviors (Molnar et al., 2012). However, this association was no longer statistically significant after the effect of PS perfectionism was taken into account. Interestingly, PC perfectionism was unrelated to the measure of health-risk behaviors, suggesting that the previous studies that used mixed health behavior measures may have underestimated the relations of this perfectionism dimension with health-promoting behaviors.

For PS perfectionism, the evidence is much less straightforward. In two of the four studies, this perfectionism dimension was positively associated with the health behavior measures (Andrews et al., 2014; Williams & Cropley, 2014). However, only one of the three subscales of PS perfectionism was associated with the mixed health behavior measure in the study by Chang et al. (2008). In the study by Molnar and colleagues (2012), PS perfectionism, measured as self-oriented perfectionism, was unrelated to health-promoting behaviors, but was negatively associated with health risk behaviors both in the bivariate analyses and in the multivariate model tested. What becomes clear from these findings is that PS perfectionism, often referred to as a healthier form of perfectionism, is not consistently associated with the practice of behaviors known to promote health. However, whether this is due to issues in how health behaviors were measured, how perfectionism was measured, or both, is unknown given the small number of studies.

Results from a small-scale meta-analysis of unpublished community and student data sets may bring some clarity to these issues by providing a more comprehensive picture of the nature of the associations between perfectionism dimensions and health-promoting behaviors. In particular, this study addressed several of the methodological issues in the published research by using a theoretically derived, well-validated measure of wellness maintenance behaviors based on the guidelines proposed by Vickers et al. (1990) across the seven samples ($N=2213$) in the meta-analysis, and by including three community samples (Sirois, 2013). The findings revealed that PC perfectionism was significantly associated with fewer health-promoting behaviors (average $r=-0.21$, $p<0.01$), whereas PS perfectionism was not significantly related to positive health behaviors (average $r=0.09$, *ns*; see Table 3.1).

Although these findings generally converge with those from the published studies, they should be considered preliminary for several reasons. Only two measures of perfectionism were included—the MPS-HF Scale (Hewitt & Flett, 1991), and the Almost Perfect Scale, revised (APSR; Slaney et al., 2001)—with the former used in two of the seven samples. It is unclear, therefore, whether the same findings would hold for the MPS-F (Frost et al., 1990), a measure used in two of the published studies reviewed. The small-scale meta-analysis approach is appropriate for culling

Table 3.1 Demographic characteristics, measures used, and effect sizes for the associations of perfectionism dimensions with health-promoting behaviors for the seven samples meta-analyzed ($N=2213$)

				Age (years)			Effect size (r)	
Sample	N	Type	Percent female	M	SD	Perfectionism measure	Perfectionistic concerns	Perfectionistic strivings
1	314	Student	71.4	21.03	4.27	MPS-HF	−0.20**	−0.08
2	70	Community	76.8	32.64	14.07	MPS-HF	−0.31**	−0.11
3	189	Student	74.2	22.4	2.12	APSR	−0.25**	0.16*
4	113	Community	73.5	31.16	15.16	APSR	−0.30**	0.07
5	339	Student	81.7	21.68	4.93	APSR	−0.27**	0.22**
6	208	Student	82.9	22.6	5.57	APSR	−0.16*	0.11
7	980	Community	36.3	32.60	9.94	APSR	−0.17**	0.16**

*$p<0.05$, **$p<0.01$

MPS-HF Multidimensional Perfectionism Scale by Hewitt & Flett, 1991; *APSR* The Almost Perfect Scale-Revised; Slaney et al., 2001

findings to advance knowledge within an area that is under-researched (Cumming, 2014). However, it is not without its limitations. For example, the number of studies in this small-scale meta-analysis did not permit moderator analyses to formally test whether the magnitude of the associations of perfectionism dimensions with health behaviors obtained with the two perfectionism scales differed significantly from one another. Given that the effect sizes obtained from samples using the MPS-HF were negative for PC perfectionism, whereas they were positive for samples using the APSR, this is an issue that future research will need to address. This is a noteworthy issue as others have argued that there is less conceptual overlap in the measurement of perfectionism dimensions among different perfectionism scales than what might be expected (Chang et al., 2008).

In summary, the research to date, though limited, provides suggestive evidence for differential associations between the perfectionism dimensions and health-promoting behaviors. Across multiple studies and measures of perfectionism, PC perfectionism is consistently related to less practice of health-promoting behaviors. Across these same studies, however, PS perfectionism is either positively related or unrelated to health behaviors, perhaps due to the way this dimension of perfectionism was measured. Given this limited evidence, researchers have not yet begun to explore the reasons why different perfectionism dimensions may pose risk or resilience for health-promoting behaviors. This next section will discuss the potential value of examining perfectionism and health behaviors from a self-regulation lens by reviewing how current theory on self-regulation intersects with what we know about the cognitive and emotional processes that characterize perfectionism.

Perfectionism and Self-Regulation

Conceptually, there are a number of reasons to expect that perfectionism should play a role in self-regulation, for better or worse, and that this may have consequences for the performance of health behaviors. If we consider that as a process self-regulation involves three components—standards, monitoring, and strength (Baumeister & Heatherton, 1996; Carver & Scheier, 1982; Tice & Bratslavsky, 2000), then the potential relationships become clearer. This *cybernetic* or feedback loop model of self-regulation (Carver & Scheier, 1982) suggests that self-monitoring is central for assessing whether the standards, or abstract notions of how things should be (Tice & Bratslavsky, 2000), are being met, so that necessary adjustments can be made to align one's behavior with set standards. For example, setting a self-regulatory goal such as sticking to a diet implies setting a particular standard of behavior (eating healthy foods, resisting unhealthy foods), and monitoring one's thoughts, emotions, and behavior to stay in line with this goal (Tice & Bratslavsky, 2000). Researchers have noted that self-regulatory strength is also important insomuch that keeping behavior consistent with these standards requires exerting effort toward controlling and overriding impulses that conflict with one's longer range or overarching goals (Baumeister, Vohs, & Tice, 2007a). From this perspective, resisting tempting, but less healthy food choices, therefore requires self-regulatory strength, which when depleted can result in self-regulation failure and thus breaking one's diet (Baumeister & Heatherton, 1996; Baumeister, Vohs, et al., 2007a).

Central to most conceptualizations of perfectionism is a focus on setting and striving to reach high standards. These "shoulds" regarding personal performance and meeting goals can become the overriding focus of one's self-regulatory efforts, often at the cost of tolerating single lapses in self-regulation, adapting one's goals to changing circumstances, or to heeding feedback indicating a low chance of success. From this perspective, self-regulation can fail due to misregulation of the self-regulatory process (Baumeister & Heatherton, 1996). Unrealistically, high goals may also be accompanied by unrealistically high standards for what constitutes success. As Wagner and Heatherton (2015) note, taking this zero-tolerance policy can mean that single lapses are viewed as indications of a complete failure resulting in abandonment of the goal. In the context of health behavior goals, this would suggest that certain perfectionists may be more prone to what is commonly termed the "what the hell" effect, whereby a single-diet transgression results in subsequent unrestrained eating (e.g., Polivy, Herman, & Deo, 2010). Not surprisingly, perfectionism is related to problems with body image and eating disorders (e.g., Antony & Swinson, 2009; Bardone-Cone et al., 2007), a topic that is discussed in-depth by Wade, O'Shea, and Shafran (2016) in Chap. 8 of this volume.

One form of misregulation particularly relevant for our discussion of perfectionism involves what Baumeister and Heatherton (1996) refer to as misunderstood contingencies, whereby people fail at self-regulation because of setting unrealistically high goals that have a greater likelihood of not being met (e.g., trying to lose 20 pounds in 2 weeks). Thus, individuals prone to this form of misregulation persist in pursuing unrealistic goals despite poor goal progress, rather than adaptively disengaging from or altering such goals (Wrosch, Scheier, Miller, Schulz, & Carver, 2003). As Baumeister and Heatherton (1996) note, such futile persistence often has emotional costs including frustration and increased distress because one's goals were not met. For perfectionists, these costs may be further exacerbated by ruminative tendencies (see Flett, Hewitt, & Nepon, 2016, Chap. 6) that contribute to both an inability to disengage from fruitless goals, and a pre-occupation with poor goal progress at the cost of taking instrumental corrective action (e.g., Campbell & Di Paula, 2002; Sirois et al., 2010). As will be discussed in the next section, these negative emotional states may further short-circuit adaptive self-regulation of behavior by depleting the resources necessary to follow through with intended actions (e.g., Tice et al., 2001; Wagner & Heatherton, 2015).

Given the implications of standard setting and monitoring for self-regulation, it is not surprising that several researchers have suggested that perfectionism may be a liability for self-regulation (e.g., Rudolph, Flett, & Hewitt, 2007), and goal regulation in particular (Eddington, 2013; Sirois et al., 2010). Indeed, one particular form of PC perfectionism, discrepancy as measured by the APSR, is characterized by perceiving large gaps between one's current and desired states (Slaney et al., 2001). Nonetheless, there are a limited number of studies examining how different perfectionism dimensions relate to self-regulation processes and the emotional consequences of these processes. What little research exists indicates that PC perfectionism is associated with ineffective self-regulation strategies. Using a self-regulatory framework, Eddington (2013) found that participants scoring high on PC perfectionism, measured as socially prescribed perfectionism (Hewitt & Flett, 1991), viewed their goals as less likely of being successful, yet were also less likely to disengage from such goals: which, in turn, predicted poorer coping and greater depression, but only during a stressful two-week period. In contrast, those scoring high on PS perfectionism, measured as self-oriented perfectionism (Hewitt & Flett, 1991), were more optimistic about their goal success and were less likely to disengage from those goals, but were more emotionally invested in the success or failure of their goals. The link between PS perfectionism and feelings of sadness due to goal failure among self-oriented perfectionists may thus reflect a greater sense of investment in these goals that further fuels the misregulation of self-regulatory resources. Aside from the difficulty in disengaging from set goals, what these findings highlight is that both forms of perfectionism are associated with emotional costs related to an inflexible approach to goal regulation (Eddington, 2013).

Strategies that might normally bolster self-regulation may also backfire for those scoring high on PC perfectionism, possibly because they provide opportunities for self-reflection and monitoring that amplify the self-critical and hyper-vigilant tendencies associated with this perfectionism dimension. For example, Powers, Koestner, and Topiciu (2005) examined whether perfectionism moderated the effectiveness of implementation intentions for goal progress across two studies. Implementation intentions are a type of goal intention that specify the when, where, and how of taking actions toward reaching a goal (Gollwitzer, 1999), and are particularly effective strategies for achieving goals (Gollwitzer & Sheeran, 2006), including health goals (Adriaanse, Vinkers, De Ridder, Hox, & De Wit, 2011; Ziegelmann, Luszczynska, Lippke, & Schwarzer, 2007). However, those scoring high on socially prescribed perfectionism reported worse goal progress over time when they made implementation intentions compared to when they did not. Relevant for our discussion of health behaviors, one of these studies examined progress toward New Year's resolutions, which included health behavior goals (Powers et al., 2005). Results indicated that formulating implementation intentions elicited negative affect for socially prescribed perfectionists, possibly because focusing on goals aroused negative self-evaluative thoughts about their chances of attaining these goals (Powers et al., 2005). It is important to note that the backfiring effects of implementation intentions were not found for self-oriented perfectionists.

Further evidence of differential self-regulatory responses distinguishing PC perfectionism and PS perfectionism comes from two experimental studies examining the self-regulatory role of counterfactuals for perfectionists (Sirois et al., 2010). Upward counterfactuals, or thoughts about how negative outcomes could have been better, can serve a behavior-regulating function by activating specific intentions to take corrective actions to improve future outcomes (Epstude & Roese, 2008), similar to implementation intentions (Gollwitzer, 1999). Thinking about how one could have avoided negative outcomes elicits negative affect which, for most individuals, fuels motivation for corrective future behavior. Across both studies, PC perfectionism was associated with making a greater number of negative affect generating counterfactuals in response to past failures (Sirois et al., 2010). However, rather than being functional, the upward counterfactuals generated by those scoring high on PC perfectionism were associated with greater distress; which, in turn, had no effect on motivation, possibly because the distress short-circuited the behavior-regulation loop (Sirois et al., 2010).

Collectively, contemporary theory and research on perfectionism and self-regulation provides promising foundational evidence to support the value of using a self-regulation framework for understanding why and how different perfectionism dimensions may be linked to the practice of health-promoting behaviors. In particular, the aforementioned research indicates that PC perfectionism may be a liability for effective self-regulation possibly because the excessive self-evaluative cognitions and high levels of associated negative affect short-circuit adaptive self-regulatory strategies and processes.

The following section will expand on these conclusions by articulating a new conceptual framework for understanding the differential associations between perfectionism dimensions and health-promoting behaviors, and provide some preliminary evidence to illustrate its application. Given the paucity of research on this topic, this new model has the potential to provide the basis for theoretically driven research on when and why certain perfectionism dimensions may help or hinder the practice of health-promoting behaviors.

A Self-Regulation Resource Model of Perfectionism and Health Behaviors

Several key ideas emerge from the theory and research reviewed to this point. First, initiating and maintaining health-promoting behaviors requires focusing on distal rather than immediate rewards to help regulate current behavior (de Ridder & de Wit, 2008). Second, although setting and striving toward certain standards of behavior or goals are necessary initial steps in the process of self-regulation, setting standards alone does not guarantee effective self-regulation, and may in fact be detrimental to achieving self-regulation goals if they are excessively high or unrealistic. According to cybernetic models of self-regulation (Carver & Scheier, 1982), bringing thoughts, feelings, and behavior in line with one's intentions and goals also requires self-monitoring to ensure the alignment of behavior with goals. Third, energy or strength models posit that self-regulation is a limited resource that when depleted, increases the likelihood of giving in to goal-derailing distractions and temptations (Baumeister, Vohs, et al., 2007a). Lastly, perfectionism (and PC perfectionism in particular) is associated with qualities that may interfere with self-regulation processes such as setting unrealistically high standards, a tendency toward vigilant monitoring coupled with rumination over perceived discrepancies between desired and actual states, and high levels of negative affect which can deplete self-regulatory resources (Baumeister, Zell, & Tice, 2007b; Wagner & Heatherton, 2015).

The self-regulation resource model (SRRM) integrates these key findings to provide a new conceptual framework for describing, explaining, and clarifying the differential relations and processes that link perfectionism dimensions to health-promoting behaviors (see Figs. 3.1 and 3.2). As suggested by its name, the SRRM focuses on the central role of resources in facilitating a successful self-regulation of health behaviors, and the increased likelihood of misregulation when resources are absent or diminished. Ostensibly, the term *resource* reflects the view that there is a common reservoir of energy to be used for self-regulation that, when depleted, can contribute to lapses in self-regulation (Baumeister, Muraven, & Tice, 2000; Muraven, Tice, & Baumeister, 1998). The exact nature of what comprises this self-regulation resource, and whether such a limited resource exists, is a source of much

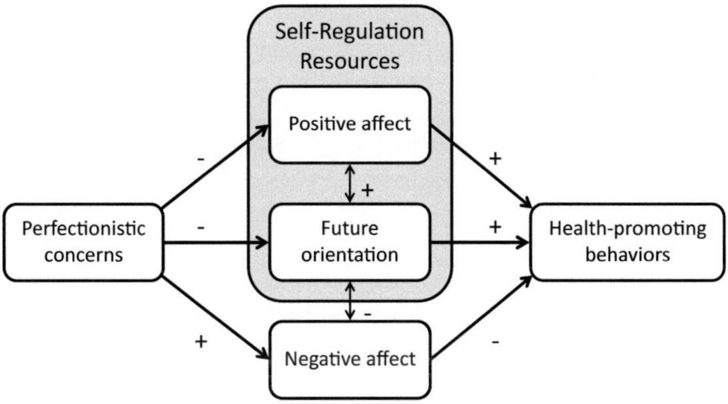

Fig. 3.1 *Conceptual Diagram of the Self-Regulation Resource Model Linking Perfectionistic Concerns to Health-Promoting Behaviours Through Associations With Future Orientation, and Positive and Negative Affect.*

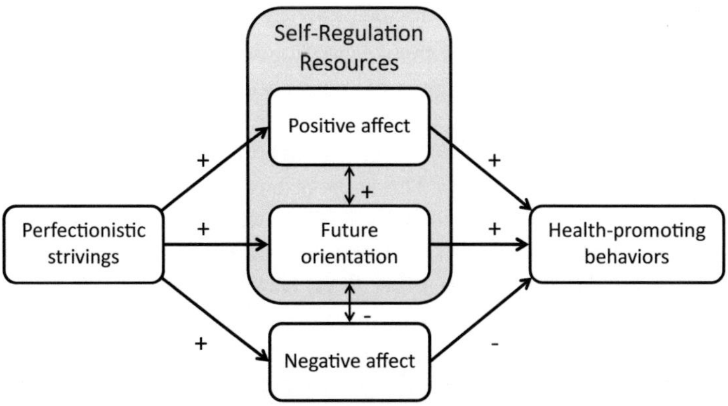

Fig. 3.2 *Conceptual Diagram of the Self-Regulation Resource Model Linking Perfectionistic Strivings to Health-Promoting Behaviours Through Associations With Future Orientation, and Positive and Negative Affect.*

debate and speculation (e.g., Chatzisarantis & Hagger, 2015). Rather than concurring with the yet-to-be settled view of self-regulation as a finite resource, the term *resource* in the context of the SRRM was chosen to reflect those factors which act as aids, supports, or tools that can be drawn upon and used in times of need to bolster self-regulation, and especially when self-regulation, or willpower as it is often referred to (Job, Dweck, & Walton, 2010), is low.

Despite the issues with the strength model of self-control, taking a resource view of self-regulation, broadly defined, has some clear advantages. For example, researchers have identified a number of factors that can facilitate or impair self-regulation by replenishing or taxing self-regulatory capacity. However, there are three factors in particular that may be relevant for understanding how perfectionism relates to health-promoting behaviors: negative emotions, positive emotions, and future time orientation. Several researchers have proposed and tested how emotions play a role in self-regulation (Baumeister, Zell, et al., 2007b). Yet, the role of temporal focus in bolstering self-regulatory capacity has remained more or less implicit. The SRRM extends previous theory and research by emphasizing the role of emotions as self-regulation resources or liabilities and by also making explicit the role of future time orientation with respect to health behaviors (see Figs. 3.1 and 3.2). Importantly, the SRRM articulates the potential for dynamic and reciprocal relations among positive and negative emotional states and temporal focus.

Perfectionism, Affect, and the Self-Regulation of Health Behaviors

According to the SRRM, emotions or affective states are potential self-regulation resources or liabilities that distinguish PC from PS perfectionism in relation to the performance of health-promoting behaviors. This proposition is informed by two lines of research. One demonstrates that these two broad dimensions of perfectionism are differentially associated with positive and negative affect. The other demonstrates how negative states can undermine self-regulation, whereas positive affect has a restorative effect on depleted self-regulation capacity.

A number of studies have found that PS perfectionism is associated with higher levels of state positive affect, whereas PC perfectionism is associated with lower levels of state positive affect (e.g., Damian, Stoeber, Negru, & Băban, 2014; Flett, Blankstein, & Hewitt, 2009; Gaudreau & Thompson, 2010; Gaudreau & Verner-Filion, 2012; Molnar et al., 2006). The associations of perfectionism dimensions with state negative affect are less consistent. Some studies have found that PC perfectionism is linked to higher levels of negative affect, and PS perfectionism is linked to lower levels of negative affect (e.g., Damian et al., 2014; Gaudreau & Thompson, 2010; Molnar et al., 2006), whereas other studies have found that only PC perfectionism, but not PS perfectionism is linked to state negative affect (e.g., Flett et al., 2009). When negative affect is construed as depression, anxiety, and anger (e.g., Hewitt & Flett, 2004; Stoeber, Schneider, Hussain, & Matthews, 2014), or as chronic negative emotionality (Shanmugasegaram et al., 2014), positive associations have been noted for both perfectionism dimensions, with stronger associations noted for PC perfectionism than PS perfectionism (e.g., Hewitt & Flett, 2004), especially after repeated failures (Stoeber et al., 2014).

Although a full discussion of the reasons why PC perfectionism is related to higher levels of negative affect is beyond the scope of this chapter, important insights regarding the source of negative affect for this form of perfectionism come from a daily diary study. Dunkley, Zuroff, and Blankstein (2003) tracked the daily affect and coping responses of individuals over a 7-day period and found that the link between PC perfectionism and negative affect was fully explained by the use of avoidant coping strategies and daily hassles. These findings suggest that the negative affect associated with PC perfectionism may result not only from their negative self-evaluations regarding performance as discussed previously (Powers et al., 2005), but also from the use of ineffective strategies for regulating stress (see also Dunkley et al., Chap. 7, this volume). As noted by Flett, Hewitt, and Nepon (2016) in Chap. 6, the rumination associated with perfectionism may further exacerbate negative affect by increasing both its intensity and duration.

The significance of these findings for the practice of health-promoting behaviors becomes clear when we consider the central role of negative affect in self-regulation failure. Negative affect is well-known to impair effective self-regulation (Tice, 2009; Wagner & Heatherton, 2015), making people more susceptible to immediately gratifying, yet distally costly, unhealthy behaviors (Sirois & Pychyl, 2013; Tice et al., 2001) and thus derailing the best of intentions to follow through with health goals (e.g., Sirois & Giguère, 2013). Although researchers have suggested a number of potential theories to explain why negative affect may thwart self-regulation, many of these reasons can be viewed as falling into two broad, but related camps: (1) short-term mood regulation; that is, finding ways to replace or eclipse immediate negative affect with feelings of positive affect (e.g., Sirois & Pychyl, 2013; Tice, 2009), or (2) narrowing of temporal focus, such that immediate concerns take precedence over long-term goals, making it easier to prioritize and consider the short-term rewards of unhealthy behaviors over their future consequences (e.g., Sirois, 2014; Tice, 2009; Wagner & Heatherton, 2015). In the first instance, negative affect shifts the priority away from regulating immediate behavior. In the second instance, negative affect shifts the temporal focus toward more immediate rather than distal concerns. Consistent with this view, and a growing body of evidence, the SRRM positions positive affect and temporal focus as key resources that can bolster or counteract the effects of self-regulation depletion, and therefore promote effective health behavior regulation.

Several lines of research converge to support a role for positive affect as a resource for the self-regulation of health behaviors. In one experimental study, watching a comedy (and therefore increasing positive affect) helped replenish the self-regulation capacity of participants whose self-regulation had been depleted by having to resist eating cookies and candies (Tice, Baumeister, Shmueli, & Muraven, 2007). Several studies have also demonstrated that positive affect is associated with the practice of health-promoting behaviors both cross-sectionally and longitudinally (Conner, 2013; Pressman & Cohen, 2005; Sirois, Kitner, & Hirsch, in press; Steptoe, 2010). Collectively, this evidence and that presented previously linking PC perfectionism to both lower levels of positive affect and lower levels of health-promoting behaviors suggests that positive affect is a potentially important self-regulation resource for understanding the differential relations of PC and PS perfectionism with health behaviors.

Temporal Focus as a Self-Regulation Resource

A second self-regulation resource that may provide insight into the connections between PC and PS perfectionism and health behaviors is temporal focus. As discussed previously, one of the reasons negative affect may impair self-regulation is because it narrows the temporal focus, placing more emphasis on immediate rather than distal concerns (Tice, 2009; Wagner & Heatherton, 2015). In most cases, the choice to engage in health-promoting behaviors presents a temporal dilemma: giving in to immediate desires and needs (including mood-regulating ones such as eating pleasurable foods) or focusing instead on the larger and often more lasting goals, such as making healthier eating choices to feel more fit. The resolution of this type of response conflict (Gillebaart & de Ridder, 2015) may therefore require shifting to a more distal temporal focus. Not surprisingly, future temporal orientation has been linked to the practice of health-promoting behaviors (Joireman, Shaffer, Balliet, & Strathman, 2012; Sirois, Shucard, & Hirsch, 2014; Strathman, Gleicher, Boninger, & Edwards, 1994), whereas a present and hedonistic temporal orientation has been linked to engaging in less healthy behaviors (e.g., Zimbardo & Boyd, 1999).

Unfortunately, there has been little if any research examining the possible links between perfectionism and temporal orientations. On the basis of the known distinctions between PC perfectionism and PS perfectionism for negative affect, it may be reasonable to assume that the higher levels of negative affect consistently linked to PC perfectionism may translate into less focus on the future, and more focus on immediate concerns. The clear distinctions on positive affect between the two dimensions of perfectionism similarly suggest a lack of future orientation associated with PC perfectionism. Positive affect is linked to having a future time orientation (Sirois, 2014; Zimbardo & Boyd, 1999), possibly because positive emotional states can broaden the scopes of cognition and attention (Fredrickson, 2001), which can foster a future-oriented perspective (Sirois, 2014). However, it is also possible that temporal focus feeds back into affective states, such that narrow or more local views reinforce negative states, whereas broader and more distal views enhance positive states, perhaps through increasing perceptions of control (Haase, Poulin, & Heckhausen, 2012; Trope & Liberman, 2003). When viewed from the framework of the SRRM, this and the preceding evidence regarding temporal orientation and health behaviors suggest that differing levels of future orientation may explain why PC perfectionism, but not PS perfectionism is associated with less engagement in health-promoting behaviors.

Preliminary Evidence for a SRRM View of Perfectionism and Health Behaviors

As presented in Figs. 3.1 and 3.2, the SRRM provides a theoretical framework suggesting that the differential relations between PC and PS perfectionism with health behaviors can be understood in terms of their links to three factors which are implicated in either depleting or replenishing self-regulation capacity. From this perspective, PS perfectionism may provide some impetus for practicing health-promoting behaviors through associations with the self-regulation boosting effects of positive affect and future orientation. However, the associations with negative affect may attenuate or even counteract these effects given the depleting role of negative affect. This may be one reason why the evidence to date regarding PS perfectionism and negative affect is less consistent than that for PC perfectionism. For PC perfectionism, the SRRM provides a clear conceptual map for understanding why this form of perfectionism may be a liability for the practice of health-promoting behaviors. Combined, the associations of PC perfectionism with high levels of negative affect, low levels of positive affect, and less future orientation are posited to result in a depletion of self-regulation resources without the opportunity to replenish the resources necessary to successfully follow through with health behavior goals. Current evidence provides some support for the proposed links between perfectionism and positive and negative affect. However, what is missing is empirical support for how perfectionism dimensions might relate to temporal orientation, and more importantly whether all three factors combined may explain the proposed differential associations with health-promoting behaviors.

Data collected in my laboratory from a community sample of adults trying to make health behavior changes provide some preliminary evidence to address this gap. In this cross-sectional, naturalistic study, 181 people completed a survey including a measure assessing a range of health promoting behaviors, the MPS-HF (Hewitt & Flett, 1991), a measure of state negative affect, and a brief measure of future orientation. The results of the correlation analyses presented in Table 3.2

Table 3.2 Bivariate correlations among the self-regulation resource model variables in community adults ($N=181$)

Variable	1	2	3	4	5	6
Self-oriented perfectionism	–	–	–	–	–	–
Socially prescribed perfectionism	0.37**	–				–
Positive affect	0.14[a]	−0.20**	–			–
Negative affect	0.27**	0.41**	0.19	–		–
Future time perspective	0.40**	−0.13	0.29**	0.01	–	–
Wellness behaviors	−0.08	−0.34**	0.20**	−0.34**	0.23**	–
Mean	4.35	3.47	2.89	1.88	3.55	3.81
Standard deviation	1.04	0.80	0.66	0.79	0.61	0.59

[a] $p=0.06$*$p<0.05$, **$p<0.01$

Table 3.3 Indirect effects from a multiple mediation model of socially prescribed perfectionism on health behaviors through positive affect (PA), negative affect (NA), and future time perspective (FTP) in a sample of community adults (N=181)

Effect	B (*SE*)	*CI*	Model R^2	*F* (*df*)
Indirect effect PA	−0.03 (0.01)	[−0.06, −0.01]		
Indirect effect NA	−0.09 (0.03)	[−0.14, −0.04]		
Indirect effect FTP	−0.02 (0.01)	[−0.05, 0.00]		
Total indirect effects	−0.13 (0.03)	[−0.20, −0.07]		
Total effect	−0.25 (0.05)	[−0.35, −0.15]	0.24	15.43** (4, 176)
Direct effect	−0.12 (0.05)	[−0.23, −0.01]		
Contrasts of indirect effects	*z*			
FTP—NA	−1.17			
FTP—PA	−2.85**			
NA—PA	−1.57			

Note: CI=95% confidence intervals; Bootstrapping analyses were conducted with 5000 resamples; all effects are unstandardized

*$p<0.05$, **$p<0.01$

Note: Analyses were also run with age and education level as covariates, and the results remained the same

are generally consistent with the predictions of the SRRM. PC perfectionism as assessed by socially prescribed perfectionism (Hewitt & Flett, 1991) was associated with lower positive affect, higher negative affect, and fewer health-promoting behaviors. The association with future orientation was in the predicted direction (negative), but was not statistically significant. For PS perfectionism, there was the expected moderately sized positive association with future time perspective, but no significant association with health behaviors. In addition, there was a marginally significant correlation with positive affect and a significant correlation with negative affect.

A more direct test of the SRRM via multiple mediation analyses yielded similarly promising results. In multiple mediation analyses, all three proposed mediators are tested simultaneously, thereby controlling for the effects of the other mediators while at the same time providing an estimate of the total effects through all mediators (Hayes, 2013). The analyses revealed significant indirect effects of socially prescribed perfectionism on health behaviors through both negative affect and positive affect, but not through future time orientation (see Table 3.3). Although the magnitude of the effects appeared to be different, the contrast test found that there was no difference. Together, these preliminary findings provide some promising initial evidence supporting the potential value of the SRRM for understanding how perfectionism is linked to health behaviors. However, given that not all of the predictions were fully supported, further research with different measures of perfectionism and future orientation, and using experimental or longitudinal designs is needed for a more thorough test of the SRRM.

Conclusions and Future Research

The aim of this chapter was to present a self-regulation resource perspective to elucidate the differential associations and underlying mechanisms linking PC and PS perfectionism to health behaviors. The theoretical foundations of the SRRM together with evidence-linking perfectionism to different affective states, and preliminary evidence noting associations with future time perspective, support the potential value of this conceptual framework for understanding why perfectionism may or may not contribute to the practice of health-promoting behaviors. Although the research to date indicates that there are clear distinctions between PC and PS perfectionism on the basis of positive affect and, to a lesser degree negative affect, further research is needed to verify the proposed links to future time orientation suggested by the SSRM. In the absence of this evidence, research indicating that PS is positively and PC is negatively associated with conscientiousness (Molnar et al., 2012; Parker & Stumpf, 1995; Stumpf & Parker, 2000) indicates that it is reasonable to assume that the links to future orientation may follow a similar pattern. For example, conscientiousness is characterized by planful, future-oriented thinking (Costa, McCrae, & Dye, 1991), which has positive consequences for health (Löckenhoff, Terracciano, Ferrucci, & Costa, 2012).

There are several potential avenues of investigation that would provide further support for the SRRM and its account of the potentially dynamic and reciprocal interactions among affective states and future orientation. First, process models of self-regulation highlight the changeable nature of emotional states during goal pursuit in response to perceived goal progress (Carver & Scheier, 1982). Perceived progress can contribute to positive emotions such as pride, whereas perceived lack of goal progress can elicit negative emotions such as frustration. From the lens of the SRRM, the ongoing assessment of health goal progress becomes another important source of emotion that can either deplete or replenish self-regulation capacity. Perfectionism may play a particular pivotal role here by coloring the perceptions of whether satisfactory progress toward reaching health behavior goals is being made. Considering the previous discussion noting that perfectionism is characterized by setting often unrealistically high goals and thus a tendency toward misregulation, it is likely that the threshold for perceived goal progress may be set very high, putting some perfectionists at risk for a cyclical increase in negative affect and subsequent self-regulatory depletion as they struggle to achieve potentially unachievable health behavior goals. To the extent that increases in negative affect further narrows temporal scope and/or foreshortens the temporal horizon, a zero-tolerance approach for small self-regulatory shifts may also be more likely. Daily diary and other approaches that are sensitive to capturing this dynamic and ongoing shifting of emotional states are clearly needed to provide a more accurate view of when and why perfectionism may be particularly detrimental for engaging in health-promoting behaviors.

The SRRM could also be valuable for understanding how perfectionism may influence health behaviors in at-risk or vulnerable populations. For individuals living with a chronic illness, engaging in health-promoting behaviors is essential for disease self-management and prevention of disease progression (Daskalopoulou et al., 2012; Gulliksson et al., 2011). In the context of living with the ongoing stress associated with chronic illness, one or both perfectionism dimensions may compromise the practice of these key behaviors by draining self-regulatory resources. Emerging adults, (i.e., young adults aged 18–25; Arnett, 2000), are another potentially important group to study with respect to perfectionism and the self-regulation of health-promoting behaviors. During this unique transition period, shifting interpersonal influences and ongoing identity development can put this developmental group at particular risk for declines in both diet and physical activity levels (Nelson, Story, Larson, Neumark-Sztainer, & Lytle, 2008). Taken together with evidence suggesting differential development of brain areas governing self-regulation which favor emotion driven rather than rational behavior in this group (Casey et al., 2008), it becomes clear that the proposed negative effects of PC perfectionism on health behaviors may be particularly pronounced in emerging adults. This evidence also highlights the importance of studying these issues in college students.

In closing, the SRRM presents a new way of conceptualizing how and why PC and PS perfectionism might be differentially linked to the practice of health-promoting behaviors. By highlighting the central and potentially reciprocal and dynamic roles of affective and temporal self-regulation resources and liabilities, it provides a promising framework to guide researchers and clinicians in their quest to understand why being a perfectionist may take one further away from, rather than closer to, the goal of perfect health.

References

Adriaanse, M. A., Vinkers, C. D. W., De Ridder, D. T. D., Hox, J. J., & De Wit, J. B. F. (2011). Do implementation intentions help to eat a healthy diet? A systematic review and meta-analysis of the empirical evidence. *Appetite, 56*(1), 183–193.

Andrews, D., Burns, L., & Dueling, J. (2014). Positive perfectionism: Seeking the healthy "should", or should we? *Open Journal of Social Sciences, 2,* 27–34.

Antony, M. M., & Swinson, R. P. (2009). *Perfecti, dieting, and body image When perfect isn't good enough: Strategies for coping with perfectionism* (2nd ed., pp. 245–260). Oakland: New Harbinger Publications.

Arnett, J. J. (2000). Emerging adulthood: A theory of development from the late teens through the twenties. *American Psychologist, 55,* 469–480.

Aruguete, M. S., Edman, J. L., & Yates, A. (2012). The relationship between anger and other correlates of eating disorders in women. *North American Journal of Psychology, 14*(1), 139–148.

Ashby, J. S., Noble, C. L., & Gnilka, P. B. (2012). Multidimensional perfectionism, depression, and satisfaction with life: Differences among perfectionists and tests of a stress-mediation model. *Journal of College Counseling, 15*(2), 130–143.

Bardone-Cone, A. M., Wonderlich, S. A., Frost, R. O., Bulik, C. M., Mitchell, J. E., Uppala, S., & Simonich, H. (2007). Perfectionism and eating disorders: Current status and future directions. *Clinical Psychology Review, 27*(3), 384–405.

Baumeister, R. F., & Heatherton, T. F. (1996). Self-regulation failure: An overview. *Psychological Inquiry, 7*(1), 1–15.

Baumeister, R. F., Muraven, M., & Tice, D. M. (2000). Ego depletion: A resource model of volition, self-regulation, and controlled processing. *Social Cognition, 18*(2), 130–150.

Baumeister, R. F., Vohs, K. D., & Tice, D. M. (2007a). The strength model of self-control. *Current Directions in Psychological Science, 16*(6), 351–355.

Baumeister, R. F., Zell, A. L., & Tice, D. M. (2007b). How emotions facilitate and impair self-regulation. In A. L. Zell & D. M. Tice (Eds.), *Handbook of emotion regulation* (pp. 408–426). New York: Guilford Press.

Bieling, P. J., Israeli, A. L., & Antony, M. M. (2004). Is perfectionism good, bad, or both? Examining models of the perfectionism construct. *Personality and Individual Differences, 36*(6), 1373–1385.

Bogg, T., & Roberts, B. W. (2013). The case for conscientiousness: Evidence and implications for a personality trait marker of health and longevity. *Annals of Behavioral Medicine, 45*(3), 278–288.

Buxton, O. M., & Marcelli, E. (2010). Short and long sleep are positively associated with obesity, diabetes, hypertension, and cardiovascular disease among adults in the United States. *Social Science & Medicine, 71*(5), 1027–1036.

Campbell, J. D., & Di Paula, A. (2002). Perfectionistic self-beliefs: Their relation to personality and goal pursuit. In G. L. Flett & P. L. Hewitt (Eds.), *Perfectionism: Theory, research, and treatment* (pp. 181–198). Washington, DC: American Psychological Association.

Carver, C. S., & Scheier, M. F. (1982). Control theory: A useful conceptual framework for personality-social, clinical, and health psychology. *Psychological Bulletin, 92*(1), 111–135.

Casey, B. J., Jones, R. M., Hare, T. A. (2008). The adolescent brain. *Ann. N. Y. Acad. Sci. 1124,* 111–126.

Chang, E. C., & Rand, K. L. (2000). Perfectionism as a predictor of subsequent adjustment: Evidence for a specific diathesis-stress mechanism among college students. *Journal of Counseling Psychology, 47*(1), 129–137.

Chang, E. C., Ivezaj, V., Downey, C. A., Kashima, Y., & Morady, A. R. (2008). Complexities of measuring perfectionism: Three popular perfectionism measures and their relations with eating disturbances and health behaviors in a female college student sample. *Eating Behaviors, 9*(1), 102–110.

Chatzisarantis, N. L. D., & Hagger, M. S. (2015). Unsuccessful attempts to replicate effects of self control operations and glucose on ego-depletion pose an interesting research question that demands explanation. *Appetite, 84*(0), 328–329.

Cohen, S., Janicki-Deverts, D., Doyle, W. J., Miller, G. E., Frank, E., Rabin, B. S., & Turner, R. B. (2012). Chronic stress, glucocorticoid receptor resistance, inflammation, and disease risk. Proceedings of the National Academy of Sciences.

Conner, M. (2013). Health cognitions, affect and health behaviors. *The European Health Psychologist, 15*(2), 33–39.

Costa, P. T. J., McCrae, R. R., & Dye, D. A. (1991). Facet scales for agreeableness and conscientiousness: A revision of the NEO Personality Inventory. *Personality and Individual Differences, 12,* 887–898.

Cumming, G. (2014). The new statistics: Why and how. *Psychological Science, 25*(1), 7–29.

Damian, L. E., Stoeber, J., Negru, O., & Băban, A. (2014). Positive and negative affect in adolescents: An investigation of the 2 × 2 model of perfectionism. *Cognition, Brain, Behavior. An Interdisciplinary Journal, 18,* 1–16.

Daskalopoulou, S. S., Khan, N. A., Quinn, R. R., Ruzicka, M., McKay, D. W., Hackam, D. G., Rabkin, S. W., Rabi, D. M., Gilbert, R. E., Padwal, R. S., Dawes, M., Touyz, R. M., Campbell, T. S., Cloutier, L., Grover, S., Honos, G., Herman, R. J., Schiffrin, E. L., Bolli, P., Wilson, T., Feldman, R. D., Lindsay, M. P., Hemmelgarn, B. R., Hill, M. D., Gelfer, M., Burns, K. D., Vallée, M., Prasad, G. V. R., Lebel, M., McLean, D., Arnold, J. M. O., Moe, G. W., Howlett, J. G., Boulanger, J.-M., Larochelle, P., Leiter, L. A., Jones, C., Ogilvie, R. I., Woo, V., Kaczorowski, J., Trudeau, L., Bacon, S. L., Petrella, R. J., Milot, A., Stone, J. A., Drouin, D., Lamarre-Cliché, M., Godwin, M., Tremblay, G., Hamet, P., Fodor, G., Carruthers, S. G., Pylypchuk, G., Burgess, E., Lewanczuk, R., Dresser, G. K., Penner, B., Hegele, R. A., McFarlane, P. A., Sharma, M., Campbell, N. R. C., Reid, D., Poirier, L., & Tobe, S. W. (2012). The 2012 Canadian Hypertension Education Program recommendations for the management of hypertension:

Blood pressure measurement, diagnosis, assessment of risk, and therapy. *Canadian Journal of Cardiology, 28*(3), 270–287.
de Ridder, D. T. D., & de Wit, J. B. F. (2008). Self-regulation in health behavior: Concepts, theories, and central issues. In D. T. D. de Ridder & J. B. F. de Wit (Eds.), *Self-regulation in health behavior* (pp. 1–23). Chichester: Wiley.
Dunkley, D. M., & Blankstein, K. R. (2000). Self-critical perfectionism, coping, hassles, and current distress: A structural equation modeling approach. *Cognitive Therapy and Research, 24*(6), 713–730.
Dunkley, D. M., Zuroff, D. C., & Blankstein, K. R. (2003). Self-critical perfectionism and daily affect: Dispositional and situational influences on stress and coping. *Journal of Personality & Social Psychology, 84,* 234–252.
Eddington, K. M. (2013). Perfectionism, goal adjustment, and self-regulation: A short-term follow-up study of distress and coping. *Self and Identity, 13*(2), 197–213.
Epstude, K., & Roese, N. J. (2008). The functional theory of counterfactual thinking. *Personality and Social Psychology Review, 12*(2), 168.
Flett, G. L., Hewitt, P. L., Blankstein, K. R., & Gray, L. (1998). Psychological distress and the frequency of perfectionistic thinking. *Journal of Personality and Social Psychology, 75,* 1363–1381.
Flett, G. L., Madorsky, D., Hewitt, P. L., & Heisel, M. J. (2002). Perfectionism cognitions, rumination, and psychological distress. *Journal of Rational-Emotive & Cognitive Behavior Therapy, 20*(1), 33–47.
Flett, G. L., Blankstein, K. R., & Hewitt, P. L. (2009). Perfectionism, performance, and state positive affect and negative affect after a classroom test. *Canadian Journal of School Psychology, 24*(1), 4–18.
Flett, G. L., Hewitt, P. L., & Nepon, T. (2016). Perfectionism, worry, and rumination in health and mental health: A review and a conceptual framework for a cognitive theory of perfectionism. In F. M. Sirois & D. S. Molnar (Eds.), *Perfectionism, health and well-being*. New York: Springer.
Forgas, J. P., Baumeister, R. F., & Tice, D. M. (2009). The psychology of self-regulation: An introductory review. In J. P. Forgas, R. F. Baumeister, & D. M. Tice (Eds.), *The psychology of self-regulation* (pp. 1–17). New York: Psychology Press.
Fredrickson, B. L. (2001). The role of positive emotions in positive psychology: The broaden-and-build theory of positive emotions. *American Psychologist, 56*(3), 218–226.
Frost, R. O., Marten, P. A., Lahart, C., & Rosenblate, R. (1990). The dimensions of perfectionism. *Cognitive Therapy and Research, 14,* 449–468.
Fugelli, P. (2006). The Zero-vision: Potential side effects of communicating health perfection and zero risk. *Patient Education and Counseling, 60*(3), 267–271.
Gaudreau, P., & Thompson, A. (2010). Testing a 2 × 2 model of dispositional perfectionism. *Personality and Individual Differences, 48*(5), 532–537.
Gaudreau, P., & Verner-Filion, J. (2012). Dispositional perfectionism and well-being: A test of the 2 × 2 model of perfectionism in the sport domain. *Sport, Exercise, and Performance Psychology, 1*(1), 29–43.
Gillebaart, M., & de Ridder, D. T. D. (2015). Effortless self-control: A novel perspective on response conflict strategies in trait self-control. *Social and Personality Psychology Compass, 9*(2), 88–99.
Gollwitzer, P. M. (1999). Implementation intentions: Strong effects of simple plans. *American Psychologist, 54,* 493–503.
Gollwitzer, P. M., & Sheeran, P. (2006). Implementation intentions and goal achievement: A meta-analysis of effects and processes. *Advances in Experimental Social Psychology, 38,* 69–119.
Goodwin, H., Haycraft, E., Willis, A. M., & Meyer, C. (2011). Compulsive exercise: The role of personality, psychological morbidity, and disordered eating. *International Journal of Eating Disorders, 44*(7), 655–660.
Gulliksson, M., Burell, G., Vessby, B., Lundin, L., Toss, H., & Svärdsudd, K. (2011). Randomized controlled trial of cognitive behavioral therapy vs standard treatment to prevent recurrent

cardiovascular events in patients with coronary heart disease: Secondary prevention in Uppsala primary health care project (SUPRIM). *Archives of Internal Medicine, 171*(2), 134–140.

Haase, C. M., Poulin, M. J., & Heckhausen, J. (2012). Happiness as a motivator: Positive affect predicts primary control striving for career and educational goals. *Personality and Social Psychology Bulletin, 38*(8), 1093–1104.

Hampson, S. E., Goldberg, L. R., Vogt, T. M., & Dubanoski, J. P. (2007). Mechanisms by which childhood personality traits influence adult health status: Educational attainment and healthy behaviors. *Health Psychology, 26*(1), 121–125.

Hayes, A. F. (2013). *An introduction to mediation, moderation, and conditional process analysis: A regression-based approach*. New York: Guilford Press.

Hewitt, P. L., & Flett, G. L. (1991). Perfectionism in the self and social contexts: Conceptualization, assessment, and association with psychopathology. *Journal of Personality and Social Psychology, 60,* 456–470.

Hewitt, P. L., & Flett, G. L. (2002). Perfectionism and stress processes in psychopathology. In G. L. Flett, & P. L. Hewitt (Eds.), *Perfectionism: Theory, research, and treatment* (pp. 255–284). Washington, DC: American Psychological Association.

Hewitt, P. L., & Flett, G. L. (2004). *Multidimensional perfectionism scale (MPS): Technical manual*. Toronto: Multi-Health Systems.

Job, V., Dweck, C. S., & Walton, G. M. (2010). Ego depletion—Is it all in your head?: Implicit theories about willpower affect self-regulation. *Psychological Science, 21*(11), 1686–1693.

Joireman, J., Shaffer, M. J., Balliet, D., & Strathman, A. (2012). Promotion orientation explains why future-oriented people exercise and eat healthy: Evidence from the two-factor Consideration of Future Consequences-14 Scale. *Personality and Social Psychology Bulletin, 38*(10), 1272–1287.

Lee, I. M., Shiroma, E. J., Lobelo, F., Puska, P., Blair, S. N., & Katzmarzyk, P. T. (2012). Effect of physical inactivity on major non-communicable diseases worldwide: An analysis of burden of disease and life expectancy. *The Lancet, 380*(9838), 219–229.

Löckenhoff, C. E., Terracciano, A., Ferrucci, L., & Costa, P. T. (2012). Five-factor personality traits and age trajectories of self-rated health: The role of question framing. *Journal of Personality, 80*(2), 375–401.

McLaren, L., Gauvin, L., & White, D. (2001). The role of perfectionism and excessive commitment to exercise in explaining dietary restraint: Replication and extension. *International Journal of Eating Disorders, 29*(3), 307–313.

Molnar, D. S., Reker, D. L., Culp, N. A., Sadava, S. W., & DeCourville, N. H. (2006). A mediated model of perfectionism, affect, and physical health. *Journal of Research in Personality, 40*(5), 482–500.

Molnar, D. S., Sadava, S. W., Flett, G. L., & Colautti, J. (2012). Perfectionism and health: A mediational analysis of the roles of stress, social support and health-related behaviours. *Psychology & Health, 27*(7), 846–864.

Muraven, M., Tice, D. M., & Baumeister, R. F. (1998). Self-control as a limited resource: Regulatory depletion patterns. *Journal of Personality and Social Psychology, 74*(3), 774–789.

Nelson, M. C., Story, M., Larson, N. I., Neumark-Sztainer, D., & Lytle, L. A. (2008). Emerging adulthood and college-aged youth: An overlooked age for weight-related behavior change. *Obesity, 16*(10), 2205–2211.

Parker, W. D., & Stumpf, H. (1995). An examination of the Multidimensional Perfectionism Scale with a sample of academically talented children. *Journal of Psychoeducational Assessment, 13*(4), 372–383.

Polivy, J., Herman, C. P., & Deo, R. (2010). Getting a bigger slice of the pie. Effects on eating and emotion in restrained and unrestrained eaters. *Appetite, 55*(3), 426–430.

Powers, T. A., Koestner, R., & Topciu, R. A. (2005). Implementation intentions, perfectionism, and goal progress: Perhaps the road to hell is paved with good intentions. *Personality and Social Psychology Bulletin, 31*(7), 902–912.

Pressman, S. D., & Cohen, S. (2005). Does positive affect influence health? *Psychological Bulletin, 131*(6), 925–971.

Rudolph, S. G., Flett, G. L., & Hewitt, P. L. (2007). Perfectionism and deficits in cognitive emotion regulation. *Journal of Rational-Emotive & Cognitive-Behavior Therapy, 25*(4), 343–357.

Schulze, M., & Hu, F. (2002). Dietary patterns and risk of hypertension, type 2 diabetes mellitus, and coronary heart disease. *Current Atherosclerosis Reports, 4*(6), 462–467.

Shanmugasegaram, S., Flett, G. L., Madan, M., Oh, P., Marzolini, S., Reitav, J., Hewitt, P. L., & Sturman, E. D. (2014). Perfectionism, Type D personality, and illness-related coping styles in cardiac rehabilitation patients. *Journal of Health Psychology, 19*(3), 417–426.

Sirois, F. M. (2013). Perfectionism, stress, and health: A meta-analytic approach. Paper presented at the 14th Annual Meeting of the Society for Personality and Social Psychology, New Orleans, LA.

Sirois, F. M. (2014). Out of sight, out of time? A meta-analytic investigation of procrastination and time perspective. *European Journal of Personality, 28,* 511–520.

Sirois, F. M., & Giguère, B. (2013). When resistance isn't futile: Task enjoyment as a protective factor against health procrastination in the face of temptation. Paper presented at the 8th Biennial Procrastination Research conference, Sherbrooke, QC.

Sirois, F. M., & Pychyl, T. (2013). Procrastination and the priority of short-term mood regulation: Consequences for future self. *Social and Personality Psychology Compass, 7*(2), 115–127.

Sirois, F. M., Kitner, R., & Hirsch, J. K. (in press). Self-compassion, affect, and health behaviors. Health Psychology.

Sirois, F. M., Monforton, J., & Simpson, M. (2010). "If only I had done better": Perfectionism and the functionality of counterfactual thinking. *Personality and Social Psychology Bulletin, 36,* 1675–1692.

Sirois, F. M., Shucard, H., & Hirsch, J. K. (2014). Procrastination and perceptions of the future self: Implications for health and well-being. Paper presented at the 2nd International Conference on Time Perspective, Warsaw, Poland.

Slaney, R. B., Rice, K. G., Mobley, M., Trippi, J., & Ashby, J. S. (2001). The revised almost perfect scale. *Measurement and Evaluation in Counseling and Development, 34*(3), 130–145.

Smith, T. W. (2006). Personality as risk and resilience in physical health. *Current Directions in Psychological Science, 15*(5), 227–231.

Steptoe, A. (2010). Positive well-being and health. In A. Steptoe (Ed.), *Handbook of behavioral medicine* (pp. 185–195). New York: Springer.

Stoeber, J., & Otto, K. (2006). Positive conceptions of perfectionism: Approaches, evidence, challenges. *Personality and Social Psychology Review, 10,* 295–319.

Stoeber, J., Hutchfield, J., & Wood, K. V. (2008). Perfectionism, self-efficacy, and aspiration level: Differential effects of perfectionistic striving and self-criticism after success and failure. *Personality and Individual Differences, 45*(4), 323–327.

Stoeber, J., Schneider, N., Hussain, R., & Matthews, K. (2014). Perfectionism and negative affect after repeated failure: Anxiety, depression, and anger. *Journal of Individual Differences, 35*(2), 87–94.

Strathman, A., Gleicher, F., Boninger, D. S., & Edwards, C. S. (1994). The consideration of future consequences: Weighing immediate and distant outcomes of behavior. *Journal of Personality and Social Psychology, 66*(4), 742–752.

Stumpf, H., & Parker, W. D. (2000). A hierarchical structural analysis of perfectionism and its relation to other personality characteristics. *Personality and Individual Differences, 28*(5), 837–852.

Tice, D. M. (2009). How emotions affect self-regulation. In J. P. Forgas, R. F. Baumeister, & D. M. Tice (Eds.), *The psychology of self-regulation: Cognitive, affective, and motivational processes* (pp. 201–215). New York: Psychology Press.

Tice, D. M., & Bratslavsky, E. (2000). Giving in to feel good: The place of emotion regulation in the context of general self-control. *Psychological Inquiry, 11,* 149–159.

Tice, D. M., Bratslavsky, E., & Baumeister, R. F. (2001). Emotional distress regulation takes precedence over impulse control: If you feel bad, do it! *Journal of Personality and Social Psychology, 80*(1), 53–67.

Tice, D. M., Baumeister, R. F., Shmueli, D., & Muraven, M. (2007). Restoring the self: Positive affect helps improve self-regulation following ego depletion. *Journal of Experimental Social Psychology, 43*(3), 379–384.

Trope, Y., & Liberman, N. (2003). Temporal construal. *Psychological Review, 110*(3), 403–421.

Vickers, R. R., Conway, T. L., & Hervig, L. K. (1990). Demonstration of replicable dimensions of health behaviors. *Preventive Medicine, 19,* 377–401.

Wagner, D. D., & Heatherton, T. F. (2015). Self-regulation and its failure: The seven deadly threats to self-regulation. In M. Mikulincer, P. R. Shaver, E. Borgida, & J. A. Bargh (Eds.), *APA handbook of personality and social psychology, Volume 1: Attitudes and social cognition. APA handbooks in psychology* (pp. 805–842). Washington, DC: American Psychological Association.

Williams, C. J., & Cropley, M. (2014). The relationship between perfectionism and engagement in preventive health behaviours: The mediating role of self concealment. *Journal of Health Psychology, 19,* 1211–1221.

Wrosch, C., Scheier, M. F., Miller, G. E., Schulz, R., & Carver, C. S. (2003). Adaptive self-regulation of unattainable goals: Goal disengagement, goal reengagement, and subjective well-being. *Personality and Social Psychology Bulletin, 29*(12), 1494–1508.

Ziegelmann, J. P., Luszczynska, A., Lippke, S., & Schwarzer, R. (2007). Are goal intentions or implementation intentions better predictors of health behavior? A longitudinal study in orthopedic rehabilitation. *Rehabilitation Psychology, 52*(1), 97–102.

Zimbardo, P. G., & Boyd, N. (1999). Putting time in perspective: A valid, reliable, individual-differences metric. *Journal of Personality and Social Psychology, 17,* 1271–1288.

Chapter 4
Trying to Be Perfect in an Imperfect World: Examining the Role of Perfectionism in the Context of Chronic Illness

Danielle S. Molnar, Fuschia M. Sirois and Tabitha Methot-Jones

In order to go on living one must try to escape the death involved in perfectionism.

Hannah Arendt

For the past 25 years, considerable effort has been directed toward increasing our understanding of perfectionism, a personality trait that is broadly defined as the setting of excessively high standards for performance, accompanied by harsh self-criticism (Frost, Marten, Lahart, & Rosenblate, 1990). Significant strides have been made with respect to our understanding of perfectionism. Research, for instance, has confirmed that perfectionism is a significant vulnerability factor for an extensive array of psychopathologies including anxiety, depression, suicidal ideation, and eating disorders (e.g., Bardone-Cone et al., 2007; Flett, Madorsky, Hewitt, & Heisel, 2002; Frost & DiBartolo, 2002), and has outlined conceptual models for understanding how perfectionism may be involved (e.g., Hewitt & Flett, 1991, 2002). Although we have made important theoretical and empirical advances into elucidating perfectionism's role in the etiology and maintenance of various forms of psychological problems, we are only beginning to understand how perfectionism may relate to health and illness. The relative paucity of contemporary research in this area is remarkable since the notion that perfectionism contributes to illness is not new (see Flett, Hewitt, & Molnar, Chap. 2, this volume) and given the recent

D. S. Molnar (✉)
Research Institute on Addictions, University at Buffalo, The State University of New York, Buffalo, NY, USA
e-mail: dmolnar@ria.buffalo.edu

D. S. Molnar · T. Methot-Jones
Department of Psychology, Brock University, St. Catharines, ON, Canada

F. M. Sirois
Department of Psychology, University of Sheffield, 309 Western Bank, S10 2TP Sheffield, UK
e-mail: f.sirois@sheffield.ac.uk

Centre for Research on Aging, Sherbrooke, QC, Canada

F. M. Sirois, D. S. Molnar (eds.), *Perfectionism, Health, and Well-Being*,
DOI 10.1007/978-3-319-18582-8_4

rekindling of interest in studying the robust relationship between personality and health (e.g., Christensen et al., 2002; Friedman et al., 1993; Ozer & Benet-Martinez, 2006; Roberts, Kuncel, Shiner, Caspi, & Goldberg, 2007; Roberts, Walton, & Bogg, 2005).

In this chapter, we argue that perfectionism is important to consider not only when examining the etiology of health problems, but also when studying adjustment to illness. Indeed, we believe that whether perfectionism is implicated in the etiology of an illness or not, perfectionism undermines and hinders coping and recovery processes once perfectionistic individuals confront chronic health problems. We begin by considering the definition of perfectionism and issues concerning its measurement. Next, we present our Stress and Coping Cyclical Amplification Model of Perfectionism in Illness (SCCAMPI) as a potentially useful framework to elucidate how perfectionism may serve as a potential risk factor for poor adjustment and unfavorable health outcomes in chronic disease and critically review the research to date on perfectionism in chronic illness. Finally, we address the implications of the SCCAMPI and possible future directions for investigation in this exciting area of research.

What is Perfectionism?

Prior to considering the role of perfectionism in health problems, we must first define what we mean by perfectionism and admit that this continues to be a point of contention in the field (see Sirois & Molnar, Chap. 1, this volume). Perfectionism is a multifarious personality construct that has been defined in various ways over the years by different groups of researchers. Consequently, several measures that assess perfectionism at the trait level are currently available for use (Enns & Cox, 2002). Further adding to the complexity are measures that have been developed to capture other potentially relevant aspects of perfectionism such as individual differences in the frequency with which individuals experience automatic perfectionistic thoughts concerning the need to be perfect (e.g., Perfectionistic Cognitions Inventory (PCI); Flett, Hewitt, Blankstein, & Gray, 1998a; Multidimensional Perfectionism Cognitions Inventory–English (MPCI-E); Kobori, 2006; Stoeber, Kobori, & Tanno, 2010) and individual differences in the tendency to engage in perfectionistic self-presentational behaviour (e.g., Perfectionistic Self-Presentation Scale (PSPS); Hewitt, Flett, Besser, Sherry, & McGee, 2003).

Although there are numerous models of trait perfectionism that continue to be widely used in the field (see Sirois & Molnar, Chap. 1, this volume), there is a growing consensus among researchers that the existing measures of trait perfectionism may actually gauge two underlying higher-order factors, which are commonly referred to in the literature as Perfectionistic Strivings (PS) and Perfectionistic Concerns (PC) (Dunkley & Blankstein, 2000; Frost, Heimberg, Holt, Mattia, & Neubauer, 1993; Stoeber & Otto, 2006). PS is a higher-order factor that consists of the setting and compulsive striving toward excessively high standards, whereas

PC is a higher-order construct that includes harsh self-scrutiny, undue concern over mistakes and others' evaluations, beliefs that others demand perfection, the perception that one is not meeting his/her exacting standards, and excessive reactions to perceived failures.

Importantly, research has established that each of these factors is differentially related to consequential outcomes. PC, for example, is considered to be maladaptive, as ample evidence indicates that it is a vulnerability factor for numerous adjustment difficulties that seem to pervade essentially all aspects of living including poor health, psychopathology, and interpersonal problems (Frost et al., 1993; Hewitt, Flett, & Ediger, 1996; Mackinnon et al., 2012; Molnar, Reker, Culp, Sadava, & DeCourville, 2006). Research suggests that PS is associated with both desirable (e.g., positive affect, achievement motivation) and undesirable outcomes (e.g., neuroticism, depression; Cox, Enns, & Clara, 2002; Enns, Cox, Sareen, & Freeman, 2001; Parker, 1997; Rice & Dellwo, 2002). These conflicting findings have created considerable debate among researchers regarding the relative adaptiveness of this higher-order construct (see Stoeber & Otto, 2006 for review). It appears that most researchers are willing to concede that PS is relatively less harmful than PC. However, in the next section, we question whether this conclusion is valid when examining PS within the context of health outcomes.

Perfectionism in the Context of Chronic Illness

According to the Centers for Disease Control and Prevention (CDC) as of the year 2012, chronic diseases such as arthritis, cancer, chronic fatigue syndrome, and heart disease affect approximately 117 million adults and are the leading cause of death and disability in the USA (CDC, 2013; Ward, Schiller, & Goodman, 2014). Apart from these very real costs to functioning and longevity, chronic illness can also take a toll on the individual in other significant ways. Being diagnosed with a chronic illness can threaten existing goals and plans for the future by creating uncertainty about the viability of such goals under potentially challenging circumstances. Pain, fatigue, and decreased daily functioning are symptoms, among many others, that can threaten goal attainment and psychological well-being (e.g., Hamilton, Karoly, & Kitzman, 2004). The process of adjusting to chronic illness may, therefore, require a renegotiation of identity as one assesses the discrepancy between the present ill self and the former illness-free self and what this identity transformation may mean for attaining future personally relevant goals (Asbring, 2001; Dickson, 2008). To the extent that symptoms fluctuate and change, this renegotiation may be an ongoing process (Sirois & Hirsch, 2013). Thus, living with a chronic illness can be a stressful and potentially traumatic experience associated with both physical and psychological downturns.

Understanding the factors and processes that impact how people with chronic illness perceive and respond to disease-related challenges and stressors can have important implications for disease management and adjustment. To this end, personality has emerged in recent years as an important epidemiological factor that can confer risk or resilience for health trajectories and outcomes (Bogg & Roberts, 2013; Hampson, Goldberg, Vogt, & Dubanoski, 2007). For example, research has convincingly demonstrated a great deal of heterogeneity in adjustment to chronic illness (e.g., Dew et al., 2005; Helgeson, Snyder, & Seltman, 2004) and indicated that individual differences, such as optimism (Contrada et al., 2004; Scheier & Carver, 1985; Shnek, Irvine, Stewart, & Abbey, 2001) and neuroticism (Brickman, Yount, Blaney, Rothberg, & De-Nour,1996; Boye et al., 2008), play an important role in the adjustment process.

Although perfectionism in chronic illness is a particularly underdeveloped area of research, there are some indications that perfectionism is a crucial dispositional factor to consider for understanding adjustment to a number of chronic diseases. Indeed, a growing body of research indicates that perfectionism is not only implicated as an important etiological factor in chronic fatigue syndrome, but also undermines adjustment efforts (Kempke, van Houdenhove, Claes, & Luyten, Chap. 5, this volume; Sirois & Molnar, 2014). In addition to case accounts (e.g., Risor, 2009), empirical studies also document how perfectionism complicates the ability to cope with chronic conditions such as fibromyalgia (Molnar, Flett, Sadava, & Colautti, 2012), chronic tinnitus (Andersson, Airikka, Buhrman, & Kaldo, 2005), and Crohn's disease (Flett, Baricza, Gupta, Hewitt, & Endler, 2011). More alarming is that perfectionism has been identified as a critical factor associated with poor adjustment and emotional difficulties in patients with cardiovascular disease (Parker et al., 2006; Shanmugasegaram et al., 2014; Stafford, Jackson, & Berk, 2009). Yet, despite this research suggesting that perfectionism may be a liability for those with chronic illness, there is also some evidence that PS may promote health, possibly by facilitating timely engagement in important disease management behaviors in the context of other chronic diseases such as type 2 diabetes (Fry & Debats, 2011). Clearly disentangling the potentially differential associations between different perfectionism dimensions and health outcomes for those with chronic illness is no easy undertaking. Indeed, the research to date on this topic does not offer evidence of a clear distinction between the supposed "adaptive" (i.e., PS) and "maladaptive" forms (i.e., PC) of perfectionism, as numerous studies have established that both PS and PC may complicate adjustment to chronic illness.

As we will discuss in more detail in the next sections, current research on perfectionism and adjustment suggests that certain forms of perfectionism are robustly associated with higher levels of stress and poor coping, which may, in turn, exacerbate important health outcomes for individuals living with chronic illness, such as physical symptoms and health-promoting behaviors. This research further hints at important factors that may contribute to health outcomes in chronic illness because of their association with adjustment in general. Impoverished social support networks, perceptions of loss of control, negative self-evaluations, and self-concealment each have the potential to elucidate how and why perfectionism is related to greater stress, poorer coping, and more negative health outcomes in the context of chronic illness.

Unfortunately, apart from a few notable exceptions, investigations aimed at elucidating the role of perfectionism in adjustment to chronic illness have been predominantly atheoretical. This is surprising in light of the number of proposed models aimed at explaining the linkages of personality in general to health (Smith, 2006; Vollrath, 2006) and theoretical models linking perfectionism to key determinants of health such as stress (e.g., Stress-Diathesis Model of Perfectionism; Flett, Hewitt, Clankstein, & Mosher, 1995a), coping (Dunkley, Ma, Lee, Preacher, & Zuroff, 2014a, see also Dunkley, Solomon-Krakus, and Moroz, Chap. 7, this volume), affect (Molnar et al. 2006), and social support (e.g., the Social Disconnection Model; see Sherry, Mackinnon, and Gautreau, Chap. 10, this volume). Research focused on perfectionism and health outcomes in the context of chronic illness should reflect conceptual models that link perfectionism with consequential health outcomes and elucidate the associated processes. Accordingly, in the next section, we present the SCCAMPI as a new conceptual framework for understanding how and why perfectionism dimensions may be differentially linked to adjustment and health outcomes in chronic illness.

The Stress and Coping Cyclical Amplification Model of Perfectionism in Illness (SCCAMPI)

There is no doubt that coping with the challenges of chronic illness is difficult for most people. However, we contend that perfectionists in particular are at increased risk for experiencing poorer adjustment to chronic illness owing to their heightened stress response and their proclivity to engage in maladaptive coping responses. As indicated by its name, the SCCAMPI highlights the intrapsychic (i.e., perceptions of control and self-evaluative tendencies) and interpersonal processes (i.e., social support and self-concealment) that link perfectionism to important health outcomes (i.e., physical symptoms and health behaviors) through the amplification of stress and maladaptive coping (see Fig. 4.1). Understanding the intrapsychic and

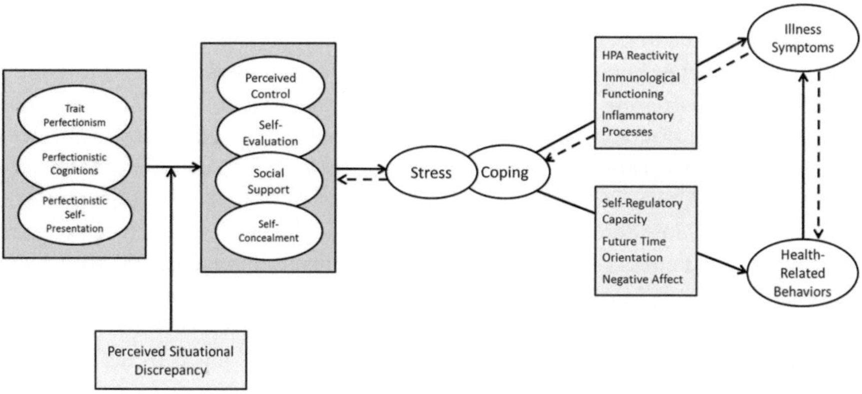

Fig. 4.1 The stress and coping cyclical amplification model of perfectionism in illness (SCCAMPI)

interpersonal dynamics of individuals with elevated perfectionism, who are struggling with chronic illness, may enhance our ability to develop specific interventions for this particularly vulnerable population.

In the following sections, we describe and summarize current research on four factors suggested by the SCCAMPI which may be particularly important for understanding how and why perfectionism creates risk for experiencing greater stress and poorer health outcomes in the context of chronic illness. Given the limited research on perfectionism in chronic illness, our review focuses on the interpersonal and intrapsychic factors that have demonstrated links with perfectionism and with greater stress and poorer coping in general populations. We argue that if these factors create increased risk for poor coping and stress in everyday circumstances, they have the potential to be that much more harmful for perfectionists who are living with the daily challenges and ongoing stress of chronic illness. In short, each of these factors reflects a pathway through which perfectionism may amplify the stressful effects of an already stressful situation and therefore contribute to greater risk for poor health outcomes.

Perceptions of Control

It is well documented in general that low perceived control is a risk factor for health problems (see Johnson & Krueger, 2005; Taylor, Kemeny, Reed, Bower, & Gruenewald, 2000) and poor adjustment to chronic health conditions (Sirois, Davis, & Morgan, 2006). Indeed, living with a chronic illness can be viewed as living in low control circumstances insomuch that the chronic illness cannot be cured or controlled and is often unpredictable (Thompson, Sobolew-Shubin, Galbraith, Schwankovsky, & Cruzen, 1993). However, increased perceptions of control in the context of chronic illness can compensate for other coping deficits including poor social support (Thompson et al., 1993). A recent long-term longitudinal study of "control trajectories" illustrated the health consequences and mortality risk for those people who are unable to develop an increasing sense of personal control over time (Infurna, Ram, & Gerstorf, 2013).

Despite approaching the study of perfectionism from different theoretical orientations, classic theorists such as Karen Horney (1950) and Albert Ellis (1962) both observed that perfectionists do not permit themselves the luxury of accepting life's little ambiguities or any level of uncertainty, for that matter, because rather than simply having a desire to perform well, perfectionists must guarantee themselves absolute perfection and therefore must demand personal control. It is our contention that perfectionists are particularly impacted when in threatening life contexts characterized by low perceived control (e.g., chronic illness), especially if exposure is prolonged and creates the states of helplessness that Seligman (1975) implicated in severe illness and death. Flett et al. (1995) posited and demonstrated empirically that potentially adaptive forms of perfectionism (i.e., self-oriented and other-oriented perfectionism (OOP)) are associated with elevated levels of the desire for control. Presumably, the sense of being unable to control life circumstances violates a central need and this is exponentially stressful and distressing for perfectionists who are highly focused on being in control and who also need to project an image of having things under control. A sense of not being able to overcome this lack of control should have profound health implications for perfectionists.

Perceptions of control represent one intrapsychic pathway linking perfectionism to stress and to later consequential health outcomes. Poor adjustment to chronic illness may be especially likely in individuals with elevated levels of perfectionism because these individuals have a strong need for control and are highly stressed by events, such as chronic illness, that are beyond their control (Flett, Hewitt, Blankstein, & Mosher, 1995a; Hewitt & Flett, 2002). The importance of perceived control has been underscored in both the perfectionism and the chronic illness literatures. With regard to perfectionism, research has established that PS and OOP are associated with a greater need for control (Flett et al., 1995). Chronic illness would violate this need for control and predictability, as chronic disease can challenge the perceptions of control in several life domains including daily schedules, bodily integrity, daily functioning, and the ability to meet the demands of work and social roles. Indeed, a central feature inherent in chronic illness is that the course and outcomes of the illness are not directly modified by the actions of the individual (Stanton & Revenson, 2011).

Research has demonstrated that PC is associated with a lack of interpersonal control (Flett et al., 1995), general perceptions of a lack of perceived control (Buhr & Dugas, 2006), and low self-control (Tangney, Baumeister, & Boone, 2004). Research by Flett, Hewitt, Blankstein, and Pickering (1998b) has also demonstrated that PC is associated with a pervasive tendency toward attributing both successes and failures to external causes. Overall, these results are in keeping with the view that a sense of personal helplessness is a core feature of PC. The sense of low personal control and helplessness that accompanies PC (Hewitt & Flett, 1991) could set the stage for greater stress and poorer health outcomes among people with elevated PC.

Self-Evaluation

The second intrapsychic pathway in the SCCAMPI that may be particularly salient for understanding how perfectionism is linked to stress and later health-related outcomes in people with chronic illness is negative self-evaluation. It is relatively common for individuals who develop a chronic illness to be critical of their earlier self for contributing to the illness or failing to proactively prevent its onset (Sirois et al., 2006). Now imagine how much more self-deprecating the perfectionist would be when he or she can no longer tenaciously strive toward his or her uncompromising standards due to health problems. We expect perfectionists with chronic illness to have a particularly harsh view of themselves because they often fail to take into account external conditions (e.g., suffering from a chronic disease) that would prevent them from reaching their excessively high standards. Horney (1950) referred to this aspect of perfectionism as “disregard for the conditions under which they [demands, high standards] could be fulfilled (p. 66).” This aspect of perfectionism could be particularly devastating in the context of chronic illness where individuals frequently experience “illness intrusions” (i.e., lifestyle disruptions caused by illness that hamper participation in activities that are deemed to be important by the individual; Devins, 1989). For instance, think of a father suffering from IBD who may have to miss going on fun outings with his children because he is experiencing gastrointestinal difficulties or the employee with CFS who is too tired to fulfill his or her work obligations. Furthermore, from the lens of Social Identity Theory, which posits that our social roles, such as being an employee, romantic partner, friend, or parent, provide the foundation of our self-concept (Thoits, 1997), it is easy to see how these “illness intrusions” can be problematic. Indeed, research has supported how illness intrusion can undermine psychosocial adjustment in the context of rheumatoid arthritis (Abraido-lanza & Revenson, 2006). We expect that these illness intrusions will be particularly threatening for perfectionists’ self-concept because they do not make any allowances for these intrusions, therefore equating their loss of social roles with personal failure.

Negative self-evaluation has long been emphasized in the perfectionism literature (Blatt, 1995; Frost et al., 1990; Hewitt & Flett, 1991). Adler (1956), for instance, postulated that perfectionism is generally motivated by a sense of inferiority and low self-esteem, whereas Ellis (1962) highlighted the centrality of negative self-evaluation when he described perfectionists’ belief systems as follows:

> A person should be thoroughly competent, adequate, talented, and intelligent in all possible respects; the main goal and purpose of life is achievement and success; incompetence in anything whatsoever is an indication that a person is inadequate or valueless (p. 89).

Indeed, strong empirical support confirms this observation. In a series of five studies, Flett, Hewitt, Blankstein, and Gray (1998a) found that perfectionists frequently engage in self-disparagement and perseverate on their failures when they have perceived that they have not attained their lofty standards. Furthermore, it appears that not only do perfectionists experience more frequent negative automatic cognitions, but they are also less likely to experience positive thoughts about themselves (Flett et al., 2011). This of course puts perfectionists doubly at risk for distress by limiting their ability to partake in the immense benefits of having positive illusions built around finding meaning and self-enhancement, which Taylor defines as “illusions that protect them psychologically from the threats they face and enable them to cope and make progress toward restoring good psychological functioning (Taylor, 2015, p. 342).”

Perfectionism is so entwined with self-criticism that some researchers have expanded the higher-order construct of PC to include self-criticism, as measured by the Depressive Experiences Questionnaire (DEQ, Blatt, D’Afflitti, & Quinlan, 1976) and/or the Dysfunctional Attitudes Scale (DAS; Weissman & Beck, 1978), and refer to this factor as self-critical perfectionism (e.g., Dunkley, Zuroff, & Blankstein, 2003, 2006, and see Dunkley, Solomon-Krakus, & Moroz, Chap. 7, this volume). This body of work has demonstrated not only that self-critical perfectionism prospectively predicts maladjustment over varying lengths of time (Dunkley, Mandel, & Ma, 2014b; (e.g., Rice, Leever, Christopher, & Porter, 2006; Sherry, Mackinnon, Macneil, & Fitzpatrick, 2013), but that self-criticism largely accounts for the associations between PC and distress (Dunkley et al., 2003, 2006). Although limited, converging evidence from the self-compassion literature suggests that perfectionism is associated with low self-compassion, reflecting a tendency to be harshly self-critical and unkind to oneself in situations of failure (Neff, 2003). Sirois and Pascual-Leone (2013) in their meta-analysis of 13 studies provide compelling evidence that both PS and PC are associated with lower levels of self-compassion.

Finally, research examining associations between perfectionism and self-esteem also indicates that self-evaluative tendencies are key processes linking perfectionism to distress. Flett et al. (1991) found that socially prescribed perfectionism was associated with lower self-esteem, whereas self-oriented perfectionism was associated with higher self-esteem. Other investigators have also documented links between PC and self-esteem (e.g., Ashby & Rice, 2002; Flett, Hewitt, Blankstein, Solnik, & Van Brunschot, 1996; Grzegorek, Slaney, Franze, & Rice, 2004; Klibert, Langhinrichsen-Rohling, & Saito, 2005; Mobley, Slaney, & Rice, 2005; Preusser, Rice, & Ashby, 1994; Rice, Ashby, & Preusser, 1996; Rice & Dellwo, 2002; Slaney, Rice, Mobley, Trippi, & Ashby, 2001; Stumpf & Parker, 2000). Interestingly, although the link between PS and higher levels of self-esteem has been replicated in some studies (e.g., Grzegorek et al. 2004), it has not in others (e.g., Flett et al. 1996).

In the context of chronic illness, there are several downstream effects of negative self-evaluation. Empirical evidence indicates that negative self-evaluations compromise coping ability and promote the use of noninstrumental and avoidance-based responses to stressors in people with chronic illness (Sirois, Molnar, & Hirsch, 2015). Importantly, self-criticism has been linked to stress-induced negative changes in biochemistry (Gruen, Silva, Ehrlich, Schweitzer, & Friedhoff, 1997). Further, self-blame is associated with poor adjustment outcomes in individuals with chronic tinnitus (Sirois et al., 2006) and has been linked to low psychological well-being in IBD patients (Voth & Sirois, 2009). Taken together, the research clearly indicates that the self-evaluative tendencies associated with perfectionism exacerbate stress and impede adaptive coping and may therefore be a liability for health outcomes in individuals with chronic illness.

Social Support

Social support is well known to be a critical resource for dealing with stressful circumstances in general and in chronic illness, specifically. The functional limitations associated with many chronic health conditions make social support a particularly important coping resource. For example, low levels of social support have been implicated in long-term functional disability and pain (Evers, Kraaimaat, Geenen,

Jacobs, & Bijlsma, 2003a) and psychological distress shortly after diagnosis (Evers, Kraaimaat, Geenen, & Bijlsma, 1997) and longitudinally over several years (Benka et al., 2012; Evers, Kraaimaat, Geenen, Jacobs, & Bijlsma, 2003b; Gafvels, Hagerstrom, Nordmark, & Wandell, 2014) in people with chronic illness. Relationship concerns and difficulties are also known to negatively impact adjustment to chronic illness (Gick & Sirois, 2010; Sirois & Gick, in press), whereas the provision of social support is associated with better quality of life (Janke, Klump, Gregor, Meisner, & Haeuser, 2005) and adjustment over time (Oliveira et al., 2007).

Consistent with this evidence, Fig. 4.1 illustrates that social support represents a critical interpersonal pathway linking perfectionism to stress and to later health outcomes. Perfectionists are at risk for experiencing greater distress and poorer health, in part, because they are socially disconnected. Sherry, Law, Hewitt, Flett, and Besser (2008) have found evidence to support their Social Disconnection Model (see Sherry, Mackinnon, & Gautreau, Chap. 10, this volume), which posits that perfectionism engenders a host of negative health and well-being outcomes through the experience of subjective social disconnection (i.e., perfectionists feel unwanted and rejected by others). Indeed, Flett, Blankstein, Hewitt, and Obertynski (1994) found that PS (as measured by self-oriented perfectionism from the MPS-HF) and OOP were each associated with reporting less social support from friends, whereas PC (as measured by socially prescribed perfectionism from the MPS-HF) was linked with less social support from family, friends, and intimate partners.

Although research on perfectionism and social support in chronic illness is lacking, evidence from healthy samples suggests that the impoverished social networks of perfectionists may be a liability for health. Molnar et al. (2012) found that PC was associated with poorer health via lower levels of social support in a sample of university students, whereas PS was associated with experiencing better health via higher levels of social support. However, the findings concerning PS were the result of classical suppression, as the initial association between PS and social support was not statistically significant and only became positive when PC was accounted for in the analyses.

Perfectionism may have a particularly salient role in the context of chronic illness because support from intimate partners is an important predictor of patients' adaption to illness (Revenson & Delongis, 2011). Indeed, both OOP and PC have been linked with maladaptive relational outcomes, such as poor relationship adjustment (Haring, Hewitt, & Flett, 2003; Lopez, Fons-Scheyd, Morúa, & Chaliman, 2006). Moreover, perfectionists behave in ways that are detrimental to either attaining or maintaining a satisfying relationship (Flett, Hewitt, Garshowitz, & Martin , 1997). Individuals with higher levels of OOP, for example, use more other-directed blame and are more dominant, exploitive, hostile, competitive, vindictive, impatient, and authoritarian than those with lower levels of OOP (Flett et al., 1994).

PC, as measured by socially prescribed perfectionism, is also related to poorer relationship outcomes, such as lower dyadic adjustment (Hewitt, Flett, & Mikail, 1995), and more frequent negative social interactions (Flett et al., 1997). Interestingly, the partners of those with higher levels of PC are also more likely to engage in conflictual coping when encountering marital difficulties (Haring et al., 2003), which speaks to the dyadic effects of perfectionism. In short, the negative relational styles associated with perfectionism may strain the necessary social support resources of those living with chronic illness, creating further risk for stress and poor coping.

Self-Concealment

The importance of the self-concealment pathway linking perfectionism to stress and later health problems derives from models of perfectionism that underscore the importance of the self-presentational aspects of perfectionism (e.g., Hewitt et al., 2003) and is consistent with the suggested functions of self-presentation for health concerns (Leary, Tchividjian, & Kraxberger, 1994). Perfectionistic self-presentation is an interpersonal expression of perfectionism in which an individual compulsively strives toward appearing flawless when in the presence of others. Consequently, individuals who adhere to this defensive impression management style work tirelessly to hide their perceived mistakes from others and to ensure that they do not disclose any potential shortcomings to anyone (see Hewitt et al., 2003; 2011). Individuals who engage in perfectionistic self-presentation are motivated by an incessant fear of negative evaluation, feeling compelled to conceal their self-loathing behind a mask of stoicism (Blatt, 1995).

Although there is clearly some overlap between facets of perfectionistic self-presentation and self-concealment, which measures the extent to which individuals actively hide information that could be seen as embarrassing, distressing, or negative, it should be noted that these constructs are not redundant (Hewitt et al., 2003). Evidence suggests that individuals higher in PS, OOP, and PC are more likely to use perfectionistic self-presentation as a strategy to hide any unappealing characteristics from others, with bivariate correlations ranging from 0.20 to 0.66 (Hewitt et al., 2003). Analogously, Frost and associates (1995, 1997) found that perfectionists are overly concerned that others will evaluate them negatively because of their mistakes and, thus, demonstrate a strong preference for nondisclosure of their mistakes.

Although this self-impression strategy may provide perfectionists with a reprieve from negative evaluation in the short term, it may be associated with significant costs later on through the protraction and exacerbation of stress (Hewitt & Flett, 2002). For example, Kawamura and Frost (2004) found an indirect link between PC and experiencing greater psychological distress via higher levels of self-concealment. Relevant for the proposed links between perfectionism and key health outcomes suggested by the SCCAMPI, Williams and Cropley (2014) found that self-concealment mediated the associations of PC with psychological distress and with less engagement in preventive health behaviors. In sum, the pattern of results from these intriguing studies suggests that PC is not only a risk factor for heightened psychological distress and antithetical to appropriate self-care, but that self-concealment is a critical factor that requires consideration when examining these associations.

Perfectionists' penchant for self-concealment may be particularly harmful in the context of chronic illness, as the need to appear perfect may cause some perfectionists to actively hide their symptoms and participate in activities that may actually exacerbate physical symptoms and conditions. Perhaps the most poignant example comes from Kelly Morgan Dempewolf's blog (i.e., http://asmybodyattacksitself.com) in which she describes how her perfectionism affects her daily adjustment and health functioning in the context of autoimmune disease and chronic fatigue syndrome. In one particular post (i.e., http://asmybodyattacksitself.com/but-you-were-able-to-do-that-why-cant-you-do-this), she discusses how she successfully used perfectionistic self-presentation skills to hide her pain and functional limitations by "sucking it up," by "putting on her happy face," and by maintaining her active engagement in all of the activities of her family vacation so that she would not let down her children and husband. Yet, she very insightfully illustrates how the benefits from this strategy were short-lived and ended up resulting in long-term consequences by causing her greater pain and a prolonged recovery period. Further, she points out how her false façade ironically caused her greater frustration and stress not only from causing her poorer health, but also because it created social constraints (i.e., perceiving that others are unreceptive to emotional self-disclosures; Lepore & Revenson, 2007). In other words, she was so successful at hiding her pain and discomfort that when she finally had to admit that she needed to rest and could no longer meet the situational demands, her family could not understand why because she appeared "fine" before.

There is also empirical evidence that perfectionistic self-presentation has negative consequences in the context of chronic illness. For example, Flett et al. (2011) found that after accounting for the effects of neuroticism and optimism, trait perfectionism, and perfectionistic self-presentation were each associated with greater sickness impact ratings in individuals with inflammatory bowel disease (IBD). Moreover, both trait perfectionism and perfectionistic self-presentation were associated with a maladaptive emotional preoccupation form of coping with this chronic illness. However, the results for perfectionistic self-presentation were more robust than those for trait perfectionism, suggesting that projecting a false façade is particularly detrimental to coping efforts in the context of IBD.

A primary concern is that by hiding behind a mask of invulnerability, perfectionists suffering from chronic illness may exacerbate their health problems and prolong their stress because potential support providers may never know the stress and physical limitations that they are actually struggling with. Thus, perfectionism may be especially detrimental for individuals with stigmatized yet hidden chronic illnesses, such as IBD, in part, because self-disclosure can be a risky and vulnerable act with negative consequences which may reinforce concealment (Defenbaugh, 2012). This is a serious issue in light of evidence suggesting that individuals with chronic illness who believe that their social networks are unreceptive as opposed to receptive are more likely to experience poorer adjustment (Danoff-Burg, Revenson, Trudeau, & Paget, 2004; Manne & Badr, 2008). Indeed, self-disclosure to others appears to be a crucial factor in adjustment to illness, as Lepore (2001) reported that self-disclosure allows individuals who are struggling with chronic illness to better understand and manage their emotions, to better understand their illness, and to restore their sense of identity.

The Role of Situational Discrepancy

Although the research discussed previously supports direct links between perfectionism and the intrapsychic and interpersonal pathways presented in the SCCAM-PI, we maintain that each of these pathways will be intensified when situational discrepancies between the present ill self and the former illness-free self are made particularly salient. The process of adjusting to chronic illness often requires the renegotiation of identity as one struggles to maintain or to reestablish a positive self-concept, which only serves to amplify perceptions of discrepancy between his or her current state of chronic illness and his or her fundamental goal of being perfect. For instance, many chronic illnesses are characterized by symptoms such as pain, fatigue, and reduced daily functioning that can jeopardize perfectionists' ability to engage in their relentless goal pursuit (e.g., Hamilton et al., 2004). Perfectionists with chronic illness can therefore be confronted on a daily basis with the knowledge that they are falling short of their incredibly high standards. Evidence indicates that perfectionists are generally highly committed to their goals and often quite reluctant to give them up because they are a key aspect of the perfectionist's identity (Flett, Sawatzky, & Hewitt, 1995b; Hewitt & Flett, 1991). Consequently, it is easy to see how the constant reminder of not meeting goals could potentially reinforce feelings of helplessness, intensify self-scrutiny and punitive self-evaluations, and increase feelings of alienation from others to the point where perfectionists suffering from chronic illness may further disengage from important self-disclosures. This is in keeping with findings illustrating that continual striving for goals in spite of making progress in those goals is associated with greater psychological distress (Carver & Scheier, 1990; Pomerantz, Saxon, & Oishi, 2000) and studies demonstrating that individuals who are able to let go of goals for which they can longer make progress toward are healthier (see Wrosch, Miller, Scheier, & Brun de Pontet, 2007).

The process of adjusting to chronic illness necessitates flexibly renegotiating goals so that they are more realistic in the context of living with illness (Hamilton et al., 2004). Yet, for some perfectionists, disengaging from unproductive goals is both difficult and costly and can result in poor coping and adjustment (Eddington, 2014). Perhaps, for individuals who believe that they must be and seem perfect, having to make goal adjustments in this context is viewed more as a failure to meet one's standards than as an adaptive and realistic response to illness imposed limitations. This is consistent with indications that some perfectionists demonstrate cognitive biases and tend to interpret a vast array of stimuli across diverse contexts in an overly negative fashion, often to the point of catastrophizing relatively innocuous situations (Ellis, 2002; Sherry & Hall, 2009). This can have particularly detrimental consequences, given that Horney (1950) observed that perfectionists experience low self-esteem as a result of perceiving a discrepancy between their ideal and actual self. Other characteristics of perfectionism such as the tendency for perfectionists to be chronically dissatisfied (see Pacht, 1984) and to perseverate on the uncontrollable aspects of failed goals (Sirois, Monforton, & Simpson, 2010) may be especially problematic for those perfectionists with an illness that impairs their ability to engage in relentless goal pursuit.

The Central Roles of Stress and Coping

The previous sections highlighted four key pathways linking perfectionism to higher levels of stress. If we acknowledge that living with a chronic health condition is akin to living with an ongoing stressor insomuch that chronic disease reflects both an unpredictable and an essentially uncontrollable circumstance (Taylor & Sirois, 2014), then it becomes clear that the stress associated with perfectionism via these routes has the potential to strain already thin coping resources to adaptively deal with this additional stress. In this respect, stress and coping are dynamically and reciprocally linked such that effective coping can downregulate the stress response and its consequences, including the need to engage further coping resources, whereas ineffective coping may exacerbate and amplify stress; which, in turn, can activate the need to engage more coping efforts. In the latter case, a cyclic amplification of stress through the interplay of stress and coping can put the perfectionist at even further risk for the harmful effects of stress.

This view is consistent with models of coping and stress which emphasize the transactional nature of stress and the importance of coping responses. Lazarus and Folkman's (1984) cognitive transaction model of stress emphasizes the central role of cognitive and behavioral coping responses in exacerbating or attenuating the stress response. From this perspective, maladaptive coping responses are those which fail to remove or reduce the stressor because they do not cognitively change its appraisal, or they do not result in instrumental action directed toward addressing the stressor (Lazarus & Folkman, 1984). Individuals with chronic illness face a variety of daily and ongoing stressors, including pain and functional limitations, which often require using different coping strategies depending on the demand (Gignac, Cott, & Badley, 2000). Thus, problems in flexibly responding to the demands of different stressors can also contribute to less successful coping.

Collectively, the research to date on coping in perfectionism characterizes perfectionists as being more vulnerable to experiencing greater stress and experiencing heightened stress responses, but also as being more poorly equipped to deal with stress (Flett & Hewitt, 2002). Indeed, a large and growing body of work now confirms that perfectionists are more likely to engage in maladaptive coping strategies, such as denial, suppression, and behavioral disengagement, and are less likely to employ adaptive coping strategies, such as information seeking, seeking social support, and problem solving (see Dunkley, Solomon-Krakus, & Moroz, Chap. 7, and Flett, Hewitt, & Nepon, Chap. 6, this volume). In the context of chronic illness, coping strategies can be targeted at either approaching or avoiding the illness (Suls & Fletcher, 1985). Broadly, individuals elevated in PC tend to engage in avoidant coping because they view themselves as being incapable of meeting the demands of stressful situations (see Dunkley, Blankstein, Halsall, Williams, & Winkworth, 2000; Flett et al., 1996). Moreover, perfectionists' proclivity to engage in avoidant coping strategies also prevents them from employing more adaptive coping strategies, which further exacerbates and prolongs their experience of stress. When confronted with chronic illness, perfectionists tend to rely on an emotion-oriented style that can exacerbate health problems (Flett et al., 2011).

Among the few studies that have examined how perfectionism is linked to coping and adjustment in chronic illness, perfectionism consistently is associated with poorer coping outcomes. Molnar et al. (2012), for example, examined the associations between dimensions of perfectionism as measured by the MPS-HF and health functioning in a sample of 489 women with fibromyalgia. Their findings revealed that both socially prescribed perfectionism (PC) and self-oriented perfectionism (PS) were associated with poorer health functioning. Moreover, these associations were maintained after accounting for the effects of broader personality traits related to both perfectionism and health such as conscientiousness, extraversion, and neuroticism. These data suggest that women with fibromyalgia who are characterized by exceptionally high levels of PS or PC experience immense pressure that undermines their adjustment efforts. These women are most likely highly vulnerable and should feel overwhelmed when other life stressors and setbacks are experienced.

Perfectionism's role in adjustment has also been established in the context of other chronic diseases. Andersson, Airikka, Buhrman, and Kaldo (2005), for instance, found that each of the MPS-F dimensions of perfectionism was positively related to tinnitus distress and anxiety among a large sample of tinnitus patients and that all of the dimensions, with the exception of organization, were positively related to depression. Research also suggests that perfectionism hinders the ability to cope with chronic illness in patients with colitis or Crohn's disease (Flett et al., 2011). These findings accord with the broader literature that has established links between perfectionism and maladaptive coping (see Dunkley et al., Chap. 7, this volume).

Calling into question the notion that PS will inevitably undermine coping efforts in the context of ongoing health limitations is the work of Fry and Debats (2011). Contrary to their previous findings relating PS to early all-cause mortality (Fry & Debats, 2009), they found in their prospective study of older adults with type 2 diabetes that PS was associated with greater longevity. They explained this unexpected finding by speculating that PS can foster longevity among older adults with diabetes by helping them better manage the strict medical regimen that must be followed by individuals coping with diabetes, such as consistently monitoring their blood glucose levels and following a stricter diet.

Yet, with the same participants, perfectionism was associated with greater mortality risk when it was operationally defined as dysfunctional perfectionistic attitudes that stress harsh self-criticism, stringent self-evaluation, extreme fear of evaluation, and unrealistic standard setting. Although some may dismiss these inconsistent findings as simply reflecting a measurement artifact, we believe that these results also illustrate the paradoxical nature of perfectionism in the context of chronic illness. That is, to the extent that PS is associated with conscientiousness, it may aid self-management of the illness which would result in better health-related outcomes. Nevertheless, for people who feel that they must be and seem perfect, having to make goal adjustments in this context may be viewed more as a failure to meet one's standards than as an adaptive and realistic response to illness imposed limitations. Other attributes such as the tendency for perfectionists to make their self-worth contingent upon meeting their unrealistically high standards may be especially problematic for those perfectionists who have an illness that undermines their ability to engage in relentless goal pursuit (e.g., Hamilton et al., 2004). Indeed, Anderson and Wolpert (2004) suggested that having perfectionistic goals may result in "diabetes burnout" for young adults.

Noteworthy findings have also emerged from studies examining perfectionism's role in recovery from cardiac illness. Parker et al. (2006) studied 489 Australian patients with acute coronary syndrome. They performed diagnostic interviews to classify patients into one of two groups: a group of patients who currently met clinical criteria for depression ($n=52$) versus a group of patients who did not presently meet diagnostic criteria for depression ($n=437$). They also evaluated the patients' lifetime histories of depression and uncovered two groups of patients: 187 patients with a lifetime history of clinical depression and 302 patients without a history of clinical depression. These researchers assessed perfectionism via a measure of self-oriented perfectionism developed by Parker and his associates that would conceptually fit under the umbrella of PS. Results indicated that PS and self-criticism were significantly elevated in those patients with a lifetime history of depression compared to patients without a history of depression. Moreover, the patients who currently met clinical criteria for depression reported higher levels of PS and self-criticism than those who did not presently meet clinical criteria for depression. These findings indicate that self-critical individuals elevated in PS are particularly likely to experience depression during the recovery period for acute coronary syndrome.

An investigation conducted by Shanmugasegaram and associates (2014) with a sample of 100 patients in cardiac recovery not only draws attention to the need to consider trait perfectionism in adjustment to chronic illness, but also points to the value of studying the potentially important role of perfectionistic self-presentation in chronic illness. As noted, perfectionistic self-presentation represents individual differences in the extent to which people portray an image suggesting that they need to appear perfect when in the presence of others (Hewitt et al., 2003). More specifically, Shanmugasegaram et al. (2014) examined the extent to which trait perfectionism and perfectionistic self-presentation are associated with the Type D personality (i.e., a distress-prone orientation characterized by chronic negative affect and social inhibition) and coping styles specific to illness. Intriguingly, their results revealed that all of the MPS-HF dimensions of trait perfectionism were associated with the Type D dimension assessing chronic negative emotionality and elevated levels of emotional preoccupation with their cardiac illness.

Findings from this study demonstrated that perfectionistic self-presentation was also associated with the Type D chronic negative emotionality component and with emotional preoccupation as a maladaptive coping style. As predicted, socially prescribed perfectionism and perfectionistic self-presentation were also associated with the Type D facet tapping social inhibition. In sum, these results indicate that elevated levels of PS and PC impede adjustment in patients with cardiac illness and implicate persistent emotional difficulties and possible impoverished social support networks due to social avoidance, as probable contributing factors.

Further evidence of the risk associated with perfectionism for people with cardiac illness has been provided by Stafford, Jackson, and Berk (2009) who conducted a longitudinal study of depression among hospitalized patients with coronary artery disease. Their data indicate that self-oriented perfectionism (as measured by a subscale included in a multidimensional measure of autonomy) predicts persistently higher levels of depression. Stafford et al. (2009) were also able to speak to the incremental predictive utility of perfectionism in the context of adjusting to chronic illness by demonstrating that perfectionism was the best predictor of depression at Time 1 (3 months post-discharge) and at Time 2 (9 months post-discharge) relative to autonomy and sociotropy. Thus, it appears that patients experiencing cardiac illness who have elevated levels of PS and PC have a proclivity to engage in coping and recovery efforts that are not conducive to adjustment.

Stress, Health Behaviors, and Illness Symptoms

The importance of managing stress in the context of chronic illness cannot be overstated. The deleterious effects of stress for individuals with chronic illness span multiple outcomes that can, in turn, amplify each other. With respect to the SC-CAMPI, we focus on two such mutually reinforcing outcomes that may be especially problematic for perfectionists: physical symptoms and the practice of health-promoting behaviors.

Stress, and chronic stress in particular, is implicated in the development and exacerbation of illness and disease through its impact on the immune system and its contributions to the dysregulation of inflammatory processes, known precursors of major chronic diseases (Cohen et al., 2012; Juster, McEwen, & Lupien, 2010; McEwen, 2007). Stress is therefore particularly problematic for diseases that involve underlying inflammatory processes, such as arthritis (e.g., Evers et al., 2013), IBD (e.g., Jaghulta et al., 2013), and cardiovascular disease (e.g., Rod, Grønbæk, Schnohr, Prescott, & Kristensen, 2009). Chronic stress can also result in compromised functioning of the hypothalamus–pituitary–adrenal (HPA) axis (one of the major human stress response systems) from overactivation, which can contribute to illness-related symptoms in certain conditions such as CFS (see Kempke et al., Chap. 5 this volume). Despite the well-established links from stress to compromised immune system functioning, inflammatory processes, HPA activation, and illness symptoms, other routes may also be involved. Researchers have noted that for particular inflammatory diseases, stress influences pain and other symptoms via non-immunological (Hassett & Clauw, 2010) and non-HPA linked mechanisms (Evers et al., 2013) which can nonetheless lead to a vicious circle of stress, pain, and inflammation (Straub & Kalden, 2009).

For many chronic diseases, physical symptoms, such as pain and fatigue, can be stressful and debilitating. Moreover, the anticipation of pain and other symptoms are stressful simply because they are unpredictable and uncontrollable (Taylor & Sirois, 2014). Stressful illness symptoms can disrupt personal goals and social and daily functioning (Graff et al., 2009; Wolfe & Sirois, 2008) and contribute to further stress, which can, in turn, exacerbate symptoms, and contribute to disease progression for certain diseases (Cámara et al., 2011; Dimsdale, 2008; Maunder, 2005; Maunder & Levenstein, 2008). For example, in one prospective study of rheumatoid arthritis patients, the experience of daily stressors and stress vulnerability factors, including a tendency to excessively worry, were predictive of fatigue, self-reported disease activity, swollen joint count, and pain 1 month later (Evers et al., 2013). Given the robust links between perfectionism and worry noted by Flett, Hewitt, and Nepon (Chap. 6, this volume), it is likely that such tendencies to ruminantly perseverate would be particularly harmful for perfectionists with chronic illness.

Perfectionism has also been associated with a wide variety of physical health symptoms including asthma (Morris, 1961), chronic pain (Van Houdenhove, 1986), headaches (Stout, 1984), and migraines (Kowal & Pritchard, 1990). When examining the links between perfectionism using multidimensional models of perfectionism, we see that there are sometimes differential associations between the different facets of perfectionism and symptoms. For example, Molnar et al. (2006) found that higher levels of PC (as measured by socially prescribed perfectionism from the MPS-HF) were associated with experiencing more frequent health symptoms via higher levels of negative affect and lower levels of positive affect, whereas PS (as measured by self-oriented perfectionism) was associated with experiencing fewer symptoms via higher levels of positive affect and lower levels of negative affect. Yet, the distinction between PS and PC is not always so clear in the context of health outcomes, as others have found evidence to support that both PS and PC are associated with experiencing more frequent psychosomatic symptoms (e.g., Martin, Flett, Hewitt, Krames, & Szanto, 1996) Saboonchi, & Lundh, 2003). We maintain that perfectionism should confer an even greater risk in the context of a chronic stressor such as chronic illness, given the links to heightened stress reactivity, and a proclivity for engaging in maladaptive coping strategies that exacerbate and extend stress responses.

Less frequent practice of health-promoting behaviors is another outcome related to stress that can further aggravate illness symptoms. Not only are poor health behaviors, such as poor diet and lack of exercise, implicated in the development and exacerbation of a number of major chronic and life-threatening diseases including hypertension, cardiovascular disease (Dimsdale, 2008; Rod et al., 2009), and diabetes (Green et al., 2007), but they also interfere with disease management. Moreover, as stress levels increase, the practice of health-promoting behaviors tends to decrease (Cohen et al., 1983; Sirois et al., 2009). Health behaviors are therefore particularly important in the context of chronic illness because they can play a central role in disease management. Although there may be some variations across different illnesses, in general maintaining a healthy diet, staying fit, getting adequate sleep, managing stress, and engaging in other health maintenance behaviors are important for weight management and behavioral control to manage symptoms and, in some cases, slow disease progression. Also critical is taking medication and getting frequent diagnostic testing.

Research linking perfectionism to the practice of health-promoting behaviors is sparse and to date has only focused on healthy samples. As noted by Sirois in Chap. 3 of this volume, the limited research on this topic is atheoretical and plagued by several methodological and conceptual issues regarding both how perfectionism and health behaviors are assessed. With only four published studies to date on this topic (Andrews, Burns, & Dueling, 2014; Chang et al., 2008; Molnar et al., 2012; Williams & Cropley, 2014), and no strong consensus regarding the differential relations of perfectionism dimensions to health behaviors, it is difficult to predict from this research whether and how perfectionism may relate to health behaviors in the context of chronic illness. Nonetheless, a small-scale meta-analysis of seven healthy samples showing that PC, but not PS perfectionism, was significantly associated with less frequent practice of a set of health behaviors (Sirois, 2013), provides suggestive evidence that may also apply to chronic illness samples.

To address this issue, Sirois (Chap. 3, this volume) proposes a self-regulation resource perspective for understanding how perfectionism may help or hinder the practice of health-promoting behaviors. Grounded in recent theory and research on self-regulation and the reciprocal influence of emotions on time perspectives, the Self-Regulation Resource Model (SRRM) posits that PC perfectionism is associated with poor practice of health behaviors because of its association with self-regulation depleting negative affect, whereas this is not always the case for PS perfectionism. However, in the context of living with a stressful and often frustrating chronic illness, it is reasonable to expect that levels of negative affect will be higher in general and that PS perfectionism may be more robustly associated with negative affect, which in turn, can disrupt the regulation of health behaviors. With respect to positive affect, research demonstrates that PC perfectionism is linked to low levels of positive affect, a potential resource for replenishing self-regulation capacity, whereas PS perfectionism is associated with higher levels of positive affect (e.g., Damian, Stoeber, Negru, & Băban, 2014; Flett, Blankstein, & Hewitt, 2009; Gaudreau & Verner-Filion, 2012; Molnar et al., 2006). The final self-regulation resource suggested by the SRRM as key for the practice of health-promoting behaviors is a future time orientation (Joireman, Shaffer, Balliet, & Strathman, 2012; Sirois, Shucard, & Hirsch, 2014; Strathman, Gleicher, Boninger, & Edwards, 1994).

According to the SRRM, high levels of stress and/or negative affect activate threat detection areas of the brain, which narrows temporal focus to more immediate concerns, thus reducing future-oriented focus (Tice, 2009; Wagner & Heatherton, 2015). Although there is little empirical evidence on how perfectionism may relate to temporal orientations, preliminary evidence presented by Sirois (Chap. 3, this volume) suggests that PS perfectionism is associated with a focus on the future, whereas PC perfectionism is not.

To summarize, current theory and research with healthy populations suggest that PC perfectionism is a liability for the practice of health-promoting behaviors in general that may also apply to individuals with chronic illness. The higher stress of living with chronic illness in combination with the stress generated from PC perfectionism may shift temporal focus away from future concerns, compromising health behaviors. Moreover, heightened negative affect linked to both perfectionism and the daily challenges of chronic illness may interfere with the timely engagement of necessary health-promoting and disease management behaviors that can further compromise physical health and symptoms in individuals with chronic illness.

Conclusions and Future Directions

The goal of this chapter was to present a new theoretical model to understand how perfectionism may serve as a risk factor for poor adjustment and unfavorable health outcomes in the context of chronic illness. The SCCAMPI underscores the importance of both intrapsychic (i.e., perceptions of control and self-evaluative tendencies) and interpersonal processes (i.e., social support and self-concealment) that link perfectionism to important health outcomes (i.e., physical symptoms and health behaviors) through the amplification of stress and maladaptive coping. Despite contemporary thinking on perfectionism suggesting that PS and PC can be distinguished from one another on the basis of their relative *(mal)*adaptiveness, we have not made this distinction in the SCCAMPI because theoretical accounts highlight the negative implications of both forms of perfectionism when individuals are under duress (Hewitt & Flett, 1991, 1993, 2002; Shafran et al., 2002) and empirical studies offer little distinction for these constructs in the context of chronic illness. We, therefore, propose that even in circumstances when perfectionism gives rise to actual benefits, such as greater achievement motivation and higher levels of personal achievement, there is often a huge price to pay for compulsively pursuing exorbitant standards in the context of chronic illness. However, this remains to be an open question given the relative dearth of research on this topic. Consequently, further research is required to test the proposition that both PS and PC will render perfectionists who live with chronic health problems at greater risk for poor adjustment and greater health problems.

It is important to note that the SCCAMPI not only emphasizes the central roles of stress and poor coping when examining the associations between perfectionism and consequential health outcomes, but also underscores the dynamic nature of these associations. Indeed, the pathways linking the intrapsychic and interpersonal processes to stress and coping along with the pathways linking stress and coping to health symptoms are considered to be fluid, mutually influencing one another, rather than static. This feature of the model coincides with transactional and interactional models of personality and health that highlight the multiple routes through which personality can directly and indirectly influence important health outcomes (Smith, 2006). The dynamic nature of our model is also consistent with the notion that adjustment to chronic disease is itself dynamic and in constant flux, waxing and waning with daily symptoms, functional disability, treatment demands, and changes in prognosis. Hence, the transactional nature of this model lends itself nicely to daily process and momentary assessment technologies, coupled with multilevel statistical techniques, which would allow researchers a more detailed understanding of how these processes unfold over time along with the twists and turns inherent in chronic illness.

Another issue that deserves empirical attention is whether the pathways in the SCCAMPI will vary according to demographic considerations such as age, cultural differences, socioeconomic status, and biological sex. This calls for research aimed at identifying important moderators of the delineated pathways above, which would serve to identify the circumstances or conditions under which these associations are most likely to be strengthened or weakened. Indeed, despite a general paucity of literature addressing sex-related differences in the area of perfectionism, we acknowledge the possibility that many of the processes in the SCCAMPI may function differently for men and women. Ample evidence suggests that women tend to report higher rates of both minor daily stressors and chronic stress compared to men, most likely due to the multiple roles that women fulfill, and that women tend to appraise their life events as more adverse and less controllable than men (e.g., Matud, 2004). Furthermore, research indicates that men and women differ in how they cope with stress, with women demonstrating greater use of avoidance and emotion-focused coping than men and reporting greater reliance on their social support networks than men (e.g., Matud, 2004; Taylor, 2006).

Very little research has addressed sex-related differences in adjustment to chronic illness. However, of the research that has been completed, there are hints that sex-related differences warrant further investigation, as studies indicate that women are more likely than men to report poorer psychological adjustment to chronic illness and this finding is present whether the woman is the patient or the caregiver (Hagedoorn, Sanderman, Bolks, Tuinstra, & Coyne, 2008; Revenson, 2003; Revenson, Abraido-Lanza, Majerovitz, & Jordan, 2005). In fact, it has been suggested that women tend to experience greater stress, poorer physiological functioning, and poorer adjustment to chronic illness because they tend to hold onto their caregiving roles in spite of their illness because these roles are essential to their self-concept (Abraido & Revenson, 2006; Stanton & Revenson, 2011). Consequently, female perfectionists who perceive that they are failing to meet their role obligations (which includes meeting their often unrealistically high standards) should be at the highest risk for experiencing poor adjustment to illness including the downstream negative health implications because they will invariably fail to permit themselves the allowance of illness intrusions which will threaten their self-concept.

A final issue to be addressed centers on the extent to which the proposed effects of perfectionism on health outcomes outlined by the SCCAMPI vary across different chronic illnesses. Although many chronic illnesses share several common symptoms such as fatigue, pain, and functional limitations (Hamilton et al., 2004), the trajectories of these symptoms can fluctuate significantly across different chronic conditions. Because circumstances which are more unpredictable and uncontrollable are also more stressful (Taylor & Sirois, 2014), illnesses characterized by greater symptom fluctuations (e.g., inflammatory bowel disease (IBD) and rheumatoid arthritis (RA)) and unpredictable disease progression (multiple sclerosis (MS)) may be especially problematic for perfectionists. As noted previously, perfectionism appears to be particularly detrimental for the health and well-being of people with IBD (Flett et al., 2011), fibromyalgia (Molnar et al., 2012), and CFS (Kempke et al., Chap. 5 this volume). Further research into the perils of perfectionism across and between different chronic illnesses would help bring clarity to these issues and further verify the predictions of the SCCAMPI.

References

Abraido-Lanza, A. F., & Revenson, T. A. (2006). Illness intrusion and psychological adjustment to rheumatic diseases: A social identity framework. *Arthritis and Rheumatism. Arthritis Care & Research, 55,* 224–232. doi:10.1002/art.21849.

Adler, A., Ansbacher, H. L., & Ansbacher, R. R. (1956). *The individual psychology of Alfred Adler: A systematic presentation in selections from his writings*. New York: Basic Books.

Anderson, B. J., & Wolpert, H. A. (2004). A developmental perspective on the challenges of diabetes education and care during the young adult period. *Patient Education and Counseling, 53,* 347–352. doi:10.1016/j.pec.2003.03.001.

Andersson, G., Airikka, M.-L., Buhrman, M., & Kaldo, V. (2005). Dimensions of perfectionism and tinnitus distress. *Psychology, Health, and Medicine, 10,* 78–87. doi:10.1080/13548500512331315389.

Andrews, D., Burns, L., & Dueling, J. (2014). Positive perfectionism: Seeking the healthy "should", or should we? *Open Journal of Social Sciences, 2,* 27–34.

Asbring, P. (2001). Chronic illness—a disruption in life: Identity-transformation among women with chronic fatgue syndrome and fibromyalgia. *Journal of Advanced Nursing, 34*(3), 312–319.

Ashby, J. S., & Rice, K. G. (2002). Perfectionism, dysfunctional attitudes, and self-esteem: A structural equations analysis. *Journal Of Counseling & Development, 80,* 197–203.

Bardone-Cone, A. M., Wonderlich, S. A., Frost, R. O., Bulik, C. M., Mitchell, J. E., Uppala, S., & Simonich, H. (2007). Perfectionism and eating disorders: Current status and future directions. *Clinical Psychology Review, 27*(3), 384–405. doi:10.1016/j.cpr.2006.12.005.

Benka, J., Nagyova, I., Rosenberger, J., Calfova, A., Macejova, Z., Middel, B., Lazurova, I., van Dijk, J. P., & Groothoff, J. W. (2012). Social support and psychological distress in rheumatoid arthritis: A 4-year prospective study. *Disability and Rehabilitation, 34*(9), 754–761. doi:10.3109/09638288.2011.619618.

Blatt, S. J. (1995). The destructiveness of perfectionism: Implications for the treatment of perfectionism. *American Psychologist, 50,* 1003–1020.

Blatt, S. J., D'Afflitti, J. P., & Quinlan, D. M. (1976). Experiences of depression in normal young adults. *Journal of Abnormal Psychology, 85,* 383–389. doi:10.1037/0021-843X.85.4.383.

Bogg, T., & Roberts, B. W. (2013). The case for conscientiousness: Evidence and implications for a personality trait marker of health and longevity. *Annals of Behavioral Medicine, 45*(3), 278–288. doi:10.1007/s12160-012-9454-6.

Boye, B., Lundin, K. E. A., Leganger, S., et al (2008). The INSPIRE study: Do personality traits predict general quality of life (short form-36) in distressed patients with ulcerative colitis and Crohn's disease? *Scandinavian Journal of Gastroenterology, 43,* 1505–1513.

Brickman, A. L., Yount, S. E., Blaney, N. T., Rothberg, S. T., & De-Nour, A. K. (1996). Personality traits and long-term health status: The influence of neuroticism and conscientiousness on renal detrioration in Type-1 diabetes. *Psychosomatics, Journal of Consultation Liason Psychiatry, 37,* 459–468.

Buhr, K., & Dugas, M. J. (2006). Investigating the construct validity of intolerance of uncertainty and its unique relationship with worry. *Journal of Anxiety Disorders, 20,* 222–236. doi:10.1016/j.janxdis.2004.12.004.

Cámara, R. J. A., Schoepfer, A. M., Pittet, V., Begré, S., von Känel, R., & the Swiss Inflammatory Bowel Disease Cohort Study Group. (2011). Mood and nonmood components of perceived stress and exacerbation of Crohn's disease. *Inflammatory Bowel Diseases, 17,* 2358–2365. doi:10.1002/ibd.21623.

Carver, C. S., & Scheier, M. F. (1990). Origins and functions of positive and negative affect: A control-process view. *Psychological Review, 97,* 19–35.

Centers for Disease Control and Prevention. (2013). Death and Mortality. NCHS FastStats Web site: http://www.cdc.gov/nchs/fastats/deaths.htm. Accessed 20 Dec 2013.

Chang, E. C., Ivezaj, V., Downey, C. A., Kashima, Y., & Morady, A. R. (2008). Complexities of measuring perfectionism: Three popular perfectionism measures and their relations with eating disturbances and health behaviors in a female college student sample. *Eating Behaviors, 9*(1), 102–110. doi:10.1016/j.eatbeh.2007.06.003.

Christensen, A. J., Ehlers, S. L., Wiebe, J. S., Moran, P. J., Raichle, K., Ferneyhough, K., & Lawton, W. J. (2002). Patient personality and mortality: A 4-year prospective examination of chronic renal insufficiency. *Health Psychology, 21,* 315–320. doi:10.1037//0278-6133.21.4.315.

Cohen, S., Kamarck, T., & Mermelstein, R. (1983). A global measure of perceived stress. *Journal of Health and Social Behavior, 24*(4), 385–396.

Cohen, S., Janicki-Deverts, D., Doyle, W. J., Miller, G. E., Frank, E., Rabin, B. S., & Turner, R. B. (2012). Chronic stress, glucocorticoid receptor resistance, inflammation, and disease risk. *Proceedings of the National Academy of Sciences, 109*(16), 5995–5999.

Contrada, R. J., Goyal, T. M., Cather, C., Rafalson, L., Idler, E. L., & Krause, T. J. (2004). Psychosocial factors in outcomes of heart surgery: The impact of religious involvement and depressive symptoms. *Health Psychology, 23,* 227–238. doi:10.1037/0278-6133.23.3.227.

Cox, B. J., Enns, M. W., & Clara, I. P. (2002). The multidimensional structure of perfectionism in clinically distressed and college student samples. *Psychological Assessment, 14,* 365–373. doi:10.1037//1040-3590.14.3.365.

Damian, L. E., Stoeber, J., Negru, O., & Băban, A. (2014). Positive and negative affect in adolescents: An investigation of the 2 × 2 model of perfectionism. *Cognition, Brain, Behavior. An Interdisciplinary Journal, 18,* 1–16.

Danoff-Burg, S., Revenson, T. A., Trudeau, K. J., & Paget, S. A. (2004). Unmitigated communion, social constraints, and psychological distress among women with rheumatoid arthritis. *Journal of Personality, 72,* 29–46. doi:10.1111/j.0022-3506.2004.00255.x.

Defenbaugh, N. L. (2012). Revealing and concealing ill identity: A performance narrative of IBD disclosure. *Health Communication, 28,* 159–169.

Devins, G. M. (1989). Enhancing personal control and minimizing illness intrusiveness. In N. G. Kutner, D. D. Cardenas, & J. D. Bower (Eds.), *Maximizing rehabilitation in chronic renal disease*. New York: PMA.

Dew, M. A., Myaskovsky, L., Switzer, G. E., DiMartini, A. F., Schulberg, H. C., & Kormos, R. L. (2005). Profiles and predictors of the course of psychological distress across four years of heart transplantation. *Psychological Medicine, 35,* 1215–1227.

Dickson, A. (2008). 'That was my old life; it's almost like a past-life now': Identity crisis, loss and adjustment amongst people living with chronic fatigue syndrome. *Psychology & Health, 1,* 1–16. doi:10.1080/08870440701757393.

Dimsdale, J. E. (2008). Psychological stress and cardiovascular disease. *Journal of the American College of Cardiology, 51*(13), 1237–1246.

Dunkley, D. M., & Blankstein, K. R. (2000). Self-critical perfectionism, coping, hassles, and current distress: A structural equation modeling approach. *Cognitive Therapy and Research, 24,* 713–730.

Dunkley, D. M., Blankstein, K. R., Halsall, J., Williams, M., & Winkworth, G. (2000). The relation between perfectionism and distress: Hassles, coping, and perceived social support as mediators and moderators. *Journal of Counseling Psychology, 47,* 437–453.

Dunkley, D. M., Zuroff, D. C., & Blankstein, K. R. (2003). Self-critical perfectionism and daily affect: Dispositional and situational influences on stress and coping. *Journal of Personality and Social Psychology, 84,* 234–252. doi:10.1037/0022-3514.84.1.234.

Dunkley, D. M., Zuroff, D. C., & Blankstein, K. R. (2006). Specific perfectionism components versus self-criticism in predicting maladjustment. *Personality and Individual Differences, 40,* 40665–40676. doi:10.1016/j.paid.2005.08.008.

Dunkley, D. M., Ma, D., Lee, I. A., Preacher, K. J., & Zuroff, D. C. (2014a). Advancing complex explanatory conceptualizations of daily negative and positive affect: Trigger and maintenance coping action patterns. *Journal of Counseling Psychology, 61,* 93–109. doi:10.1037/a0034673.

Dunkley, D. M., Mandel, T., & Ma, D. (2014b). Perfectionism, neuroticism, and daily stress reactivity and coping effectiveness 6 months and 3 years later. *Journal of Counseling Psychology, 61,* 616–633. doi:10.1037/cou0000036.

Eddington, K. M. (2014). Perfectionism, goal adjustment, and self-regulation: A short-term follow-up study of distress and coping. *Self & Identity, 13,* 197–213.

Ellis, A. (1962). *Reason and emotion in psychotherapy*. New York: Stuart.

Ellis, A. (2002). The role of irrational beliefs in perfectionism. In G. L. Flett & P. L. Hewitt (Eds.), *Perfectionism: Theory, research, and treatment* (pp. 217–229). Washington, DC: American Psychological Association Press. doi:10.1037/10458-009.

Enns, M. W., & Cox, B. J. (2002). The nature and assessment of perfectionism: A critical analysis. In G. L. Flett, P. L. Hewitt, G. L. Flett, & P. L. Hewitt (Eds.), *Perfectionism: Theory, research, and treatment* (pp. 33–62). Washington, DC: American Psychological Association. doi:10.1037/10458-002.

Enns, M. W., Cox, B. J., Sareen, J., & Freeman, P. (2001). Adaptive and maladaptive perfectionism in medical students: A longitudinal investigation. *Medical Education, 35,* 1034–1042.

Evers, A. W. M., Kraaimaat, F. W., Geenen, R., & Bijlsma, J. W. J. (1997). Determinants of psychological distress and its course in the first year after diagnosis in rheumatoid arthritis patients. *Journal of Behavioral Medicine, 20*(5), 489–504.

Evers, A. W., Kraaimaat, F. W., Geenen, R., Jacobs, J. W., & Bijlsma, J. W. (2003a). Pain coping and social support as predictors of long-term functional disability and pain in early rheumatoid arthritis. *Behavior Research and Therapy, 41*(11), 1295–1310. doi:10.1016/S0005-7967(03)00036-6.

Evers, A. W., Kraaimaat, F. W., Geenen, R., Jacobs, J. W., & Bijlsma, J. W. (2003b). Stress-vulnerability factors as long-term predictors of disease activity in early rheumatoid arthritis. *Journal of Psychosomatic Research, 55*(4), 293–302. doi:10.1016/S0022-3999.

Evers, A. W. M., Verhoeven, E. W. M., van Middendorp, H., Sweep, F. C. G. J., Kraaimaat, F. W., Donders, A. R. T., Eijsbouts, A. E., van Laarhoven, A. I. M., de Brouwer, S. J. M., Wirken, L., Radstake, T. R. D. J., & van Riel, P. L. C. M. (2013). Does stress affect the joints? Daily stressors, stress vulnerability, immune and HPA axis activity, and short-term disease and symptom fluctuations in rheumatoid arthritis. *Annals of the Rheumatic Diseases, 73,* 6.

Flett, G. L., & Hewitt, P. L. (2002). *Perfectionism: Theory, research, and treatment*. Washington, DC: American Psychological Association.

Flett, G. L., Hewitt, P. L., Blankstein, K. R., & Obrien, S. (1991). Perfectionism and learned resourcefulness in depression and self-esteem. *Personality And Individual Differences, 12,* 61–68.

Flett, G. L., Blankstein, K. R., Hewitt, P. L., & Obertynski, M. (1994, November). Personality and coping in depression: A comparison of sociotropy, autonomy, and perfectionism. Paper presented at the annual convention of the Association for the Advancement of Behavior Therapy, San Diego, CA.

Flett, G. L., Hewitt, P. L., Blankstein, K. R., & Mosher, S. W. (1995a). Perfectionism, life events, and depressive symptoms: A test of diathesis-stress model. *Current Psychology, 14,* 112–128.

Flett, G. L., Sawatzky, D. L., & Hewitt, P. L. (1995b). Dimensions of perfectionism and goal commitment: A further comparison of two perfectionism measures. *Journal of Psychopathology and Behavioral Assessment, 17,* 111–124. doi:10.1007/BF02229013.

Flett, G. L., Hewitt, P. L., Blankstein, K. R., Solnik, M., & Van Brunschot, M. (1996). Prfectionism, social problem-solving ability, and psychological distress. *Journal of Rational—Emotive and Cognitive—Behavior Therapy, 14,* 245–274.

Flett, G. L., Hewitt, P. L., Garshowitz, M., & Martin, T. R. (1997). Personality, negative social interactions, and depressive symptoms. *Canadian Journal of Behavioural Science, 29,* 28–37.

Flett, G. L., Hewitt, P. L., Blankstein, K., & Gray, L. (1998a). Psychological distress and the frequency of perfectionistic thinking. *Journal of Personality and Social Psychology, 75,* 1363–1381.

Flett, G. L., Hewitt, P. L., Blankstein, K. R., & Pickering, D. (1998b). Perfectionism in relation to attributions for success and failure. *Current Psychology, 17,* 249–262.

Flett, G. L., Madorsky, D., Hewitt, P. L., & Heisel, M. J. (2002). Perfectionism cognitions, rumination, and psychological distress. *Journal of Rational-Emotive & Cognitive Behavior Therapy, 20*(1), 33–47.

Flett, G. L., Blankstein, K. R., & Hewitt, P. L. (2009). Perfectionism, performance, and state positive affect and negative affect after a classroom test. *Canadian Journal of School Psychology, 24,* 4–18.

Flett, G. L., Baricza, C., Gupta, A., Hewitt, P. L., & Endler, N. S. (2011). Perfectionism, psychosocial impact and coping with irritable bowel disease: A study of patients with Crohn's disease and ulcerative colitis. *Journal of Health Psychology, 16,* 561–571. doi:10.1177/1359105310383601.

Friedman, H. S., Tucker, J. S., Tomlinson-Keasey, C., Schwartz, J. E., Wingard, D. L., & Criqui, M. H. (1993). Does childhood personality predict longevity? *Journal of Personality and Social Psychology, 65,* 176–185.

Frost, R. O., & DiBartolo, P. M. (2002). Can cognitive restructuring reduce the disruption associated with perfectionistic concerns? In G. L. Flett & P. L. Hewitt (Eds.), *Perfectionism: Theory, research, and treatment* (pp. 341–371). Washington, DC: American Psychological Association.

Frost, R. O., Marten, P., Lahart, C., & Rosenblate, R. (1990). The dimensions of perfectionism. *Cognitive Therapy and Research, 14,* 449–468.

Frost, R. O., Heimberg, R. G., Holt, C. S., Mattia, J. I., & Neubauer, A. L. (1993). A comparison of two measures of perfection. *Personality and Individual Differences, 14,* 119–126.

Frost, R., Turcotte, T., Heimberg, R., Mattia, J., Holt, C., & Hope, D. (1995). Reactions to mistakes among subjects high and low in perfectionistic concern over mistakes. *Cognitive Therapy and Research, 19,* 195–205.

Frost, R. O., Trepanier, K. L., Brown, E. J., Heimberg, R. G., Juster, H. R., Makris, G. S., & Leung, A. W. (1997). Self-monitoring of mistakes among subjects high and low in perfectionistic concern over mistakes. *Cognitive Therapy & Research, 21,* 209–222.

Fry, P. S., & Debats, D. (2009). Perfectionism and the five-factor personality traits as predictors of mortality in older adults. *Journal of Health Psychology, 14,* 513–524. doi:10.1177/1359105309103571.

Fry, P. S., & Debats, D. L. (2011). Perfectionism and other related trait measures as predictors of mortality in diabetic older adults: A six-and-a-half-year longitudinal study. *Journal of Health Psychology*. doi:10.1177/1359105311398684.

Gafvels, C., Hagerstrom, M., Nordmark, B., & Wandell, P. (2014). What predicts negative effects of rheumatoid arthritis? A follow-up two years after diagnosis. *SpringerPlus, 3,* 118.

Gaudreau, P., & Verner-Filion, J. (2012). Dispositional perfectionism and well-being: A test of the 2 × 2 model of perfectionism in the sport domain. *Sport, Exercise, and Performance Psychology, 1,* 29–43.

Gick, M. L., & Sirois, F. M. (2010). Insecure attachment moderates women's adjustment to inflammatory bowel disease severity. *Rehabilitation Psychology, 55,* 170–179. doi:10.1037/a0019358.

Gignac, M. A. M., Cott, C., & Badley, E. M. (2000). Adaptation to chronic illness and disability and its relationship to perceptions of independence and dependence. *Journals of Gerontology Series B: Psychological Sciences and Social Sciences, 55*(6), 362–372.

Green, A. J., Bazata, D. D., Fox, K. M., Grandy, S., & for the, S. S. G. (2007). Health-related behaviours of people with diabetes and those with cardiometabolic risk factors: Results from SHIELD. *International Journal of Clinical Practice, 61*(11), 1791–1797. doi:10.1111/j.1742-1241.2007.01588.x.

Gruen, R. J., Silva, R., Ehrlich, J., Schweitzer, J. W., & Friedhoff, A. J. (1997). Vulnerability to stress: Self-criticism and stress-induced changes in biochemistry. *Journal of Personality, 65*(1), 33–47.

Grzegorek, J. L., Slaney, R. B., Franze, S., & Rice, K. G. (2004). Self-criticism, dependency, self-esteem, and grade point average satisfaction among clusters of perfectionists and nonperfectionists. *Journal of Counseling Psychology, 51,* 192–200. doi:10.1037/0022-0167.51.2.192.

Hagedoorn, M., Sanderman, R., Bolks, H. N., Tuinstra, J., & Coyne, J. C. (2008). Distress in couples coping with cancer: A meta-analysis and critical review of role and gender effects. *Psychological Bulletin, 134,* 1–30. doi:10.1037/0033-2909.134.1.1.

Helgeson, V. S., Snyder, P., & Seltman, H. (2004). Psychological and physical adjustment to breast cancer over 4 years: Identifying distinct trajectories of change. *Health Psychology, 23,* 3–15.

Hamilton, N., Karoly, P., & Kitzman, H. (2004). Self-regulation and chronic pain: The role of emotion. *Cognitive Therapy and Research, 28*(5), 559–576. doi:0147-5916/04/1000-0559/0.

Hampson, S. E., Goldberg, L. R., Vogt, T. M., & Dubanoski, J. P. (2007). Mechanisms by which childhood personality traits influence adult health status: Educational attainment and healthy behaviors. *Health Psychology, 26*(1), 121–125. doi:0278-6133/13/$12.00.

Haring, M., Hewitt, P. L., & Flett, G. L. (2003). Perfectionism, coping, and quality of intimate relationships. *Journal of Marriage and Family, 65,* 143–158.

Hassett, A., & Clauw, D. (2010). The role of stress in rheumatic diseases. *Arthritis Research & Therapy, 12*(3), 123.

Hewitt, P. L., & Flett, G. L. (1991). Perfectionism in the self and social contexts: Conceptualization, assessment, and association with psychopathology. *Journal of Personality and Social Psychology, 60,* 456–470.

Hewitt, P. L., & Flett, G. L. (1993). Dimensions of perfectionism, daily stress, and depression: A test of the specific vulnerability hypothesis. *Journal of Abnormal Psychology, 102,* 58–65.

Hewitt, P. L., & Flett, G. L. (2002). Perfectionism and stress processes in psychopathology. In G. L. Flett & P. L. Hewitt (Eds.), *Perfectionism: Theory, research, and treatment* (pp. 255–284). Washington, DC: American Psychological Association.

Hewitt, P. L., Flett, G. L., & Mikail, S. (1995). Perfectionism and relationship adjustment in pain patients and their spouses. *Journal of Family Psychology, 9,* 335–347. doi:10.1037/0893-3200.9.3.335.

Hewitt, P. L., Flett, G. L., & Ediger, E. (1996). Perfectionism and depression: Longitudinal assessment of a specific vulnerability hypothesis. *Journal of Abnormal Psychology, 105,* 276–280.

Hewitt, P. L., Flett, G. L., Besser, A., Sherry, S. B., & McGee, B. (2003). Perfectionism is multidimensional: A reply to Shafran, Cooper, and Fairburn. *Behavior Research and Therapy, 41,* 1221–1236. doi:10.1016/S0005-7967(03)00021-4.

Hewitt, P. L., Blasberg, J. S., Flett, G. L., Besser, A., Sherry, S. B., Caelian, C.., et al (2011). Perfectionistic self-presentation in children and adolescents: Development and validation of the

perfectionistic self-presentation scale Junior Form. *Psychological Assessment, 23,* 125–142. doi:10.1037/a0021147.
Horney, K. (1950). *Neurosis and human growth; the struggle toward self-realization*. New York: Norton.
Infurna, F. J., Ram, N., & Gerstorf, D. (2013). Level and change in perceived control predict 19-year mortality: Findings from the Americans' changing lives study. *Developmental Psychology, 49,* 1833–1847.
Jaghulta, S., Saboonchib, F., Mollere, J., Johanssona, U.-B., Wredlinga, R., & Kapraalia, M. (2013). Stress as a trigger for relapses in IBD: A case-crossover study. *Gastroenterology Research, 6*(1), 10–16.
Janke, K. H., Klump, B., Gregor, M., Meisner, C., & Haeuser, W. (2005). Determinants of life satisfaction in inflammatory bowel disease. *Inflammatory Bowel Diseases, 11*(3), 272–286. doi:10.1097/01.MIB.0000160809.38611.f7.
Johnson, W., & Krueger, R. F. (2005). Higher perceived life control decreases genetic variance in physical health: Evidence from a national twin study. *Journal of Personality & Social Psychology, 88,* 165–173. doi:10.1037/0022-3514.88.1.165.
Joireman, J., Shaffer, M. J., Balliet, D., & Strathman, A. (2012). Promotion orientation explains why future-oriented people exercise and eat healthy: Evidence from the two-factor consideration of future consequences-14 scale. *Personality and Social Psychology Bulletin, 38,* 1272–1287.
Juster, R.-P., McEwen, B. S., & Lupien, S. J. (2010). Allostatic load biomarkers of chronic stress and impact on health and cognition. *Neuroscience & Biobehavioral Reviews, 35*(1), 2–16.
Kawamura, K. Y., & Frost, R. O. (2004). Self-concealment as a mediator in the relationship between perfectionism and psychological distress. *Cognitive Therapy & Research, 28,* 183–191.
Klibert, J. J., Langhinrichsen-Rohling, J., & Saito, M. (2005). Adaptive and maladaptive aspects of selforiented versus socially prescribed perfectionism. *Journal of College Student Development, 46,* 141–156.
Kobori, O. (2006). *A cognitive model of perfectionism: The relationship of perfectionism personality to psychological adaptation and maladaptation.* Unpublished doctoral dissertation. Tokyo: University of Tokyo.
Kowal, A., & Pritchard, D. (1990). Psychological characteristics of children who suffer from head ache: A research note. *Journal of Child Psychology and Psychiatry and Allied Disciplines, 31,* 637–649.
Lazarus, R. S., & Folkman, S. (1984). *Stress, appraisal, and coping*. New York: Springer.
Leary, M. R., Tchividjian, L. R., & Kraxberger, B. E. (1994). Self-presentation can be hazardous to your health: Impression management and health risk. *Health Psychology: Official Journal of the Division of Health Psychology. American Psychological Association, 13,* 461–470.
Lepore, S. J. (2001). A social–cognitive processing model of emotional adjustment to cancer. In A. Baum & B. Andersen (Eds.), *Psychosocial interventions for cancer* (pp. 99–118). Washington, DC: American Psychological Association.
Lepore, S. J., & Revenson, T. A. (2007). Social constraints on disclosure and adjustment to cancer. *Social & Personality Psychology Compass, 1,* 313. doi:10.1111/j.1751-9004.2007.00013.x.
Lopez, F. G., Fons-Scheyd, A., Morúa, W., & Chaliman, R. (2006). Dyadic perfectionism as a predictor of relationship continuity and distress among college students. *Journal of Counseling Psychology, 53,* 543–549.
Mackinnon, S., Sherry, S., Antony, M., Stewart, S., Sherry, D., & Hartling, N. (2012). Caught in a bad romance: Perfectionism, conflict, and depression in romantic relationships. *Journal of Family Psychology, 26,* 215–225. doi:10.1037/a0027402.
Manne, S., & Badr, H. (2008). Intimacy and relationship processes in couples' psychosocial adaptation to cancer. *Cancer, 112,* 2541–2555. doi:10.1002/cncr.23450.
Martin, T., Flett, G., Hewitt, P., Krames, L., & Szanto, G. (1996). Personality correlates of depression and health symptoms: A test of a self-regulation model. *Journal of Research in Personality, 30,* 264–277.

Matud, M. P. (2004). Gender differences in stress and coping styles. *Personality and Individual Differences, 37,* 1401–1415. doi:10.1016/j.paid.2004.01.010.
Maunder, R. G. (2005). Evidence that stress contributes to inflammatory bowel disease: Evaluation, synthesis, and future directions. *Inflammatory Bowel Diseases, 11*(6), 600–608. doi:10.1097/01.MIB.0000161919.42878.a0.
Maunder, R. G., & Levenstein, S. (2008). The role of stress in the development and clinical course of inflammatory bowel disease: Epidemiological evidence. *Current Molecular Medicine, 8*(4), 247–252.
McEwen, B. S. (2007). Physiology and neurobiology of stress and adaptation: Central role of the brain. *Physiological Reviews, 87*(3), 873–904.
Mobley, M., Slaney, R. B., & Rice, K. G. (2005). Cultural validity of the almost perfect scale-revised for African American college students. *Journal of Counseling Psychology, 52,* 629–639.
Molnar, D. S., Reker, D. L., Culp, N. A., Sadava, S. W., & DeCourville, N. H. (2006). A mediated model of perfectionism, affect, and physical health. *Journal of Research in Personality, 40,* 482–500. doi:10.1016/j.jrp.2005.04.002.
Molnar, D. S., Sadava, S. W., Flett, G. L., & Colautti, J. (2012). Perfectionism and health-related quality of life in women with fibromyalgia. *Journal of Psychosomatic Research, 73,* 295–300. doi:10.1016/j.jpsychores.2012.08.001.
Morris, R. P. (1961). Effect of the mother on goal-setting behaviour of the asthmatic child. *Annals of Allergy, 19,* 44–54.
Neff, K. D. (2003). The development and validation of a scale to measure self-compassion. *Self & Identity, 2,* 223–250. doi:10.1080/15298860390209035.
Oliveira, S., Zaltman, C., Elia, C., Vargens, R., Leal, A., Barros, R., & Fogaça, H. (2007). Quality-of-life measurement in patients with inflammatory bowel disease receiving social support. *Inflammatory Bowel Diseases, 13*(4), 470–474. doi:10.1002/ibd.20071.
Ozer, D. J., & Benet-Martinez, V. (2006). Personality and the prediction of consequential outcomes. *Annual Review of Psychology, 57,* 401–421. doi:10.1146/annurev.psych.57.102904.190127.
Pacht, A. R. (1984). Reflections on perfectionism. *American Psychologist, 39,* 386–390.
Parker, W. D. (1997). An empirical typology of perfectionism in academically talented children. *American Educational Research Journal, 34,* 545–562.
Parker, G., Heruc, G., Hilton, T., Olley, A., Brotchie, H.., et al (2006). Explicating links between acute coronary syndrome and depression: Study design and method. *Australian and New Zealand Journal of Psychiatry, 40,* 245–252. doi:10.1111/j.1440-1614.2006.01781.x.
Pomerantz, E. M., Saxon, J. L., & Oishi, S. (2000). The psychological tradeoffs of goal investment. *Journal of Personality and Social Psychology, 79,* 617–630.
Preusser, K. J., Rice, K. G., & Ashby, J. S. (1994). The role of self-esteem in mediating the perfectionism-depression connection. *Journal of College Student Development, 35,* 88–93.
Revenson, T. A. (2003). Scenes from a marriage: Examining support, coping, and gender within the context of chronic illness. In J. Suls & K. Wallston (Eds.), *Social psychological foundations of health and illness* (pp. 530–559). Oxford: Blackwell Publishing.
Revenson, T. A., & DeLongis, A. (2011). Couples coping with chronic illness. In S. Folkman (Ed.), *The Oxford handbook of stress, health, and coping* (pp. 101–123). New York: Oxford University Press.
Revenson, T. A., Abraido-Lanza, A. F., Majerovitz, S. D., & Jordan, C. (2005). Couples coping with chronic illness: What's gender got to do with it? In T. A. Revenson, K. Kayser, & G. Bodenmann (Eds.), *Couples coping with stress: Emerging perspectives on dyadic coping* (pp. 137–156). Washington, DC: American Psychological Association.
Rice, K., & Dellwo, J. P. (2002). Perfectionism and self-development: Implications for self-esteem, depression, and college adjustment. *Journal of Counseling and Development, 80,* 188–196. doi:10.1002/j.1556-6678.2002.tb00182.x.
Rice, K. G., Ashby, J. S., & Preusser, K. J. (1996). Perfectionism, relationships with parents, and self-esteem. *Individual Psychology: The Journal of Adlerian Theory, Research & Practice, 52,* 246–260.

Rice, K. G., Leever, B. A., Christopher, J., & Porter, J. D. (2006). Perfectionism, stress, and social (dis)connection: A short-term study of hopelessness, depression, and academic adjustment among honors students. *Journal of Counseling Psychology, 53,* 524–534.

Risor, M. B. (2009). Illness explanations among patients with medically unexplained symptoms: Different idioms for different contexts. *Health: An Interdisciplinary Journal for the Social Study of Health, Illness, and Medicine, 13,* 505–521.

Rod, N. H., Grønbæk, M., Schnohr, P., Prescott, E., & Kristensen, T. S. (2009). Perceived stress as a risk factor for changes in health behaviour and cardiac risk profile: A longitudinal study. *Journal of Internal Medicine, 266*(5), 467–475. doi:10.1111/j.1365-2796.2009.02124.x.

Roberts, B. W., Walton, K. E., & Bogg, T. (2005). Conscientiousness and health across the life course. *Review of General Psychology, 9,* 156–168. doi:10.1037/1089-2680.9.2.156.

Roberts, B. W., Kuncel, N. R., Shiner, R., Caspi, A., & Goldberg, L. R. (2007). The power of personality: The comparative validity of personality traits, socioeconomic status, and cognitive ability for predicting important life outcomes. *Perspectives on Psychological Science, 2,* 313–345.

Saboonchi, F., & Lundh, L. G. (2003). Perfectionism, anger, somatic health and positive affect. *Personality and Individual Differences, 35,* 1585–1599. doi:10.1016/S0191-8869(02)00382-3.

Scheier, M. F., & Carver, C. S. (1985). Optimism, coping, and health: Assessment and implications of generalized outcome expectancies. *Health Psychology, 4,* 219–247.

Seligman, M. E. P. (1975). *Helplessness*. San Francisco: W. H. Freeman.

Shafran, R., Cooper, Z., & Fairburn, C. G. (2002). Clinical perfectionism: A cognitive-behavioural analysis. *Behaviour Research and Therapy, 40,* 773–791.

Shanmugasegaram, S., Flett, G., Madan, M., Oh, P., Marzolini, S., Reitav, J., & Sturman, E. (2014). Perfectionism, Type D personality, and illness-related coping styles in cardiac rehabilitation patients. *Journal Of Health Psychology, 19,* 417–426. doi:10.1177/1359105312471571.

Sherry, S. B., & Hall, P. A. (2009). The perfectionism model of binge eating: Tests of an integrative model. *Journal of Personality and Social Psychology, 96,* 690–709. doi:10.1037/a0014528.

Sherry, S. B., Law, A., Hewitt, P. L., Flett, G. L., & Besser, A. (2008). Social support as a mediator of the relationship between perfectionism and depression: A preliminary test of the social disconnection model. *Personality and Individual Differences, 45,* 339–344. doi:10.1016/j.paid.2008.05.001.

Sherry, S. B., Mackinnon, S. P., Macneil, M. A., & Fitzpatrick, S. (2013). Discrepancies confer vulnerability to depressive symptoms: A three-wave longitudinal study. *Journal of Counseling Psychology, 60,* 112–126. doi:10.1037/a0030439.

Shnek, Z. M., Irvine, J., Stewart, D., & Abbey, S. (2001). Psychological factors and depressive symptoms in ischemic heart disease. *Health Psychology, 20,* 141–145. doi:10.1037//0278-6133.20.2.141.

Sirois, F. M. (2013). Perfectionism, stress, and health: A meta-analytic approach. Paper presented at the 14th Annual Meeting of the Society for Personality and Social Psychology, New Orleans, LA.

Sirois, F. M., & Gick, M. L. (in press). An appraisal-based coping model of attachment and adjustment to arthritis. *Journal of Health Psychology*.

Sirois, F. M., & Hirsch, J. K. (2013). Associations of psychological thriving with coping efficacy, expectations for future growth, and depressive symptoms over time in people with arthritis. *Journal of Psychosomatic Research, 75*(3), 279–286. doi:10.1016/j.jpsychores.2013.06.004.

Sirois, F. M., & Molnar, D. S. (2014). Perfectionism and maladaptive coping styles in patients with chronic fatigue syndrome, irritable bowel syndrome and fibromyalgia/arthritis and in healthy controls. *Psychotherapy and Psychosomatics, 83,* 384–385. doi:10.1159/000365174.

Sirois, F. M., Davis, C. G., & Morgan, M. S. (2006). "Learning to live with what you can't rise above": Control beliefs, symptom control, and adjustment to tinnitus. *Health Psychology, 25*(1), 119–123. doi:10.1037/0278-6133.25.1.119.

Sirois, F. M., Voth, J., & Pychyl, T. A. (2009). "I'll look after my health, later": A prospective study of the linkages of procrastination to health and well-being in undergraduate students. Paper presented at the 6th Biennial conference of Counseling the Procrastinator in Academic Settings. Toronto: York University.

Sirois, F. M., Monforton, J., & Simpson, M. (2010). "If only I had done better": Perfectionism and counterfactual thinking. *Personality and Social Psychology Bulletin, 36,* 1675–1692.

Sirois, F. M., & Pascual-Leone, A. (2013, May). A meta-analytic view of the associations of perfectionism with low self-compassion. In F. M. Sirois & G. Flett (chairs) The Emotional, Interpersonal, and Health Costs and Consequences of Perfectionism. Paper presented at the 25th Annual Convention of the Association for Psychological Science (APS), Washington, DC.

Sirois, F. M., Shucard, H., & Hirsch, J. K. (2014). Procrastination and perceptions of the future self: Implications for health and well-being. Paper presented at the 2nd International Conference on Time Perspective, Warsaw, Poland.

Sirois, F. M., Molnar, D. S., & Hirsch, J. K. (2015). Self-compassion, stress, and coping in the context of chronic illness. *Self and Identity, 13,* 1–14.

Slaney, R. B., Rice, K. G., Mobley, M., Trippi, J., & Ashby, J. S. (2001). The revised almost perfect scale. *Measurement and Evaluation in Counseling and Development, 34,* 130–145.

Smith, T. W. (2006). Personality as risk and resilience in physical health. *Current Directions in Psychological Science, 15*(5), 227–231.

Stafford, L., Jackson, H., & Berk, M. (2009). Cognitive-personality style as vulnerability to depression in patients with coronary artery disease: Roles of sociotropy and autonomy. *Psychosomatic Medicine, 71,* 63–69.

Stanton, A., & Revenson, T. A. (2011). Adjustment to chronic disease: Progress and promise in research. In H. S. Friedman (Ed.), *Oxford handbook of health psychology*. New York: Oxford University Press.

Strathman, A., Gleicher, F., Boninger, D. S., & Edwards, C. S. (1994). The consideration of future consequences: Weighing immediate and distant outcomes of behavior. *Journal of Personality and Social Psychology, 66,* 742–752.

Straub, R., & Kalden, J. (2009). Stress of different types increases the proinflammatory load in rheumatoid arthritis. *Arthritis Research & Therapy, 11*(3), 114. doi:10.1186/ar2712.

Stoeber, J., & Otto, K. (2006). Positive conceptions of perfectionism: Approaches, evidence, challenges. *Personality and Social Psychology Review, 10,* 295–319. doi:10.1207/s15327957pspr1004_2.

Stoeber, J., Kobori, O., & Tanno, Y. (2010). The multidimensional perfectionism cognitions inventory–english (MPCI-E): Reliability, validity, and relationships with positive and negative affect. *Journal of Personality Assessment, 92*(1), 16–25.

Stout, M. A. (1984). A cognitive-behavioral study of self-reported stress factors in migraine headache. *Psychopathology, 17,* 290–296.

Stumpf, H., & Parker, W. D. (2000). A hierarchical structural analysis of perfectionism and its relation to other personality characteristics. *Personality and Individual Differences, 28,* 837–852.

Suls, J., & Fletcher, B. (1985). The relative efficacy of avoidant and nonavoidant coping strategies: A meta-analysis. *Health Psychology: Official Journal of the Division of Health Psychology. American Psychological Association, 4,* 249–288.

Tangney, J. P., Baumeister, R. F., & Boone, A. L. (2004). High self-control predicts good adjustment, less pathology, better grades, and interpersonal success. *Journal of Personality, 72,* 271–324. doi:10.1111/j.0022-3506.2004.00263.x.

Taylor, S. E. (2006). Tend and befriend: Biobehavioral bases of affiliation under stress. *Current Directions in Psychological Science, 15,* 273–277. doi:10.1111/j.1467-8721.2006.00451.x.

Taylor, S. E. (2015). Social cognition and health. In M. Mikulincer, P. R. Shaver, E. Borgida, J. A. Bargh, M. Mikulincer, P. R. Shaver, & J. A. Bargh (Eds.), *APA handbook of personality and social psychology, Volume 1: Attitudes and social cognition* (pp. 339–361). Washington, DC: American Psychological Association. doi:10.1037/14341-012.

Taylor, S. E., & Sirois, F. M. (2014). *Health psychology (Third Canadian edition ed.)*. Toronto: McGraw-Hill Ryerson.

Taylor, S. E., Kemeny, M. E., Reed, G. M., Bower, J. E., & Gruenewald, T. L. (2000). Psychological resources, positive illusions, and health. *The American Psychologist, 55,* 99–109. doi:10. I037//0003-066X.55.1.99.

Thoits, P. A. (1997). Me's and we's: Forms and functions of social identities. In R. D. Ashmore & L. Jussim (Eds.), *Self and identity: Fundamental issues* (Vol. 1, pp. 106–133). New York: Oxford University Press.

Thompson, S. C., Sobolew-Shubin, A., Galbraith, M. E., Schwankovsky, L., & Cruzen, D. (1993). Maintaining perceptions of control: Finding perceived control in low-control circumstances. *Journal of Personality and Social Psychology, 64,* 293–304.

Tice, D. M. (2009). How emotions affect self-regulation. In J. P. Forgas, R. F. Baumeister, & D. M. Tice (Eds.), *The psychology of self-regulation: Cognitive, affective, and motivational processes* (pp. 201–215). New York: Psychology Press.

Van Houdenhove, B. (1986). Prevalence and psychodynamic interpretation of premorbid hyperactivity in patients with chronic pain. *Psychotherapy and Psychosomatics, 45,* 195–200.

Vollrath, M. E. (2006). *Handbook of personality and health.* West Sussex: Wiley. doi:10.1002/9780470713860.

Voth, J., & Sirois, F. (2009). The role of self-blame and responsibility in adjustment to inflammatory bowel disease. *Rehabilitation Psychology, 54,* 99–108. doi:10.1037/a0014739.

Wagner, D. D., & Heatherton, T. F. (2015). Self-regulation and its failure: The seven deadly threats to self-regulation. In M. Mikulincer, P. R. Shaver, E. Borgida, & J. A. Bargh (Eds.), *APA handbook of personality and social psychology, Volume 1: Attitudes and social cognition. APA handbooks in psychology* (pp. 805–842). Washington, DC: American Psychological Association.

Ward, B. W., Schiller, J. S., & Goodman, R. A. (2014). Multiple chronic conditions among US adults: A 2012 update. *Preventing Chronic Disease, 11,* 130389. doi:http://dx.doi.org/10.5888/pcd11.130389.

Weissman, A. N., & Beck, A. T. (1978). Development and validation of the dysfunctional attitude scale: A preliminary investigation. Paper presented at the meeting of the Association for the Advancement of Behavior Therapy, Chicago.

Williams, C. J., & Cropley, M. (2014). The relationship between perfectionism and engagement in preventive health behaviours: The bediating role of self concealment. *Journal of Health Psychology*. doi:10.1177/1359105313488971.

Wolfe, B. J., & Sirois, F. M. (2008). Beyond standard quality of life measures: The subjective experiences of living with inflammatory bowel disease. *Quality of Life Research, 17,* 877–886. doi:10.1007/s11136-008-9362-1.

Wrosch, C., Miller, G. E., Scheier, M. F., & Brun de Pontet, S. (2007). Giving up on unattainable goals: Benefits for health? *Personality and Social Psychology Bulletin, 33,* 251–265. doi:10.1177/0146167206294905.

Chapter 5
The Role of Perfectionism in Chronic Fatigue Syndrome

Stefan Kempke, Boudewijn Van Houdenhove, Stephan Claes and Patrick Luyten

Introduction

Nancy, a 42-year-old woman, has been suffering from disabling fatigue and general weakness for the past 5 years. Over the last 6 months, her symptoms have gradually become worse. She has had repeated viral throat infections and was exhausted almost all of the time, which forced her to give up her demanding job. She used to be very active (e.g. in sports) despite her fatigue complaints, but now she can only carry out simple daily tasks, and even small amounts of exercise (e.g. doing household work) typically lead to extreme exhaustion or a complete energy "crash". Her social life became severely restricted by the illness. After a comprehensive examination at the hospital including several laboratory tests, no medical (or psychiatric) condition could be identified that may explain her complaints. She was then diagnosed with chronic fatigue syndrome (CFS). Nancy's story is typical of many patients diagnosed with CFS.

CFS is a complex syndrome that is still the subject of much controversy which is in large part due to the fact that relatively little is known about the exact causes of this disorder. As illustrated by the story of Nancy, the syndrome is usually associated with severe functional impairment and social isolation. As a result, CFS places an enormous economic burden on health-care systems and society in general (Jason,

*Stefan Kempke is a postdoctoral researcher of the Research Foundation Flanders (FWO).

S. Kempke (✉) · P. Luyten
Faculty of Psychology and Educational Sciences, University of Leuven, Tiensestraat 102, 3000 Leuven, Belgium
e-mail: stefan.kempke@ppw.kuleuven.be

B. Van Houdenhove · S. Claes
Department of Psychiatry, University Hospitals Leuven, University of Leuven, Leuven, Belgium

P. Luyten
Research Department of Clinical, Educational and Health Psychology, University College London, London, UK

F. M. Sirois, D. S. Molnar (eds.), *Perfectionism, Health, and Well-Being,*
DOI 10.1007/978-3-319-18582-8_5

Benton, Valentine, Johnson, & Torres-Harding, 2008; Reynolds, Vernon, Bouchery, & Reeves, 2004). For instance, the annual productivity loss related to CFS in the USA is estimated at approximately $ 9.1 billion (Reynolds et al., 2004).

We begin this chapter with a brief description of the diagnosis of CFS. We then present a working model for the development and maintenance of CFS integrating biological and psychological research findings. Next, we specifically focus on the purported role of perfectionism in CFS, the topic of this chapter. We provide an overview of theory and research on perfectionism in CFS. After reviewing empirical studies that have investigated the role of perfectionism in CFS, we look at the mechanisms that may explain the relationship between both. We then look at the possible origins of perfectionism in CFS, including studies that have demonstrated a link between early childhood adversity and CFS. We close this chapter by a summary of treatment implications of these findings.

Chronic Fatigue Syndrome

The term chronic fatigue syndrome was coined in the 1980s, a century after George Miller Beard introduced the concept of neurasthenia to denote a similar condition of exhaustion (Wessely, Hotopf, & Sharpe, 1998). Today, CFS is seen as belonging to a spectrum of functional somatic syndromes, an umbrella term encompassing a group of syndromes characterized by persistent somatic symptoms (e.g. fatigue, musculoskeletal pain, and gastrointestinal symptoms) without any organic impairments (Wessely et al., 1998). Studies indicate that functional somatic symptoms are highly prevalent and may represent up to 30 % of all primary care consultations (Kirmayer, Groleau, Looper, & Dao, 2004). CFS involves both physical and mental exhaustion and usually develops gradually over months or years (most often between ages 40–49), although acute onset of CFS has also been reported (Boneva et al., 2011; Van Houdenhove et al., 2009). CFS is more common in females than in males in adults as well as in children and in adolescents (Farmer, Fowler, Scourfield, & Thapar, 2004; Gallagher, Thomas, Hamilton, & White, 2004; Jason et al., 1999). The diagnosis of CFS is based on consensus criteria developed by experts and involves an extensive medical and psychiatric examination to rule out other conditions that may be causing the symptoms. The most widely used diagnostic criteria are the Centers for Disease Control and Prevention (CDC) criteria (Fukuda et al., 1994), which define CFS as a condition that is characterized by unexplained prolonged fatigue for at least 6 months that is not the result of ongoing exertion and is not substantially relieved by rest, along with other symptoms such as musculoskeletal pain, sore throat, headaches, tender lymph nodes, substantial impairment of short-term memory or concentration, unrefreshing sleep, and post-exertional malaise (i.e. extreme exhaustion or flu-like feelings after physical and/or mental activity). In the recently redefined International Consensus Criteria (Carruthers et al., 2011), post-exertional exhaustion, that is, increased physical and/or cognitive fatigability in response to exertion, plays a more central role in the conceptualization of CFS. There is indeed increasing evidence that effort intolerance is one of the key diagnostic features of CFS, probably reflecting a loss of "adaptability" of the human stress response system involving a reduced tolerance for a wide range of physical and mental stressors and environmental stimuli (e.g. loud noise, bright lights, alcohol, and certain foods) (Van Houdenhove & Luyten, 2010; Van Houdenhove, Luyten, & Kempke, 2013), as discussed in greater detail below.

Comorbidity with other medical and psychiatric disorders is often observed in CFS patients. For instance, studies have demonstrated a high rate of comorbidity between CFS and chronic pain syndromes such as fibromyalgia syndrome (FMS), a condition that is mainly characterized by widespread muscle pain and tenderness (Ablin et al., 2012; Kanaan, Lepine, & Wessely, 2007). In the context of the ongoing debate as to whether medically unexplained syndromes should be considered as discrete diagnostic entities or as variants of one single functional somatic syndrome (known as the "lumpers" versus "splitters" debate) (Kanaan et al., 2007), we and others have argued that both conditions may comprise one larger cluster of fatigue and pain symptoms, particularly because studies have suggested substantial overlap in the etiology of CFS and FMS (Ablin et al., 2012; Van Houdenhove, Kempke, & Luyten, 2010; Van Houdenhove et al., 2013). However, it should be noted that not all CFS patients experience chronic pain, pointing to the need to identify subgroups of patients (Ablin et al., 2012; Kempke et al., 2013a). CFS is also associated with high rates of both lifetime and current psychiatric comorbidity, in particular depression (Arnold, 2008; Van Houdenhove & Luyten, 2006). The association between depression and CFS might be in part explained not only by shared risk factors (e.g. personality features such as perfectionism) (Luyten, Blatt, Van Houdenhove, & Corveleyn, 2006) but also by the fact that CFS itself is a risk factor for developing depression because of severe physical and mental impairments leading to social isolation and feelings of hopelessness (Arnold, 2008).

A Working Model of CFS

Although much remains to be learned about the causes of CFS, there is compelling evidence that CFS can best be conceptualized as a stress-related disorder with both psychosocial (i.e. personality and (early) life stress) and biological (i.e. neurobiological and genetic factors) factors playing a role in the etiology and maintenance of this disorder (Luyten, Kempke, Van Wambeke, Claes, Blatt, & Van Houdenhove 2011; Nater, Maloney, Heim, & Reeves, 2011; Van Houdenhove & Luyten, 2008; Van Houdenhove et al., 2013). Specifically, evidence over the past years suggests that CFS may reflect loss of resilience of the hypothalamic–pituitary–adrenal (HPA) axis, the main human stress response system, after a prolonged period of chronic stress (i.e. childhood adversity and/or cumulative life stress) or overexertion (Kempke, Luyten, Mayes, Van Houdenhove, & Claes, 2014; Luyten et al., 2011; Van Houdenhove & Luyten, 2010; Van Houdenhove et al., 2013; Van Houdenhove, Van Den Eede, & Luyten, 2009). The onset of the disorder is often triggered by acute stressors, which can be either physical (e.g. after a surgery, an infection) or psychosocial (e.g. loss experiences) or a combination of both (Van Houdenhove & Egle, 2004; Van Houdenhove et al., 2010, 2013).

There is indeed increasing evidence from neurobiological research that in at least a subgroup of patients, CFS is associated with lower cortisol levels and blunted cortisol responses to stressors, suggesting reduced HPA axis functioning in these patients (Cleare, 2003; Papadopoulos & Cleare, 2011; Tak et al., 2011; Van Houdenhove et al., 2009). This is not only congruent with the recent emphasis on effort intolerance in the diagnosis of CFS (Carruthers et al., 2011) but also with the conceptualization of "allostatic" load in explaining stress-related conditions referring to the "wear and tear" of chronic stress on stress-regulating systems (McEwen, 1998, see also Arroll, 2013). This is also congruent with more general findings showing that chronic stress may eventually result in a "switch" (or neurobiological "crash") from hyperactivity to hypoactivity of the HPA axis (Fries, Hesse, Hellhammer, & Hellhammer, 2005; Lupien, McEwen, Gunnar, & Heim, 2009; Van Houdenhove et al., 2009).

The association between chronic stress and HPA axis dysregulation in CFS may be mediated by so-called epigenetic modifications (i.e. changes in the expression and activation) of genes that have been shown to regulate the neuroendocrine system (Van Houdenhove et al., 2013). Indeed, ground-breaking advances have recently been made in our understanding of the epigenetic regulation of the HPA axis (Bick et al., 2012), but studies in CFS are currently lacking. Importantly, the HPA axis has been shown to interact with other neurobiological systems such as neurotransmitter systems, the immune system, and pain processing systems, which may explain in part the high comorbidity between fatigue, pain, and depression (Van Houdenhove & Egle, 2004). For instance, reduced HPA axis function may be responsible for the typical "sickness response" (or flu-like feelings) of many CFS patients, since hypocortisolism may lead to low-grade immune activation (Silverman, Heim, Nater, Marques, & Sternberg, 2010).

In sum, evidence is growing that CFS may reflect a neurobiologically based loss of "adaptability" because of prolonged exposure to chronic stress or overexertion in psychologically and perhaps also genetically susceptible individuals (for a review, see Van Houdenhove et al., 2013).

Perfectionism as a Precipitating and Perpetuating Factor in CFS

Elsewhere, we have put forward a theoretical model in which increased vulnerability for chronic stress and subsequent neurobiological alterations in CFS may result, in part, from elevated levels of self-critical or maladaptive perfectionism (Kempke et al., 2013a; Kempke, Luyten, Mayes et al., 2014; Kempke et al., 2013c; Luyten et al., 2011; Van Houdenhove et al., 2013). This model is depicted graphically in Fig. 5.1. Of course, perfectionism is not the only factor contributing to chronic fa-

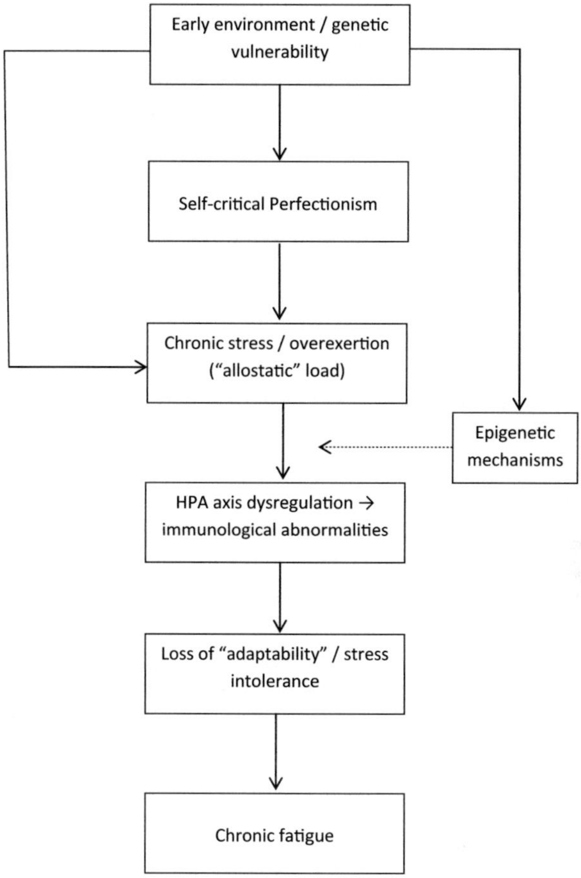

Fig 5.1 Role of perfectionism in the development of CFS

tigue conditions and certainly not involved in all cases with CFS (for an overview of risk factors see Van Houdenhove & Luyten, 2008). Further, congruent with the developmental psychopathology principle of multifinality (i.e. similar risk factors can lead to different outcomes) (Luyten, Vliegen, Van Houdenhove, & Blatt, 2008), it is clear that maladaptive perfectionism is a "transdiagnostic" vulnerability factor that is implicated in the development and maintenance of a wide range of negative outcomes (e.g. low self-esteem) and disorders, most notably affective spectrum disorders (Egan, Wade, & Shafran, 2011; Luyten & Blatt, 2013).

Clinicians and researchers have long theorized that perfectionistic attitudes are implicated in chronic fatigue and pain conditions. CFS patients have been described as overcommitted, conscientious, hard-working, overactive, and achievement oriented (van Geelen, Sinnema, Hermans, & Kuis, 2007; Van Houdenhove, Neerinckx, Onghena, Lysens, & Vertommen, 2001). Several theoretical models have been employed to measure perfectionism in CFS. Frost's two-factor model (Frost, Marten, Lahart, & Rosenblate, 1990) distinguishes between two dimensions of perfectionism, that is, adaptive or positive (i.e. normal achievement strivings) and maladaptive or negative (i.e. maladaptive evaluative concerns (MEC)) perfectionism. From a psychodynamic perspective, Blatt's conceptualization of self-criticism or self-critical perfectionism (SCP) refers to a personality style characterized by both high personal standards and overly critical self-evaluations (Blatt, 2004; Kempke et al., 2013a). Numerous studies have shown that MEC or self-criticism is indeed associated with maladaptive outcomes (Stoeber & Otto, 2006; Dunkley, Blankstein, Masheb, & Grilo, 2006).

With a few exceptions (Blenkiron, Edwards, & Lynch, 1999; Wood & Wessely, 1999), studies have revealed a positive association between perfectionism and chronic fatigue. Magnusson et al. (1996) showed that maladaptive perfectionism was significantly associated with mental and physical trait fatigue among female nurses. In a large sample of CFS patients, Kempke et al. (2011a) found evidence for a two-factor model of perfectionism in CFS, that is, maladaptive, but not adaptive, perfectionism was positively related to severity of fatigue in CFS. In accordance with a study by Deary and Chalder (2010), analyses also indicated a substantial association between both perfectionism dimensions, suggesting that both factors are interrelated in CFS patients, that is, high achievement strivings are not really "adaptive" in these patients and are coupled with MEC (i.e. self-criticism). Indeed, Luyten and colleagues (2006) found that CFS patients retrospectively reported both higher levels of adaptive and maladaptive perfectionism before illness onset.

Further, case-control studies have shown significantly increased levels of unhealthy perfectionism in CFS patients. White and Schweitzer (2000), for instance, showed higher levels of maladaptive perfectionism among CFS patients compared to non-fatigued controls. Likewise, Deary and Chalder (2010) reported higher levels of maladaptive, but not adaptive, perfectionism among CFS patients compared to healthy controls. Recently, Sirois and Molnar (2014) replicated and extended previous findings by demonstrating higher levels of maladaptive perfectionism in CFS patients relative to well controls, patients with irritable bowel syndrome, and patients with FMS or arthritis. Moreover, CFS patients showed higher levels of self-blame coping compared to normal controls, congruent with findings on the specific role of self-criticism in these patients.

Prospective studies have provided further support for cross-sectional findings on the relationship between perfectionism and fatigue (Dittner, Rimes, & Thorpe, 2011; Kempke et al., 2013a; Moss-Morris, Spence, & Hou, 2010). Of particular note is a study conducted by Moss-Morris and colleagues (2010) showing that maladaptive perfectionism predicted the onset of CFS in patients with an acute episode of infectious mononucleosis (glandular fever). Dittner et al. (2011), in turn, showed that negative perfectionism significantly predicted fatigue levels in undergraduate students following a period of academic stress. Finally, a recent diary method study by our group (Kempke et al., 2013a) demonstrated that SCP predicted daily fatigue and pain symptoms in CFS patients over a 14-day period, attesting to its important role in the course of this disorder.

Although perfectionism seems to be more closely related to CFS, congruent with its transdiagnostic status and the high rate of comorbidity between functional somatic syndromes, it is important to note that unhealthy perfectionism and related factors such as "counterdependency" (i.e. an overreliance on autonomy and self-sufficiency) and "all-or-nothing" behaviour (see below) have also been linked to chronic pain and gastrointestinal disorders such as irritable bowel syndrome and functional dyspepsia (Gregory, Manring, & Wade, 2005; Lerman, Rudich, & Shahar, 2010; Lerman, Shahar, & Rudich, 2011; Ochi et al., 2008; Spence & Moss-Morris, 2007; Rudich, Lerman, Gurevich, Weksler, & Shahar, 2008).

Finally, another important line of evidence for the role of perfectionism in CFS comes from research showing features of obsessive-compulsive personality disorder (OCPD) in CFS patients, a personality disorder that is mainly characterized by perfectionism and a strong need for control (Kempke et al., 2013c; Nater et al., 2010). For instance, we recently investigated personality features and personality disorders in CFS patients compared to well-matched control groups consisting of normal community individuals and psychiatric patients (Kempke et al., 2013c). As expected, CFS patients did not show an increased prevalence of personality disorders, but they did show elevated levels of obsessive-compulsive (and depressive) personality features, congruent with findings on the role of maladaptive perfectionism in CFS.

Perfectionism and Fatigue: Possible Mechanisms

The studies reviewed above clearly suggest a relationship between perfectionism and CFS. Importantly, research has also identified several potential mechanisms that may explain this relationship. Specifically, there is good evidence to suggest that perfectionism may be implicated in CFS because it is associated with (a) increased stress sensitivity, stress generation, and depression and (b) impairments in embodied mentalizing and emotion regulation leading to overexertion and other maladaptive behaviours that exacerbate and perpetuate symptoms. The common denominator of both pathways is that perfectionism overburdens the stress response system, thus contributing to "allostatic" load (Kempke et al., 2013a; Kempke, Luyten, Mayes et al., 2014).

Perfectionism, Stress Sensitivity/Stress Generation, and Depression

It has been shown that stress, and repeated or chronic stress in particular, may play a predisposing, precipitating (e.g. acute life stressors), and perpetuating role in CFS (Nater et al., 2011; Van Houdenhove & Luyten, 2008). There is increasing evidence to suggest that perfectionism, SCP in particular, is associated with chronic physical and/or mental stress and subsequent neurobiological alterations in CFS (Kempke, Luyten, Mayes et al., 2014; Van Houdenhove et al., 2013). Indeed, numerous studies have demonstrated that SCP is associated with both increased stress sensitivity and stress generation, making individuals vulnerable to stress-related conditions

(Blatt & Shahar, 2005; Luyten & Blatt, 2013). With regard to stress sensitivity, SCP has been related to both interpersonal- and achievement-related distress (i.e. holding excessive high standards for oneself leading to a sense of failure), suggesting that this personality dimension may reflect a general vulnerability factor to stress (Blatt & Shahar, 2005; Shahar, 2013).

Other studies have demonstrated that SCP is also associated with the "active" generation of stress, as indicated by findings that show that highly self-critical individuals experience more person-dependent (self-generated) stressors (e.g. negative interpersonal events) over time and tend to "degenerate" protective factors (e.g. social support) in their environment (Blatt & Shahar, 2005; Hammen, 2006; Luyten et al., 2006; Shahar & Porcerelli, 2006). Recently, our group (Luyten et al., 2011) replicated these findings in CFS patients by showing that SCP was associated with the generation of daily hassles over the last 2 months and with increased stress sensitivity over the course of a 14-day period. As a result, patients tended to show increased levels of depression, which has been shown to exacerbate fatigue symptoms and impede treatment response (Kempke et al., 2010; Kempke et al., 2011a). These findings are congruent with other studies showing that SCP in CFS may give rise to negative self-perceptions (i.e. lower self-esteem) and thus may increase vulnerability to depression (Kempke et al., 2011b; Kempke et al., 2011a).

Most recently, we provided evidence for the neurobiological mechanisms underlying the relationship between perfectionism and CFS. Specifically, we investigated the effect of SCP on cortisol stress response in CFS patients by using the Trier Social Stress Test (TSST) (Kirschbaum, Pirke, & Hellhammer, 1993), a widely used laboratory psychosocial stress induction paradigm involving a mathematics and public speech task in front of a video camera and an evaluative audience. Studies have shown that the TSST elicits a significant rise in cortisol (Kudielka & Wüst, 2010). CFS patients were instructed to provide saliva samples for cortisol analysis before the TSST, immediately after the test and at follow-up (i.e. 90 min relative to the onset of the TSST) to capture the complete stress process of each patient. In line with the hypotheses summarized above, we found that SCP was associated with higher subjective or self-reported stress, but with decreased cortisol stress reactivity after experimental stress induction and during recovery (Kempke, Luyten, Mayes et al., 2014). Thus, these results provided evidence that SCP may be one of the key factors that may contribute to reduced or blunted HPA axis reactivity in CFS, probably as a result of the "wear and tear" of prolonged chronic stress and/or overexertion, in combination with high subjective stress (Kempke, Luyten, Mayes et al., 2014a). Notwithstanding these promising results, further research is needed to unravel the neurobiological effects of SCP in CFS.

Perfectionism, Embodied Mentalizing/Emotion Regulation, and Overexertion

Perfectionism in CFS has also been associated with impairments in embodied mentalizing (i.e. the capacity to reflect on bodily sensations in terms of mental states) and emotion regulation, probably within the context of insecure attachment, leading to overexertion and other unhelpful behaviours, thoughts (e.g. catastrophizing), and maladaptive coping strategies (Luyten, Van Houdenhove, Lemma, Target, & Fonagy, 2012, 2013), further exacerbated by the often unbearable feelings of pain, fatigue, and resulting helplessness and worthlessness.

In particular, studies have demonstrated that CFS patients tend to have negative beliefs about the experience and expression of emotions (e.g. experiencing negative emotions as a sign of weakness or fearing that others will negatively react to displays of emotions) (Rimes & Chalder, 2010), show a tendency to emotional suppression (Hambrook et al., 2011), and are less likely to interpret physical symptoms in terms of negative emotional states (Dendy, Cooper, & Sharpe, 2001), reflecting the dismissive or avoidant attachment pattern (i.e. denial of attachment needs and emotional experiences) observed in CFS patients with high levels of SCP (Luyten et al., 2012, 2013). Dismissive attachment strategies are typically activated when confronted with increased levels of stress and are considered to be exacerbated by the disorder itself (i.e. suffering from "unexplained" symptoms), leading to impaired emotion regulation (Luyten et al., 2012, 2013).

As a result, CFS patients tend to engage in excessive physical and/or mental activities as a way to cope with negative self-feelings in an attempt to prove self-worth (Luyten et al., 2012, 2013; Van Houdenhove, Neerinckx, Onghena et al., 2001). In this regard, more than a decade ago, Van Houdenhove et al. (2001) argued that the achievement-oriented lifestyle observed in the history of many CFS patients may serve as a coping strategy to maintain self-esteem and to prevent depression. Congruent with this assumption, Nater et al. (2006), in a population-based study, reported that escape/avoidance (i.e. behavioural efforts to escape or avoid a stressor) was the most prominent coping style in CFS patients. Harvey, Wadsworth, Wessely, and Hotopf (2008), using a large prospective birth cohort, found that overactivity (i.e. excessive levels of exercise) was associated with an increased risk for CFS. Similarly, high "action-proneness", "persistence", and "all-or-nothing" behaviour have been empirically linked to chronic fatigue (Fukuda et al., 2010; Moss-Morris et al., 2010; Van Campen et al., 2009; Van Houdenhove, Bruyninckx, & Luyten, 2006).

The concept of "action-proneness" was coined by Van Houdenhove, Onghena, Neerinckx, and Hellin (1995) to describe a tendency towards direct action in CFS (and chronic pain) patients that may increase the risk of overburdening. In a series of studies, Van Houdenhove and colleagues (Van Houdenhove et al., 2006; Van Houdenhove, Neerinckx, Onghena et al., 2001; Van Houdenhove et al., 1995) found that CFS patients described themselves retrospectively as more "action-prone" compared to normal controls. Moreover, they also found a strong agreement between the patients' self-report and the judgment by significant others regarding patients' premorbid lifestyle, ruling out the possibility that patients may have idealized their premorbid situation (Van Houdenhove, Neerinckx, Onghena et al., 2001). More recently, in a qualitative study, Pemberton and Cox (2014) identified a premorbid state of constant action among CFS patients. Moreover, the concepts of "doing nothing" and "rest" were associated with negative feelings and beliefs in patients. These findings are consistent with studies showing an association between CFS and "persistence" as measured with the Temperament and Character Inventory (TCI), referring to the tendency of patients to persevere despite fatigue and frustration, pushing themselves past their limits (Fukuda et al.2010; Van Campen et al., 2009). Similarly, Moss-Morris et al. (2010) reported that "all-or-nothing" behaviour (i.e. an activity pattern characterized by cycles of overactivity and complete rest) is one of the most important predictors of developing CFS in patients with glandular fever.

Clinical experience and some empirical evidence suggest that CFS patients with high self-criticism are especially prone to "all-or-nothing" behaviour because of their inability to tolerate inactivity and rest (e.g. doing nothing is associated with feelings of guilt because of not being productive) (Kempke et al., 2013a; Luyten et al., 2011; Moss-Morris et al., 2010). Once ill self-critical patients may lower their excessive standards (Luyten et al., 2006), but may still show the tendency to exceed their mental and physical limits. Indeed, these patients often show periodic "outbursts of activity" when feeling somewhat better, followed by post-exertional malaise and complete rest, thereby exacerbating symptoms and impairments (Luyten et al., 2011; Luyten, Van Houdenhove, Pae, Kempke, & Van Wambeke, 2008; Moss-Morris et al., 2010). Although understandable as CFS can be completely incapacitating, in the long run, a "boom and bust" pattern increases the wear and tear on the stress response system (Luyten et al., 2012, 2013).

Origins of Perfectionism in CFS

Research suggests that SCP may be in part genetically determined (Moser, Slane, Alexandra Burt, & Klump, 2012) and first develops in the context of early attachment relationships (Blatt, 2004; Soenens, Vansteenkiste, & Luyten, 2010). Specifically, SCP appears to reflect an overemphasis or exaggeration of the development of the self and autonomy to the neglect of the development of the capacity for relatedness (Blatt, 2004; Luyten & Blatt, 2013) and may develop in an attempt to avoid rejection and criticism (or to seek approval from others) as a result of cold, critical, intrusive parenting characterized by conditional affection (i.e. parents make their affection conditional upon meeting high standards), and/or low emotion expressiveness (Blatt & Homann, 1992; Flett, Hewitt, Oliver, & Macdonald, 2002; Greenspon, 2008; Shahar & Henrich, 2013; Soenens et al., 2010). From this perspective, perfectionism in CFS may be a coping mechanism to compensate for feelings of worthlessness and inferiority (Kempke et al., 2013a; Kempke, Coppens, Luyten, & Van Houdenhove, in press; Van Houdenhove, Neerinckx, Onghena et al., 2001)—sometimes also reflected in excessive self-sacrificing tendencies (Van Houdenhove, Neerinckx, Onghena et al., 2001; Van Houdenhove et al., 2001; Hambrook et al., 2011).

Longitudinal research investigating these assumptions in CFS specifically is lacking, although there is evidence that CFS is related to a history of exposure to adverse childhood experiences (for a review, see Kempke et al., 2013b). For instance, a recent meta-analysis revealed a substantial relationship between self-reported psychological trauma and functional somatic syndromes, with the largest association in CFS (Afari et al., 2014). In a landmark study published in 2001, Van

Houdenhove et al. showed elevated levels of early adversity, in particular emotional trauma, in a mixed sample of CFS and fibromyalgia patients. They found that more than 60% (i.e. 64.1%) had a history of early adversity, with a considerable proportion reporting lifelong victimization (e.g. living in an abusive relationship). Similar results have been found in population-based studies conducted in the USA. Heim et al. (2006, 2009) showed that early trauma was associated with a three- to eight-fold increased risk for CFS. More recently, Kempke et al. (2013a) replicated and extended these findings in a sample of 90 well-screened CFS patients by showing that more than half of the patients (54.4%) had experienced at least one type of early childhood adversity and more than 40% multiple trauma, with the majority of these patients reporting emotional abuse and/or emotional neglect. Hence, CFS may be more closely associated with more subtle, "emotional" adverse childhood experiences rather than more "objective" or physical types of trauma, congruent with findings showing negative self-perceptions (i.e. high self-criticism) and a tendency towards overcompensation in these patients.

Clinically, CFS patients with a history of early adversity are particularly vulnerable to person-dependent stressors (e.g. daily hassles) and interpersonal difficulties, which may perpetuate and even exacerbate symptoms (Kempke et al., 2013b; Luyten et al., 2013). This is congruent with both animal and human studies suggesting that adversity, especially in early developmental stages, may have serious consequences for the developing stress system though its impact on brain structures and the epigenetic expression of genes involved in stress processing, leading to increased stress sensitivity, thereby increasing vulnerability to chronic stress and neuroendocrine dysregulation in later life (Lupien et al., 2009; Luyten et al., 2008; Uhrlass & Gibb, 2007; Van Houdenhove, Luyten, & Egle, 2009). For instance, Heim et al. (2009) found that only CFS patients with a history of early trauma showed reduced basal HPA axis activity. Recently, we demonstrated a significant association between emotional neglect and reduced HPA axis reactivity following experimental stress induction with the TSST paradigm (Kempke et al., 2015). Of note, similar results have been reported in patients with FMS (Riva, Mork, Westgaard, Ro, & Lundberg, 2010), suggesting that decreased HPA axis functioning might be implicated in both CFS and FMS and that these conditions are part of one larger spectrum of fatigue and pain conditions.

Conclusions and Clinical Implications

In this chapter, we provided evidence that self-critical or maladaptive perfectionism is implicated as a predisposing and perpetuating factor in at least a subgroup of CFS patients. Moreover, we summarized growing evidence suggesting that SCP is one of the key factors that may contribute to chronic stress and overexertion in CFS, thereby overburdening the stress response system. Finally, we discussed theory and research linking SCP to disruptions in early attachment relationships, congruent with studies demonstrating high rates of early childhood adversity in CFS patients.

Future research should concentrate on possible epigenetic mechanisms (i.e. DNA methylation) involved in the relationship between early adversity, SCP, and stress sensitivity in later life (Van Houdenhove et al., 2013), which is likely to further our understanding of the etiology of this condition and functional somatic syndromes in general. Furthermore, there is a pressing need for more longitudinal developmental studies concerning the origins of SCP, especially with regard to the emotional family environment and its interaction with genetic vulnerability including gene–environment interactions, in CFS and related conditions such as FMS (Kempke et al., 2013a; Kempke et al., 2015).

The findings reviewed in this chapter have important implications for the treatment of CFS. The most common treatment for chronic fatigue and pain conditions is cognitive behavioural therapy (CBT) and graded exercise therapy (GET) (Knoop, Prins, Moss-Morris, & Bleijenberg, 2010; Price, Mitchell, Tidy, & Hunot, 2008), although a number of other psychological treatments, including mindfulness-based treatment (Fjorback et al., 2013), acceptance and commitment therapy (Wicksell et al., 2013), and mentalization-based treatment (Luyten et al., 2012), have also been proposed. Regardless of theoretical orientation, research suggests that treatment of CFS should include a focus on perfectionism and related cognitive-behavioural factors, such as exaggerated "action-proneness" and "all-or-nothing" behaviour, in at least a subset of patients (Surawy, Hackmann, Hawton, & Sharpe, 1995; Van Houdenhove et al., 2006; Moss-Morris et al., 2010). For instance, Van Houdenhove and colleagues (2006) showed that high "action-proneness" in CFS could be changed by a multidisciplinary CBT-based group treatment. Likewise, Morlion et al. (2011) demonstrated significant changes in "action-proneness" in chronic pain patients who followed a brief cognitive-behaviourally based psycho-educational treatment.

Importantly, a number of studies on depression have shown that self-critical patients may negatively respond to brief, structured treatments because such interventions may undermine their sense of control and autonomy (Blatt, Zuroff, Hawley, & Auerbach, 2010; Luyten, Corveleyn, & Blatt 2005). Moreover, it has been shown that self-critical patients need more time to establish and maintain a therapeutic alliance and hence need more intensive treatment (Blatt et al., 2010; Luyten et al., 2005). Congruent with these findings, we recently showed that pretreatment SCP negatively predicted treatment outcome in terms of pain severity in patients with chronic pain following a brief, psycho-educational CBT-based treatment (Kempke, Luyten, Van Wambeke, Coppens, & Morlion, 2014). Also, perfectionism has been associated with lack of acceptance and the typical "boom-and-bust" activity pattern in CFS, leading to (periodic) overactivity and increased levels of depression, thereby impeding treatment response (Brooks, Rimes, & Chalder, 2011; Kempke et al., 2013a; Moss-Morris et al., 2010).

Hence, it is reasonable to suggest that CFS patients with high levels of SCP might benefit more from intensive and/or tailored treatment. In this regard, a wide range of specialized interventions exist to treat self-critical perfectionistic tendencies, including cognitive-behavioural and psychodynamic approaches (Blatt, 2004; Flett & Hewitt, 2008; Glover, Brown, Fairburn, & Shafran, 2007; Kannan &

Levitt, 2013; Luyten et al., 2012, 2013). In general, treatment for CFS patients with high levels of SCP should be aimed at helping patients change typical patterns of feeling and thinking associated with perfectionism (i.e. excessive need for the approval of others, negative beliefs about emotions) (Jason et al., 2013; Luyten & Van Houdenhove, 2013; Surawy et al., 1995; Van Houdenhove & Luyten, 2008; Van Houdenhove et al., 2013), which may facilitate behavioural and lifestyle changes.

References

Ablin, J. N., Buskila, D., Van Houdenhove, B., Luyten, P., Atzeni, F., & Sarzi-Puttini, P. (2012). Is fibromyalgia a discrete entity? *Autoimmunity Reviews, 11*(8), 585–588.

Afari, N., Ahumada, S. M., Wright, L. J., Mostoufi, S., Golnari, G., Reis, V., & Cuneo, J. G. (2014). Psychological trauma and functional somatic syndromes: A systematic review and meta-analysis. *Psychosomatic Medicine, 76*(1), 2–11.

Arnold, L. M. (2008). Understanding fatigue in major depressive disorder and other medical disorders. *Psychosomatics, 49*(3), 185–190.

Arroll, M. A. (2013). Allostatic overload in myalgic encephalomyelitis/chronic fatigue syndrome (ME/CFS). *Medical Hypotheses, 81*(3), 506–508.

Bick, J., Naumova, O., Hunter, S., Barbot, B., Lee, M., Luthar, S. S., et al. (2012). Childhood adversity and DNA methylation of genes involved in the hypothalamus–pituitary–adrenal axis and immune system: Whole-genome and candidate-gene associations. *Development and Psychopathology, 24*(4), 1417–1425.

Blatt, S. J. (2004). *Experiences of depression: Theoretical, clinical and research perspectives*. Washington, DC: APA.

Blatt, S. J., & Homann, E. (1992). Parent-child interaction in the etiology of dependent and self-critical depression. *Clinical Psychology Review, 12*(1), 47–91.

Blatt, S. J., & Shahar, G. (2005). A dialectic model of personality development and psychopathology: Recent contributions to understanding and treating depression. In J. Corveleyn, P. Luyten, & S. J. Blatt (Eds.), *The theory and treatment of depression: Towards a dynamic interactionism model* (pp. 137–162). Leuven: Leuven University Press/Lawrence Erlbaum Associates.

Blatt, S. J., Zuroff, D. C., Hawley, L. L., & Auerbach, J. S. (2010). Predictors of sustained therapeutic change. *Psychotherapy Research, 20*(1), 37–54.

Blenkiron, P., Edwards, R., & Lynch, S. (1999). Associations between perfectionism, mood, and fatigue in chronic fatigue syndrome: A pilot study. *Journal of Nervous and Mental Disease, 187*(9), 566–570.

Boneva, R. S., Maloney, E. M., Lin, J. M., Jones, J. F., Wieser, F., Nater, U. M., & Reeves, W. C. (2011). Gynecological history in chronic fatigue syndrome: A population-based case-control study. *Journal of Women's Health, 20*(1), 21–28.

Brooks, S. K., Rimes, K. A., & Chalder, T. (2011). The role of acceptance in chronic fatigue syndrome. *Journal of Psychosomatic Research, 71*(6), 411–415.

Carruthers, B. M., van de Sande, M. I., De Meirleir, K. L., Klimas, N. G., Broderick, G., Mitchell, T., et al. (2011). Myalgic encephalomyelitis: International consensus criteria. *Journal of Internal Medicine, 270*(4), 327–338.

Cleare, A. J. (2003). The neuroendocrinology of chronic fatigue syndrome. *Endocrine Reviews, 24*(2), 236–252.

Deary, V., & Chalder, T. (2010). Personality and perfectionism in chronic fatigue syndrome: A closer look. *Psychology and Health, 25*(4), 465–475.

Dendy, C., Cooper, M., & Sharpe, M. (2001). Interpretation of symptoms in chronic fatigue syndrome. *Behaviour Research and Therapy, 39*(11), 1369–1380.

Dittner, A. J., Rimes, K., & Thorpe, S. (2011). Negative perfectionism increases the risk of fatigue following a period of stress. *Psychology and Health, 26*(3), 253–268.
Dunkley, D. M., Blankstein, K. R., Masheb, R. M., & Grilo, C. M. (2006). Personal standards and evaluative concerns dimensions of "clinical" perfectionism: A reply to Shafran et al. (2002, 2003) and Hewitt et al. (2003). *Behavior Research and Therapy, 44*(1), 63–84.
Egan, S. J., Wade, T. D., & Shafran, R. (2011). Perfectionism as a transdiagnostic process: A clinical review. *Clinical Psychology Review, 31*(2), 203–212.
Farmer, A., Fowler, T., Scourfield, J., & Thapar, A. (2004). Prevalence of chronic disabling fatigue in children and adolescents. *British Journal of Psychiatry, 184,* 477–481.
Fjorback, L. O., Arendt, M., Ornbol, E., Walach, H., Rehfeld, E., Schroder, A., & Fink, P. (2013). Mindfulness therapy for somatization disorder and functional somatic syndromes: Randomized trial with one-year follow-up. *Journal of Psychosomatic Research, 74*(1), 31–40.
Flett, G. L., & Hewitt, P. L. (2008). Treatment interventions for perfectionism—introduction to the special issue. *Journal of Rational-Emotive and Cognitive-Behavior Therapy, 26,* 127–133.
Flett, G. L., Hewitt, P. L., Oliver, J. M., & Macdonald, S. (2002). Perfectionism in children and their parents: A developmental analysis. In G. L. Flett & P. L. Hewitt (Eds.), *Perfectionism: Theory, research, and treatment* (pp. 89–132). Washington, DC: American Psychological Association.
Fries, E., Hesse, J., Hellhammer, J., & Hellhammer, D. H. (2005). A new view on hypocortisolism. *Psychoneuroendocrinology, 30*(10), 1010–1016.
Frost, R. O., Marten, P., Lahart, C.M., & Rosenblate, R. (1990). The dimensions of perfectionism. *Cognitive Therapy and Research, 14,* 449–468.
Fukuda, K., Straus, S. E., Hickie, I., Sharpe, M. C., Dobbins, J. G., & Komaroff, A. (1994). The chronic fatigue syndrome: A comprehensive approach to its definition and study. International Chronic Fatigue Syndrome Study Group. *Annals of Internal Medicine, 121*(12), 953–959.
Gallagher, A. M., Thomas, J. M., Hamilton, W. T., & White, P. D. (2004). Incidence of fatigue symptoms and diagnoses presenting in UK primary care from 1990 to 2001. *Journal of the Royal Society of Medicine, 97*(12), 571–575.
Glover, D. S., Brown, G. P., Fairburn, C. G., & Shafran, R. (2007). A preliminary evaluation of cognitive-behaviour therapy for clinical perfectionism: A case series. *British Journal of Clinical Psychology, 46*(Pt 1), 85–94.
Greenspon, T. S. (2008). Making sense of error: A view of the origins and treatment of perfectionism. *American Journal of Psychotherapy, 62*(3), 263–282.
Gregory, R. J., Manring, J., & Wade, M. J. (2005). Personality traits related to chronic pain location. *Annals of Clinical Psychiatry, 17*(2), 59–64.
Hambrook, D., Oldershaw, A., Rimes, K., Schmidt, U., Tchanturia, K., Treasure, J., & Chalder, T. (2011). Emotional expression, self-silencing, and distress tolerance in anorexia nervosa and chronic fatigue syndrome. *British Journal of Clinical Psychology, 50*(3), 310–325.
Hammen, C. (2006). Stress generation in depression: Reflections on origins, research, and future directions. *Journal of Clinical Psychology, 62*(9), 1065–1082.
Harvey, S. B., Wadsworth, M., Wessely, S., & Hotopf, M. (2008). Etiology of chronic fatigue syndrome: Testing popular hypotheses using a national birth cohort study. *Psychosomatic Medicine, 70*(4), 488–495.
Heim, C., Wagner, D., Maloney, E., Papanicolaou, D. A., Solomon, L., Jones, J. F., et al. (2006). Early adverse experience and risk for chronic fatigue syndrome: Results from a population-based study. *Archives of General Psychiatry, 63*(11), 1258–1266.
Heim, C., Nater, U. M., Maloney, E., Boneva, R., Jones, J. F., & Reeves, W. C. (2009). Childhood trauma and risk for chronic fatigue syndrome: Association with neuroendocrine dysfunction. *Archives of General Psychiatry, 66*(1), 72–80.
Jason, L. A., Richman, J. A., Rademaker, A. W., Jordan, K. M., Plioplys, A. V., Taylor, R. R., et al. (1999). A community-based study of chronic fatigue syndrome. *Archives of Internal Medicine, 159*(18), 2129–2137.
Jason, L. A., Benton, M. C., Valentine, L., Johnson, A., & Torres-Harding, S. (2008). The economic impact of ME/CFS: Individual and societal costs. *Dynamic Medicine, 7,* 6.

Jason, L. A., Brown, M., Brown, A., Evans, M., Flores, S., Grant-Holler, E., & Sunnquist, M. (2013). Energy conservation/envelope theory interventions to help patients with myalgic encephalomyelitis/chronic fatigue syndrome. *Fatigue, 1*(1–2), 27–42.

Kannan, D., & Levitt, H. M. (2013). A review of client self-criticism in psychotherapy. *Journal of Psychotherapy Integration, 23*(2), 166–178.

Kanaan, R. A., Lepine, J. P., & Wessely, S. C. (2007). The association or otherwise of the functional somatic syndromes. *Psychosomatic Medicine, 69*(9), 855–859.

Kempke, S., Goossens, L., Luyten, P., Bekaert, P., Van Houdenhove, B., & Van Wambeke, P. (2010). Predictors of outcome in a multi-component treatment program for chronic fatigue syndrome. *Journal of Affective Disorders, 126,* 174–179.

Kempke, S., Van Houdenhove, B., Luyten, P., Goossens, L., Bekaert, P., & Van Wambeke, P. (2011a). Unraveling the role of perfectionism in chronic fatigue syndrome: Is there a distinction between adaptive and maladaptive perfectionism? *Psychiatry Research, 186*(2–3), 373–377.

Kempke, S., Luyten, P., Van Houdenhove, B., Goossens, L., Bekaert, P., & Van Wambeke, P. (2011b). Self-esteem mediates the relationship between maladaptive perfectionism and depression in chronic fatigue syndrome. *Clinical Rheumatology, 30*(12), 1543–1548.

Kempke, S., Luyten, P., Claes, S., Goossens, L., Bekaert, P., Van Wambeke, P., & Van Houdenhove, B. (2013a). Self-critical perfectionism and its relationship to fatigue and pain in the daily flow of life in patients with chronic fatigue syndrome. *Psychological Medicine, 43*(5), 995–1002.

Kempke, S., Luyten, P., Claes, S., Van Wambeke, P., Bekaert, P., Goossens, L., & Van Houdenhove, B. (2013b). The prevalence and impact of early childhood trauma in chronic fatigue syndrome. *Journal of Psychiatric Research, 47*(5), 664–669.

Kempke, S., Van Den Eede, F., Schotte, C., Claes, S., Van Wambeke, P., Van Houdenhove, B., & Luyten, P. (2013c). Prevalence of DSM-IV personality disorders in patients with chronic fatigue syndrome: A controlled study. *International Journal of Behavioral Medicine, 20*(2), 219–228.

Kempke, S., Luyten, P., Mayes, L., Van Houdenhove, B., & Claes, S. (2014). Self-critical perfectionism predicts lower cortisol response to experimental stress in patients with chronic fatigue syndrome. Manuscript submitted for publication.

Kempke, S., Luyten, P., Van Wambeke, P., Coppens, E., & Morlion, B. (2014). Self-critical perfectionism predicts outcome in multidisciplinary treatment for chronic pain. *Pain Practice, 14*(4), 309–314.

Kempke, S., Luyten, P., De Coninck, S., Van Houdenhove, B., Mayes, L., & Claes, S. (2015). Effects of early childhood trauma on hypothalamic-pituitary-adrenal (HPA) axis function in patients with chronic fatigue syndrome. *Psychoneuroendocrinology, 52,* 14–21.

Kempke, S., Coppens, E., Luyten, P., & Van Houdenhove, B. (in press). The self in chronic fatigue syndrome. In M. Kyrios, R. Moulding, M. Nedeljkovic, S. S. Bhar, G. Doron, & M. Mikulincer (Eds.), *The self in understanding and treating psychological disorders*. Cambridge: Cambridge University Press.

Kirmayer, L. J., Groleau, D., Looper, K. J., & Dao, M. D. (2004). Explaining medically unexplained symptoms. *Canadian Journal of Psychiatry, 49*(10), 663–672.

Kirschbaum, C., Pirke, K. M., & Hellhammer, D. H. (1993). The 'Trier Social Stress Test'—a tool for investigating psychobiological stress responses in a laboratory setting. *Neuropsychobiology, 28*(1–2), 76–81.

Knoop, H., Prins, J. B., Moss-Morris, R., & Bleijenberg, G. (2010). The central role of cognitive processes in the perpetuation of chronic fatigue syndrome. *Journal of Psychosomatic Research, 68*(5), 489–494.

Kudielka, B. M., & Wust, S. (2010). Human models in acute and chronic stress: Assessing determinants of individual hypothalamus–pituitary–adrenal axis activity and reactivity. *Stress, 13*(1), 1–14.

Lerman, S. F., Rudich, Z., & Shahar, G. (2010). Distinguishing affective and somatic dimensions of pain and depression: A confirmatory factor analytic study. *Journal of Clinical Psychology, 66*(4), 456–465.

Lerman, S. F., Shahar, G., & Rudich, Z. (2011). Self-criticism interacts with the affective component of pain to predict depressive symptoms in female patients. *European Journal of Pain, 16*(1), 115–22.

Lupien, S. J., McEwen, B. S., Gunnar, M. R., & Heim, C. (2009). Effects of stress throughout the lifespan on the brain, behaviour and cognition. *Nature Reviews Neuroscience, 10*(6), 434–445.

Luyten, P., & Blatt, S. J. (2013). Interpersonal relatedness and self-definition in normal and disrupted personality development: Retrospect and prospect. *American Psychologist, 68*(3), 172–183.

Luyten, P., & Van Houdenhove, B. (2013). Common versus specific factors in the treatment of functional somatic disorders. *Journal of Psychotherapy Integration, 23*(1), 14–27.

Luyten, P., Corveleyn, J., & Blatt, S. J. (2005). The convergence among psychodynamic and cognitive-behavioral theories of depression: A critical review of empirical research. In J. Corveleyn, P. Luyten, & S. J. Blatt (Eds.), *The theory and treatment of depression: Towards a dynamic interactionism model* (pp. 95–136). Leuven: Leuven University Press/Lawrence Erlbaum Associates.

Luyten, P., Blatt, S. J., Van Houdenhove, B., & Corveleyn, J. (2006). Depression research and treatment: Are we skating to where the puck is going to be? *Clinical Psychology Review, 26*(8), 985–999.

Luyten, P., Van Houdenhove, B., Cosyns, N., & Van den Broeck, A.-L. (2006). Are patients with chronic fatigue syndrome perfectionistic—or were they? A case-control study. *Personality and Individual Differences, 40*(7), 1473–1483.

Luyten, P., Van Houdenhove, B., Pae, C. U., Kempke, S., & Van Wambeke, P. (2008). Treatment of chronic fatigue syndrome: Findings, principles and strategies. *Psychiatry Investigation, 5*(4), 209–212.

Luyten, P., Vliegen, N., Van Houdenhove, B., & Blatt, S. J. (2008). Equifinality, multifinality, and the rediscovery of the importance of early experiences: Pathways from early adversity to psychiatric and (functional) somatic disorders. *Psychoanalytic Study of the Child, 63,* 27–60.

Luyten, P., Kempke, S., Van Wambeke, P., Claes, S., Blatt, S. J., & Van Houdenhove, B. (2011). Self-critical perfectionism, stress generation, and stress sensitivity in patients with chronic fatigue syndrome: Relationship with severity of depression. *Psychiatry, 74*(1), 21–30.

Luyten, P., van Houdenhove, B., Lemma, A., Target, M., & Fonagy, P. (2012). A mentalization-based approach to the understanding and treatment of functional somatic disorders. *Psychoanalytic Psychotherapy, 26*(2), 121–140.

Luyten, P., Van Houdenhove, B., Lemma, A., Target, M., & Fonagy, P. (2013). Vulnerability for functional somatic disorders: A contemporary psychodynamic approach. *Journal of Psychotherapy Integration, 23*(3), 250–262.

Magnusson, A. E., Nias, D. K., & White, P. D. (1996). Is perfectionism associated with fatigue? *Journal of Psychosomatic Research, 41*(4), 377–383.

McEwen, B. S. (1998). Stress, adaptation, and disease. Allostasis and allostatic load. *Annals of the New York Academy of Sciences, 840,* 33–44.

Morlion, B., Kempke, S., Luyten, P., Coppens, E., & Van Wambeke, P. (2011). Multidisciplinary pain education program (MPEP) for chronic pain patients: Preliminary evidence for effectiveness and mechanisms of change. *Current Medical Research and Opinion, 27*(8), 1595–601.

Moser, J. S., Slane, J. D., Alexandra Burt, S., & Klump, K. L. (2012). Etiologic relationships between anxiety and dimensions of maladaptive perfectionism in young adult female twins. *Depression and Anxiety, 29*(1), 47–53.

Moss-Morris, R., Spence, M. J., & Hou, R. (2011). The pathway from glandular fever to chronic fatigue syndrome: Can the cognitive behavioural model provide the map? *Psychological Medicine, 41*(5), 1099–1107.

Nater, U. M., Wagner, D., Solomon, L., Jones, J. F., Unger, E. R., Papanicolaou, D. A., Reeves, W. C., & Heim, C. (2006). Coping styles in people with chronic fatigue syndrome identified from the general population of Wichita, KS. *Journal of Psychosomatic Research, 60*(6), 567–573.

Nater, U. M., Jones, J. F., Lin, J. M., Maloney, E., Reeves, W. C., & Heim, C. (2010). Personality features and personality disorders in chronic fatigue syndrome: A population-based study. *Psychotherapy and Psychosomatics, 79*(5), 312–318.

Nater, U. M., Maloney, E., Heim, C., & Reeves, W. C. (2011). Cumulative life stress in chronic fatigue syndrome. *Psychiatry Research, 189*(2), 318–320.

Ochi, M., Tominaga, K., Iketani, T., Kadouchi, K., Tanigawa, T., Shiba, M. et al. (2008). Perfectionism underlying psychological background correlated with the symptoms of functional dyspepsia. *Journal of Gastroenterology, 43*(9), 699–704.

Papadopoulos, A. S., & Cleare, A. J. (2011). Hypothalamic-pituitary-adrenal axis dysfunction in chronic fatigue syndrome. *Nature Reviews Endocrinology, 3*(1), 22–32.

Pemberton, S., & Cox, D. L. (2014). Experiences of daily activity in chronic fatigue syndrome/myalgic encephalomyelitis (CFS/ME) and their implications for rehabilitation programmes. *Disability and Rehabilitation, 36,* 1790–1797.

Price, J. R., Mitchell, E., Tidy, E., & Hunot, V. (2008). Cognitive behaviour therapy for chronic fatigue syndrome in adults. *Cochrane Database of Systematic Review, 16*(3), CDD001027. doi:10.1002/14651858.CD001027.

Reynolds, K. J., Vernon, S. D., Bouchery, E., & Reeves, W. C. (2004). The economic impact of chronic fatigue syndrome. *Cost Effectiveness and Resource Allocation, 2*(1), 4.

Rimes, K. A., & Chalder, T. (2010). The Beliefs about Emotions Scale: Validity, reliability and sensitivity to change. *Journal of Psychosomatic Research, 68*(3), 285–292.

Riva, R., Mork, P. J., Westgaard, R. H., Ro, M., & Lundberg, U. (2010). Fibromyalgia syndrome is associated with hypocortisolism. *International Journal of Behavioral Medicine, 17*(3), 223–233.

Rudich, Z., Lerman, S. F., Gurevich, B., Weksler, N., & Shahar, G. (2008). Patients' self-criticism is a stronger predictor of physician's evaluation of prognosis than pain diagnosis or severity in chronic pain patients. *Journal of Pain, 9*(3), 210–216.

Shahar, G. (2013). An integrative psychotherapist's account of his focus when treating self-critical patients. *Psychotherapy, 50*(3), 322–325.

Shahar, G., & Henrich, C. C. (2013). Axis of criticism model (ACRIM): An integrative conceptualization of person-context exchanges in vulnerability to adolescent psychopathology. *Journal of Psychotherapy Integration, 23*(3), 236–249.

Shahar, G., & Porcerelli, J. H. (2006). The action formulation: A proposed heuristic for clinical case formulation. *Journal of Clinical Psychology, 62*(9), 1115–1127.

Silverman, M. N., Heim, C. M., Nater, U. M., Marques, A. H., & Sternberg, E. M. (2010). Neuroendocrine and immune contributors to fatigue. *PM & R, 2*(5), 338–346.

Sirois, F. M., & Molnar, D. (2014). Perfectionism and maladaptive coping styles in chronic fatigue syndrome: A comparative analysis with well controls and individuals with irritable bowel syndrome, and fibromyalgia/arthritis. *Psychotherapy and Psychosomatics, 83,* 384–385.

Soenens, B., Vansteenkiste, M., & Luyten, P. (2010). Toward a domain-specific approach to the study of parental psychological control: Distinguishing between dependency-oriented and achievement-oriented psychological control. *Journal of Personality, 78*(1), 217–256.

Spence, M. J., & Moss-Morris, R. (2007). The cognitive behavioural model of irritable bowel syndrome: A prospective investigation of patients with gastroenteritis. *Gut, 56*(8), 1066–1071.

Stoeber, J., & Otto, K. (2006). Positive conceptions of perfectionism: Approaches, evidence, challenges. *Personality and Social Psychology Review, 10*(4), 295–319.

Surawy, C., Hackmann, A., Hawton, K., & Sharpe, M. (1995). Chronic fatigue syndrome: A cognitive approach. *Behaviour Research and Therapy, 33*(5), 535–544.

Tak, L. M., Cleare, A. J., Ormel, J., Manoharan, A., Kok, I. C., Wessely, S., & Rosmalen, J. G. (2011). Meta-analysis and meta-regression of hypothalamic-pituitary-adrenal axis activity in functional somatic disorders. *Biological Psychology, 87*(2), 183–194.

Uhrlass, D. J., & Gibb, B. E. (2007). Childhood emotional maltreatment and the stress generation model of depression. *Journal of Social and Clinical Psychology, 26,* 119–130.

Van Campen, E., Van Den Eede, F., Moorkens, G., Schotte, C., Schacht, R., Sabbe, B. G., Cosyns, P., & Claes, S. J. (2009). Use of the temperament and character inventory (TCI) for assessment of personality in chronic fatigue syndrome. *Psychosomatics, 50*(2), 147–154.

van Geelen, S. M., Sinnema, G., Hermans, H. J., & Kuis, W. (2007). Personality and chronic fatigue syndrome: Methodological and conceptual issues. *Clinical Psychology Review, 27*(8), 885–903.

Van Houdenhove, B., & Egle, U. T. (2004). Fibromyalgia: A stress disorder? Piecing the biopsychosocial puzzle together. *Psychotherapy and Psychosomatics, 73*(5), 267–275.

Van Houdenhove, B., & Luyten, P. (2006). Stress, depression and fibromyalgia. *Acta Neurologica Belgica, 106*(4), 149–156.

Van Houdenhove, B., & Luyten, P. (2008). Customizing treatment of chronic fatigue syndrome and fibromyalgia: The role of perpetuating factors. *Psychosomatics, 49*(6), 470–477.

Van Houdenhove, B., & Luyten, P. (2010). Chronic fatigue syndrome reflects loss of adaptability. *Journal of Internal Medicine, 268*(3), 249–251.

Van Houdenhove, B., Onghena, P., Neerinckx, E., & Hellin, J. (1995). Does high 'action-proneness' make people more vulnerable to chronic fatigue syndrome? A controlled psychometric study. *Journal of Psychosomatic Research, 39*(5), 633–640.

Van Houdenhove, B., Neerinckx, E., Lysens, R., Vertommen, H., Van Houdenhove, L., Onghena, P., et al. (2001). Victimization in chronic fatigue syndrome and fibromyalgia in tertiary care: A controlled study on prevalence and characteristics. *Psychosomatics, 42*(1), 21–28.

Van Houdenhove, B., Neerinckx, E., Onghena, P., Lysens, R., & Vertommen, H. (2001). Premorbid "overactive" lifestyle in chronic fatigue syndrome and fibromyalgia. An etiological factor or proof of good citizenship? *Journal of Psychosomatic Research, 51*(4), 571–576.

Van Houdenhove, B., Bruyninckx, K., & Luyten, P. (2006). In search of a new balance. Can high "action-proneness" in patients with chronic fatigue syndrome be changed by a multidisciplinary group treatment? *Journal of Psychosomatic Research, 60*(6), 623–625.

Van Houdenhove, B., Luyten, P., & Egle, U.T. (2009). The role of childhood trauma in chronic pain and fatigue. In V. J. E. V. L. Banyard & K. A. Kendall-Tackett (Eds.), *Trauma and physical health. Understanding the effects of extreme stress and of psychological harm* (pp. 37–64). London: Routledge.

Van Houdenhove, B., Van Den Eede, F., & Luyten, P. (2009). Does hypothalamic-pituitary-adrenal axis hypofunction in chronic fatigue syndrome reflect a 'crash' in the stress system? *Medical Hypotheses, 72*(6), 701–705.

Van Houdenhove, B., Van Hoof, E., Becq, K., Kempke, S., Luyten, P., & De Meirleir, K. (2009). A comparison of patients with chronic fatigue syndrome in two "ideologically" contrasting clinics. *Journal of Nervous and Mental Disease, 197*(5), 348–353.

Van Houdenhove, B., Kempke, S., & Luyten, P. (2010). Psychiatric aspects of chronic fatigue syndrome and fibromyalgia. *Current Psychiatry Reports, 12*(3), 208–214.

Van Houdenhove, B., Luyten, P., & Kempke, S. (2013). Chronic fatigue syndrome/fibromyalgia: A "stress-adaptation" model. *Fatigue: Biomedicine, Health and Behavior, 1*(3), 137–147.

Wessely, S., Hotopf, M., & Sharpe, M. (1998). *Chronic fatigue and its syndromes*. Oxford: Oxford University Press.

White, C., & Schweitzer, R. (2000). The role of personality in the development and perpetuation of chronic fatigue syndrome. *Journal of Psychosomatic Research, 48*(6), 515–524.

Wicksell, R. K., Kemani, M., Jensen, K., Kosek, E., Kadetoff, D., Sorjonen, K., Ingvar, M., & Olsson, G. L. (2013). Acceptance and commitment therapy for fibromyalgia: A randomized controlled trial. *European Journal of Pain, 17*(4), 599–611.

Wood, B., & Wessely, S. (1999). Personality and social attitudes in chronic fatigue syndrome. *Journal of Psychosomatic Research, 47*(4), 385–397.

Part II
Perfectionism, Psychopathology, and Well-Being

Chapter 6
Perfectionism, Worry, and Rumination in Health and Mental Health: A Review and a Conceptual Framework for a Cognitive Theory of Perfectionism

Gordon L. Flett, Taryn Nepon and Paul L. Hewitt

This chapter examines the tendency for perfectionists to ruminate, worry, and experience various other forms of overthinking when they feel stressed and distressed because life is less than perfect and they feel less than perfect due to an abiding sense of failure. Our analysis focuses jointly on worry and rumination as comparable forms of cognitive perseveration that can impair the well-being and prolong and exacerbate the stress and emotional distress of obsessive perfectionists. Our chapter is based extensively, though not exclusively, on the seminal work on rumination and brooding by Susan Nolen-Hoeksema and her colleagues (see Nolen-Hoeksema, 1991). Indeed, this chapter is dedicated to her memory and her many exceptional contributions. Several years ago, the first author of this chapter had the exceedingly good fortune to attend a compelling keynote address by Dr. Nolen-Hoeksema; it was during the question phase of this keynote address when Dr. Nolen-Hoeksema highlighted the link between perfectionism and rumination in her answer to a challenging question about the likely developmental antecedents of rumination. Her immediate response emphasized perfectionism as a possible antecedent of rumination and the need for further exploration of this association.

Research on perfectionism and rumination and associated forms of cognitive perseveration has progressed at a steady rate. This is important because gaining a better understanding of the link between perfectionism and cognitive perseveration and associated cognitive processes is essential to illuminate the complexities inherent in perfectionism. Accordingly, in the current chapter, we summarize and analyze an existing body of research that shows consistent links between perfectionism and rumination. A key theme that emerges from our summary is that both self-oriented perfectionism (SOP) and socially prescribed perfectionism (SPP; along with other elements of evaluative concerns perfectionism) are associated consistently with

G. L. Flett (✉) · T. Nepon
York University, Toronto, Canada
e-mail: gflett@yorku.ca

P. L. Hewitt
University of British Columbia, Vancouver, Canada

F. M. Sirois, D. S. Molnar (eds.), *Perfectionism, Health, and Well-Being*,
DOI 10.1007/978-3-319-18582-8_6

worry and rumination in ways that suggest that many people with high levels of trait perfectionism are chronic overthinkers; we refer to these people as "perseverating perfectionists." The overthinking of perseverating perfectionists is highly salient and occurs frequently at a level that can impact and interfere with their lives in many significant respects. The links that worry and rumination have with SOP are particularly noteworthy because these associations qualify attempts to characterize this perfectionism dimension as adaptive. Below we outline some new evidence that links high personal standards in people with either diagnosable generalized anxiety disorder (GAD) or exceptionally high levels of worry.

Another central theme in this chapter is that perfectionism is associated with multiple forms of cognitive perseveration, including some types of cognitive operations, processes, and products that are quite unique to perfectionism (i.e., ruminating about the need to be perfect and specific mistakes) and a highly deleterious type of cognitive rumination (i.e., social comparison rumination) that has not been identified thus far in the existing literature. This overthinking of perfectionists extends quite significantly to ruminating about possible or actual failures; here, it is noteworthy that both SOP (i.e., being driven to meet extreme personal standards) and SPP (i.e., a socially imposed pressure on the self) have both been linked empirically with this type of cognitive perseveration, as reflected by agreement with such statements as "If I fail at something, I think about that particular failure for a long time afterwards" (see Hewitt, Flett, Turnbull-Donovan, & Mikail, 1991). Cognitive perseveration can occur in response to a range of stressors, and we contend that several experienced or anticipated stressors elicit cognitive perseveration among perfectionists. Moreover, among chronically stressed perfectionists, the constant pressure that emanates internally from the self or externally from the physical and social environment often translates into chronic cognitive perseveration that can occur at a level that impairs overall levels of cognitive capacity. While the automaticity of cognitive processing has not been empirically examined in controlled laboratory studies, it is reasonable to also suggest that for many vulnerable perfectionists, their cognitive activity has become largely automatic and operates at both conscious and unconscious, subliminal levels.

Finally, the third overarching theme addressed in this chapter is that the chronic cognitive perseveration that characterizes certain perfectionists is not only implicated in vulnerability to psychological distress, it also contributes to vulnerability to the onset of physical illness and it can exacerbate the impact of physical illness once it is experienced. This view of the role of heightened cognitive perseveration among perfectionists is in keeping with what is known generally about the role of overthinking and overanalyzing in mental health and health outcomes. For instance, countless studies now exist showing that ruminative brooding is associated with heightened psychological distress and vulnerability to distress (Aldao, Nolen-Hoeksema, & Schweizer, 2010; Lyubomirsky, Layous, Chancellor, & Nelson, 2015), and cognitive perseveration and negative thought intrusions heighten the impact of failure experiences and associated stressors (Ruscio, Seitchik, Gentes, Jones, & Hallion, 2011). Moreover, there is now extensive evidence that attests to the role of rumination and cognitive perseveration in health problems (see Verkuil, Brosschot, Gebhardt, & Thayer, 2011). This research is designed to test the *cognitive perseveration hypothesis*, which is the notion that rumination in response to an extensive range of stressors tends to prolong the stress response in ways than can have dire health-related consequences (see Brosschot, Gerin, & Thayer, 2006). When examined in this context, perseverative cognition is defined as "the repeated or chronic activation of the cognitive representation of one or more psychological stressors" (Brosschot et al., 2006, p. 113). Parenthetically, it should be noted that the term "cognitive perseveration" is used broadly throughout the current chapter to refer to various forms of overthinking, including types of rumination and automatic thoughts.

We emphasize the potential role of cognitive perseveration in the health problems of perseverating perfectionism given the strong empirical support obtained thus far for the cognitive perseveration hypothesis as it relates to health outcomes. Key, Campbell, Bacon, & Gerin (2008) found that rumination contributes to stress and hypertension by prolonging cardiovascular activation following a stressful experience, while a naturalistic 14-day study found that the students who ruminated extensively about an interpersonal transgression also had elevated levels of salivary cortisol (McCullough, Orsulak, Brandon, & Akers, 2007). Rumination also contributes to an impoverished immune system response (Thomsen et al., 2004), and it can exacerbate the distress of people already attempting to cope with a chronic illness (Soo, Burney, & Basten, 2009). Trait rumination is also linked with prolonged cardiovascular activation during sleep (Johnson, Key, Routledge, Gerin, & Campbell, 2014). These data suggest that perseverating perfectionists who are chronically stressed are substantially at risk for poor physical well-being.

With the exception of one investigation (see Flett, Molnar, Nepon, & Hewitt, 2012), the roles of worry and rumination as contributors to the links between perfectionism and health problems have not been explored empirically. Nevertheless, the role of rumination can be extrapolated from the findings of earlier research on perfectionism and coping with chronic illness. Separate studies with cardiac patients and with patients diagnosed with Crohn's disease or colitis revealed that both trait perfectionism and perfectionistic self-presentation tend to be accompanied by an illness-related coping style focused on emotional preoccupation (Flett, Baricza, Gupta, Hewitt, & Endler, 2011; Shanmugasegaram et al., 2014). Emotional preoccupation coping is usually seen as a pervasive style of ruminative coping that captures the tendency to cognitively perseverate. The current chapter focuses on the associations of perfectionism with worry, rumination, and other forms of overthinking due to actual or anticipated stressors. The studies described contribute to an emerging picture of the brooding, perseverating perfectionist. A central premise in our chapter is that vulnerable perfectionists exhibit multiple types of perseverative and intrusive thinking that fuel their distress and stress. These cognitive tendencies can include negative thinking in general (Macedo et al., 2015) and a tendency to experience frequent counterfactual thoughts about how fabulous life could have possibly been when recalling negative life events (Sirois, Monforton, & Simpson, 2010).

The remainder of our chapter is organized as follows. First, given our extensive focus on worry and rumination, we briefly discuss how they are similar in several respects, yet distinguishable in terms of other key features. We then examine the links that perfectionism has with both worry and rumination from a conceptual perspective. We believe that this analysis is timely given mounting interest in the links that perfectionism has with these forms of cognitive perseveration. Our analysis also includes a summary of research conducted thus far on multidimensional perfectionism and worry and rumination. Most research that will be discussed has utilized either the Frost Multidimensional Perfectionism Scale (FMPS; Frost, Marten, Lahart, & Rosenblate, 1990) or the Hewitt and Flett Multidimensional Perfectionism Scale (HFMPS; Hewitt & Flett, 1991, 2004). Our discussion of results involving the FMPS will focus mostly on three subscales—personal standards (PS), concern over mistakes (COM), and doubts about actions (DAA). The HFMPS also measures PS perfectionism in the form of SOP, but it also assesses interpersonal perfectionism in terms of other-oriented perfectionism (OOP; i.e., demanding perfection from others) and SPP, which, as noted above, is the tendency to perceive that others demand perfection from the self. Our analysis of worry and rumination and its link with the HFMPS will focus on SOP and SPP. The remainder of our chapter introduces the main tenets of our proposed perfectionism cognition theory and outlines key directions for future research. First, however, we begin by examining the nature of worry and rumination in general.

Worry and Rumination

In what ways are worry and rumination similar yet distinguishable? We will only briefly discuss this topic given that previous authors have already provided detailed, insightful analyses (e.g., Nolen-Hoeksema, Wisco, & Lyubomirsky, 2008).

Both worry and rumination are the forms of cognitive perseveration that can become chronic and obsessional in nature. It is generally accepted that worry is the cognitive component of anxiety, while rumination is best regarded as a self-reflective form of brooding that is experienced when a sad and distressed person is seeking to understand the reasons why he or she is feeling sad or distressed (Nolen-Hoeksema, 1991; Treynor, Gonzalez, & Nolen-Hoeksema, 2003). According to Nolen-Hoeksema et al. (2008), they are both repetitive, perseverative forms of thinking that are abstract and overgeneralized and involve cognitive inflexibility and difficulties in shifting attention. They share a host of negative consequences, including performance deficits and poor problem-solving, and can exacerbate and prolong anxiety and depression. Key differences reflect differences in temporal focus, with worry being focused on the future, and rumination typically being focused on current and past circumstances. Another important distinction emphasized by Nolen-Hoeksema et al. (2008) is that worry is focused on actual or anticipated threats, while rumination is "focused on issues of self-worth, meaning, themes of loss" (p. 407). The ruminator is preoccupied with personal feelings of sadness and despair and the factors that contribute to these feelings, including deficiencies in the self.

Not surprisingly, measures of worry and rumination tend to be robustly correlated, and case studies of perfectionists who engage in extensive cognitive perseveration often show both worry and rumination. Costello and Borkovec (1992) provided a detailed account of Mike, a 34-year-old married graduate student with one child, who described himself as worried all of his life and very eager to please other people, including his parents. Mike was described as a perfectionist with high performance standards. SPP was evident in terms of his feeling pressured by his family to meet high expectations. Mike had received a primary diagnosis of generalized anxiety disorder and secondary diagnoses of social phobia and simple phobia (due to his additional fears of air travel, animals, blood, and injury). His generalized anxiety was signified by a substantially elevated intake score of 66 on the Penn State Worry Questionnaire. At the root of Mike's difficulties was a steady stream of negative thoughts such as "I'm inadequate," "I will never get out of my problem," and "I'm letting my family down." His worry was fuelled by metacognitive beliefs that worrying helped him prepare for the worst possible outcome and helped him cope with his fear of losing control. Perfectionism was reflected in his repetitive, catastrophic thinking; he was cognitively preoccupied with the possibility of failing his upcoming comprehensive examination which had to be passed to satisfy his doctoral degree requirements. He anticipated "choking" and freezing up during the exam. Fortunately, Mike improved substantially over time as a result of a combined treatment that utilized relaxation training and cognitive behavioral techniques. Key factors that were identified as contributing to his improvement were a strong support system, developing a strong therapeutic alliance, and being highly motivated to improve. Unfortunately, there was no assessment of his perfectionism, and treatment was not tailored to address Mike's perfectionism and how he would react in situations involving possible failure that could activate his underlying need to be perfect.

Typically, distressed perfectionists often experience a blended form of rumination with dysfunctional attitudes and automatic thoughts involving their need to be perfect, negative automatic thoughts about themselves in general, and cognitions related to their other personality characteristics. For instance, Leahy (2002) described Tom, a 41-year-old accountant suffering from generalized anxiety disorder, co-morbid depression, and low self-esteem. He worried about a wide range of things including his clients getting angry with him, never achieving anything, and being seen as a failure. Tom had difficulties with procrastination, work, decision-making, and assertiveness to the extent that he failed to complete and file his own taxes. Assessment revealed thoughts and assumptions related to personal feelings and beliefs about the self as "defective, incompetent, and pathetic." In this instance, Tom's low self-esteem contributed to worry and rumination about anticipated mistakes in the future. The close association between negative views of the self and thoughts about perfectionism and procrastination were reflected by his cognitive preoccupation with the need to be perfect and always having to do things perfectly, along with such thoughts as "I am a total loser," and "Nothing I've done counts if I don't finish my own taxes." He also had a deficit in self-assertiveness that was underscored by chronic ruminations involving anticipated negative feedback from other people who he predicted would respond to him with anger and confrontation should he try to be more assertive with things such as demanding that an overdue client pay him for his work. Fortunately, Leahy (2002) reported that Tom responded well to cognitive behavior therapy as reflected by a substantial increase in self-esteem and reduced levels of anxiety and depression.

Why do Perfectionists Engage in Cognitive Perseveration?

The next segment of our chapter will examine perfectionism and worry from a conceptual perspective. The initial research on perfectionism and worry was conducted by Meyer, Miller, Metzger, & Borkovec (1990) as part of the initial psychometric work in developing the Penn State Worry Questionnaire (PSWQ), a 16-item self-report measure of pathological, uncontrollable worry. Meyer et al. (1990) reported a significant positive correlation between PSWQ scores and scores on the unidimensional Burns Perfectionism Scale. Although these authors did not explain why perfectionism should relate to pathological worry, they did report that perfectionism accounted for significant unique variance in pathological worry when pitted against various other predictors, including self-consciousness and need for control.

When it comes to trying to understand the nature of the link between perfectionism and cognitive perseveration in the form of worry, useful clues come from studies that examine common fears such as social evaluation fears. Borkovec, Metzger, & Pruzinsky (1986) concluded that worry is largely socially evaluative in nature and self-referent. In fact, they went so far as to suggest that "social evaluation may be the core fear of the worrier" (p. 225). This conclusion was reached after summarizing the most predominant fears of worriers. According to Borkovec et al. (1986), the five most prevalent fears are the fears related to feeling self-conscious, making mistakes, meeting someone for the first time, failing on tests, and being criticized; clearly, at least four of the top five fears are potentially relevant to perfectionism. One of our earliest studies examined the fears of trait perfectionists in a sample of university students (see Blankstein, Flett, Hewitt, & Eng, 1993) and found that both SOP and SPP were associated significantly with the fear of loss of control, fear of failure, and fear of making mistakes. In addition, SPP was linked with the fears of looking foolish and being criticized. These data suggest quite clearly that any theoretical account of the nature of worry among perfectionists should emphasize socially evaluative and self-evaluative concerns.

In all likelihood, the origins of worry among perfectionists reflect several of the proposed developmental antecedents of perfectionism outlined by Flett, Hewitt, Oliver, & MacDonald (2002) in their analysis of how perfectionism originates. They highlighted the likely role of genetic factors, an anxious temperament, and an insecure attachment style based on less than optimal parent–child interactions. Evidence was also provided linking perfectionism with a strong and active behavioral inhibition system as described by Gray (1991), and this has been supported by subsequent research (Randles, Flett, Nash, McGregor, & Hewitt, 2010). These factors are important to emphasize because they suggest that a propensity to worry and being highly anxious will be evident early on in development. Thus, it is not surprising that there is evidence attesting to the link between perfectionism and various forms of anxiety in children and adolescents (e.g., Essau, Leung, Conradt, Broeren, & Wong, 2008; Hewitt et al., 2002).

Key insights that help illuminate why perfectionists tend to worry can be gained by considering the related question, "What are the functions of the worry when worry is experienced by perfectionists?" One team of researchers have suggested that worry is perceived as useful from a metacognitive perspective as the perfectionistic worrier comes to believe that worry is adaptive (Macedo, Marques, & Pereira, 2014). While this may indeed be the case, we believe that worry stems largely from the tendency of self-doubting perfectionists to be highly attentive to worry-provoking threats, whether actual or anticipated. In addition to the safety concerns that contribute to worry in most people, evaluative cues suggesting that the self is less than perfect (e.g., unflattering social comparison information) will often provoke worry. The worry of perfectionistic individuals also reflects their dislike of and inability to tolerate uncertain and ambiguous situations that arouse concerns over lack of control, and about the need to seem perfect while often feeling like an imposter.

The worry of perfectionists can also be considered within the context of theoretical accounts that emphasize worry as a potentially adaptive way of distracting someone through cognitive avoidance, or as a way of preparing the self so that unexpected and intense negative emotions are never actually experienced in reality (e.g., Borkovec, Alcaine, & Behar, 2004). The experience of worry is functional to the extent that worry may help avert the experience of strong negative emotions, which is highly desirable for those perfectionists who have the emotional perfectionism described by David Burns (1980). Perfectionists are hypervigilant to emotional experience, and strong emotional failures can be quite threatening because they signal to oneself and others that either life failures have occurred and/or the person is a failure in terms of ability to control negative occurrences and generate positive outcomes and experiences. Viewed from this perspective, the cognitive perseveration of perfectionists can have multiple purposes (e.g., avoidance of stronger affect, making uncertain and ambiguous circumstances more predictable, gaining corrective feedback that will limit future mistakes and imperfections).

Rumination and worry activate and magnify a self-focus and concerns about being disapproved of and negatively evaluated by other people. There is a clear self-presentational element to the link between perfectionism and various forms of cognitive perseveration. Indeed, we are in the process of collecting evidence across several studies, which suggests that many perfectionists, including children and adolescents, are extensively engaged in hiding their rumination and worry. We have described this phenomenon as "perfect on the outside but brooding on the inside." This form of self-presentation has many potential negative consequences, including the following: (1) it limits access to social support due to an unwillingness and inability to self-disclose to potential support providers; and (2) it contributes to emotional inexpressiveness and expressive suppression of stress that may ultimately contribute to the development and exacerbation of health problems. Here, it is important to draw a key distinction between experiential suppression versus the suppression of emotions and stress (for a discussion, see Lemaire, El-Hage, &

Frangou, 2014). Our work has been based on the premise that perfectionists are particularly prone to experiencing stress and distress, in part due to their tendency for self-generated stress (Hewitt & Flett, 2002). But vulnerable perfectionists prone to cognitive perseveration are less able to suppress the experience of negative emotions while simultaneously being relatively low in the tendency to express these negative emotions.

Research on Perfectionism and Worry

Table 6.1 displays a select summary of 11 published studies we collected, which include at least one measure of perfectionism and one measure of worry. A few other relevant studies on perfectionism and worry that are not in Table 6.1 can be found in Table 6.2, which provides an overview of research on perfectionism and rumination and includes studies that have focused jointly on rumination and worry.

Overall, six studies shown in Table 6.1 included the FMPS. The general pattern that emerges is that there are consistent links between worry and elevated scores on the FMPS subscales assessing COM and DAA. Typically, there is also a smaller, but significant association found between worry and high PS. Note that some additional studies with the FMPS were not included in Table 6.1 because they focused on total perfectionism scores and established a strong, positive link between total FMPS scores and scores on the PSWQ (e.g., Smári, Olason, Eypórsdóttir, & Frölunde, 2007; Whiting et al., 2014) or they combined the FMPS dimensions into composite scores, but with a nonstandard version of the FMPS. For instance, Khawaja and Armstrong (2005), as part of their attempt to reduce the FMPS to 24 items, showed that PSWQ scores were linked robustly with a factor that combined COM and DAA ($r=.56$) and there was also a significant correlation between worry and the PS factor ($r=.28$).

A few illustrative examples from Table 6.1 are now provided. Santanello and Gardner (2006) examined the associations among maladaptive perfectionism, pathological worry, and experiential avoidance in a sample of 125 students. Experiential avoidance refers to the tendency for a person to avoid internal thoughts and feelings that cause discomfort by suppressing or avoiding situations that create them. In this study, maladaptive perfectionism was assessed using a factor that combines concern over mistakes and doubts (CMD), as well as parental expectations and criticism (PEC). Correlational analyses revealed that maladaptive perfectionism was associated with higher levels of pathological worry, and was also positively correlated with experiential avoidance, which was, in turn, positively related to worry. Experiential avoidance partially mediated the link between maladaptive perfectionism and worry.

A study by Chang and colleagues (2007) examined how perfectionism is associated with domains of nonpathological worry and the behavioral inhibition system (BIS) and behavioral activation system (BAS) motives. The Worry Domains Questionnaire (WDQ; Tallis, Eysenck, & Mathews, 1992) assessed the following

Table 6.1 Studies linking perfectionism and worry

Author(s)	Title	Measures	Results re: worry & perfectionism
Buhr & Dugas (2006)	Investigating the construct validity of intolerance of uncertainty and its unique relationship with worry	HFMPS and Penn State Worry Questionnaire (PSWQ)	SOP and SPP were both linked with higher levels of pathological worry as well as intolerance of uncertainty and intolerance of ambiguity
Chang (2006)	Conceptualization and measurement of adaptive and maladaptive aspects of performance perfectionism: relations to personality, psychological functioning, and academic achievement	Performance Perfectionism Scale and Worry Domains Questionnaire	Negative self-oriented and negative socially prescribed performance perfectionism were associated with higher levels of pathological worry. Positive self-oriented performance perfectionism was associated with lower levels of pathological worry
Chang, Zumberg, Sanna, Girz, Kade, et al. (2007)	Relationship between perfectionism and domains of worry in a college student population: considering the role of BIS/BAS motives	FMPS and Worry Domains Questionnaire	COM, parental criticism, and DAA were positively correlated with all six domains of nonpathological worry. PS was positively correlated with relationship and work incompetence worries. Parental expectations was positively linked with relationship, lack of confidence, and work incompetence worries
Flett, Hewitt, Endler, & Tassone (1994/1995)	Perfectionism and components of state and trait anxiety	Burns Perfectionism Scale, HFMPS, Endler Multidimensional Anxiety Scales	Unidimensional perfectionism, SOP and SPP were positively linked with the cognitive-worry and autonomic-emotional facets of state anxiety, and with the total state anxiety scores. SPP was linked with higher state anxiety in a high ego involvement condition, but not in a low ego condition
Gentes & Ruscio (2014)	Perceptions of functioning in worry and generalized anxiety disorder	FMPS and PSWQ	High worriers with generalized anxiety disorder (GAD) and high worriers without GAD had significantly higher levels of total perfectionism, relative to normal worriers
Handley, Egan, Kane, & Rees (2014)	The relationships between perfectionism, pathological worry, and generalized anxiety disorder	FMPS, Clinical Perfectionism Questionnaire, and PSWQ	COM, PS, and clinical perfectionism were all positively associated with pathological worry, even after controlling for gender and depression
Kawamura, Hunt, Frost, & Marten DiBartolo (2001)	Perfectionism, anxiety, and depression: are the relationships independent?	FMPS and PSWQ	Maladaptive perfectionism was positively associated with a social anxiety/trait anxiety/worry factor of anxiety, even after controlling for depression

Table 6.1 (continued)

Author(s)	Title	Measures	Results re: worry & perfectionism
Lakey &Tanner (2013)	Social influences in negative thinking and affect	Perfectionism Cognitions Inventory (PCI) and PSWQ	Across two studies, perfectionistic automatic thoughts were positively correlated with pathological worry
Meyer, Miller, Metzger, & Borkovec (1990)	Development and validation of the Penn State Worry Questionnaire	Burns Perfectionism Scale and PSWQ reactions to tests	Perfectionism was positively correlated with pathological worry. Pathological worry was also positively correlated with the worry subscale of the reactions to tests
Santanello & Gardner (2006)	The role of experiential avoidance in the relationship between maladaptive perfectionism and worry	FMPS and PSWQ	Maladaptive perfectionism was positively associated with pathological worry
Stöber & Joormann (2001)	Worry, procrastination, and perfectionism: differentiating amount of worry, pathological worry, anxiety, and depression	FMPS, Worry Domains Questionnaire, and PSWQ	COM and DAA, as well as parental expectations and criticism were positively correlated with both pathological and nonpathological worry. PS was positively correlated with nonpathological worry on the worry domains questionnaire

worry domains: relationship, lack of confidence, aimless future, work incompetence, financial, and sociopolitical. Analyses indicated all worry domains were linked positively with COM, doubts about action, and PEC. PS perfectionism was positively correlated with the domains of relationship and work incompetence worries. Dimensions of perfectionism also significantly predicted unique variance in all domains of worry scores, above and beyond measures tapping the motives linked with the BIS and the BAS.

In an earlier study, Stöber and Joormann (2001) explored the associations between dimensions of perfectionism and both pathological and nonpathological worry. Perfectionism was assessed using CMD and PEC, and the PS subscale. Both CMD and PEC perfectionism scores were positively correlated with pathological and nonpathological worry. There was a small positive correlation between PS and nonpathological worry. The correlations that CMD and PEC had with nonpathological worry were still significant after controlling for depression and anxiety. Only the correlation between CMD and pathological worry remained significant after controlling for depression and anxiety. A smaller number of studies have examined worry and perfectionism as assessed by the HFMPS, though the research points to the links between worry and both SOP and SPP (e.g., Blankstein and Lumley, 2008; Flett, Coulter, Hewitt, & Nepon, 2011). Buhr and Dugas (2006) found that SOP and SPP were both associated with pathological worry and that all were also positively linked with intolerance of uncertainty. After controlling for intolerance of uncertainty, SOP was still significantly linked with worry.

Another series of studies examined perfectionism and worry as part of a broader investigation of perfectionism and both state and trait anxiety in students (Flett, Hewitt, & Tassone, 1994/1995). The Endler Multidimensional Anxiety Scales (EMAS; Endler, Edwards, & Vitelli, 1991) were used in three studies to assess both state and trait anxiety, and these scales provide a separate assessment of cognitive worry. In Study 1, unidimensional perfectionism, as measured by the Burns Perfectionism Scale, was positively linked with the cognitive-worry and autonomic-emotional facets of state anxiety. Perfectionism was also linked with higher social evaluation and ambiguous trait anxiety. Study 2 used the HFMPS to assess multidimensional perfectionism and showed in the total sample that SOP and SPP were positively correlated with the cognitive-worry and autonomic-emotional components of state anxiety, and with the total score. Similar results were found in women, while only SPP was linked with higher cognitive-worry in men. In Study 3, an experiment was conducted where participants engaged in an anagram task with either a high or low level of ego involvement. The results indicated that SPP was linked with higher state anxiety including cognitive worry in a high ego involvement condition for both men and women, but not in a low ego involvement condition.

Overall, there is a paucity of research on perfectionism and worry with clinical samples, but some key data involving the FMPS have recently emerged. A study by Gentes and Ruscio (2014) is highly illuminating; their original paper included results only for total FMPS scores, but these investigators graciously provided the results for the various FMPS subscales upon request. Specifically, Gentes and Ruscio (2014) examined perfectionism, distress, and impairment among worriers with generalized anxiety disorder (GAD) and uncontrollable worry, extremely high worriers who did not qualify for a GAD diagnosis, and a subsample of normal worriers. Participants were divided into groups based on clinical interviews and self-report measures of worry. They also completed various self-report indices of distress and impairment and the FMPS. The results indicated that individuals in the GAD group and the non-GAD high worry group had significantly higher levels of global perfectionism, compared with those in the normal worry group. There were no significant differences on global perfectionism between the GAD group and the non-GAD high worry group. Moreover, individuals in the GAD group had the highest levels of distress and impairment on important life domains, followed by those in the non-GAD high worry group, and then those in the normal worry group.

The additional results involving the FMPS subscales that were provided to us paint a clear and vivid portrait of the perseverating perfectionist who either has diagnosable GAD or an exceptionally high level of worry. People in these groups, relative to participants in the control group, had exceptionally high levels of perfectionism across all FMPS dimensions, but especially on the dimensions of PS perfectionism and COM. For the GAD group, the mean on PS perfectionism was 27.04 ($SD=3.98$), while the mean on COM was 31.35 ($SD=6.43$). The mean score on PS perfectionism far exceeds the norms reported by Flett and Hewitt (2014a) in their published review of perfectionism measures. Similarly, the mean on COM far exceeds the cutoff of 25 used by Frost and associates (1995) to identify people with exceptionally high levels of COM. The overall level of perfectionism that was found calls into question the idea that PS perfectionism is adaptive among perfectionists who tend to worry and ruminate. The extreme worrier or person with GAD, who also has exceptionally high PS, should be highly attentive to any information that suggests he or she is not living up to those standards. Uncontrollable stressors that highlight a lack of personal control and/or create uncertainty and ambiguity should provoke high state levels of worry among these people. The elevated COM that was detected among the high worriers and people with GAD points clearly to a strong cognitive preoccupation with previous or anticipated mistakes.

Overall, the analyses of various other measures included by Gentes and Ruscio (2014) led them to conclude that worry reflects a tendency to evaluate oneself according to exceptionally high evaluative standards. That is, high worriers "…hold elevated standards for what constitutes adequate functioning, and may evaluate themselves according to those elevated standards" (p. 525). The authors noted that while generalized anxiety and high standards are clearly related, it is not possible to determine whether the standards preceded the extreme anxiety or vice versa.

In another study of perfectionism, pathological worry, and GAD, Handley, Egan, Kane, & Rees (2014) evaluated a clinical sample of 36 adults with elevated GAD symptoms, who had self-referred for a perfectionism treatment trial. Perfectionism was assessed with the FMPS PS, COM, and DAA (DAA) subscales, as well as with the Clinical Perfectionism Questionnaire. Participants also completed the PSWQ and the Beck Depression Inventory—II. Mean levels of perfectionism confirmed that the participants once again had substantially elevated levels of perfectionism on COM ($M=33.19$, $SD=6.47$) and PS ($M=28.61$, $SD=4.46$). Correlational results within this sample revealed that pathological worry had strong links with COM ($r=.68$), PS ($r=.49$), and clinical perfectionism ($r=.49$). All dimensions of perfectionism and worry were also linked with higher levels of depression. In addition, COM, PS, and clinical perfectionism all uniquely predicted pathological worry scores, after controlling for gender and depression. This study is unique in establishing links between dimensions of perfectionism and pathological worry in a clinical sample of individuals with elevated GAD symptoms.

Research on Perfectionism and Rumination

Table 6.2 presents a representative summary of 16 published studies that we compiled that had at least one measure of perfectionism and one measure of rumination. Three of these studies also include a measure of worry. As noted below, a similar pattern of findings emerged as well as evidence that rumination acts as a mediator of the link between perfectionism and negative psychological outcomes. The mediational role of rumination is in keeping with other evidence showing that rumination mediates the link between perfectionistic dysfunctional attitudes and distress (Ciesla & Roberts, 2007), and it plays a role in mediating the link that conceptually related factors (e.g., self-criticism) have with depression (Spasojevic & Alloy, 2001).

The vast majority of studies included in Table 6.2 used either the FMPS or the HFMPS, and some of these studies are described below. Only one study we located used the Almost Perfect Scale—Revised, which assesses high PS and the perceived discrepancy from these standards (see Slaney, Rice, Mobley, Trippi, & Ashby, 2001). This study by Sirois et al. (2010) showed that there was a robust positive relation between discrepancy and ruminative brooding ($r=.60$). There were also small positive associations between reflection and both high PS and discrepancy. Future research on perfectionism discrepancy is clearly needed given the evidence linking rumination with the size of the discrepancy between the actual self and the ideal self, as described in self-discrepancy theory, and indications that rumination and discrepancies interact to produce heightened depression (see Papadakis, Prince, Jones, & Strauman, 2006; Roelofs et al., 2007).

Studies Using the Frost MPS (FMPS)

Research involving the FMPS is now described. One study listed in Table 6.2 examined perfectionism and rumination among people being treated for post-traumatic stress disorder (PTSD) (Egan, Hattaway, & Kane, 2014). Correlational analyses revealed that PS, COM, and clinical perfectionism were all linked with higher levels of rumination. COM, clinical perfectionism, and rumination were associated with more frequent PTSD symptoms. Rumination also mediated the link between COM and PTSD symptoms. This was the first study to test rumination as a mediator of the perfectionism–PTSD link.

Table 6.2 Studies linking perfectionism and rumination

Author(s)	Title	Measures	Results: rumination and perfectionism
Besharat, Issazadegan, Etemadinia, Golssanamlou, & Abdolmanafi (2014)	Risk factors associated with depressive symptoms among undergraduate students	Tehran Multidimensional Perfectionism Scale (TMPS) and Ruminative Responses Scale	SOP was negatively correlated with rumination, while both other-oriented and SPP were positively correlated with rumination
Blankstein, & Lumley (2008)	Multidimensional perfectionism and ruminative brooding in current dysphoria, anxiety, worry, and anger	HFMPS Ruminative Brooding Checklists, adapted from Nolen-Hoeksema et al. (1993) Worry Inventory adapted from PSWQ	SPP was positively correlated with depressive brooding in men and women, while SOP was only correlated with these variables in women. Self-oriented and SPP were positively correlated with worry in men and women
Brown & Kocovski (2014)	Perfectionism as a predictor of post-event rumination in a socially anxious sample	HFMPS-SPP FMPS-COM, DAA; State Perfectionism Subscales, Rumination and Reflection Questionnaire, and Post-event Processing Questionnaire	Both trait and state facets of perfectionism were positively correlated with trait rumination. These trait and state facets of perfectionism also predicted post-event rumination 2 days following a social anxiety-inducing speech task
Burns & Fedewa (2005)	Cognitive styles: links with perfectionistic thinking	Positive and Negative Perfectionism Scale and Responses to Depression Questionnaire	Negative perfectionism, a type of evaluative concerns perfectionism, was positively linked with rumination
Egan, Hattaway, & Kane (2014)	The relationship between perfectionism and rumination in post-traumatic stress disorder	FMPS-PS, COM; Clinical Perfectionism Scale and Response Styles Questionnaire	PS, COM, and clinical perfectionism were all positively related to rumination
Flett, Coulter, Hewitt, & Nepon (2011)	Perfectionism, rumination, worry, and depressive symptoms in early adolescents	Child–Adolescent Perfectionism Scale, PCI, Children's Response Styles Questionnaire, and PSWQ for Children	SOP and perfectionism cognitions were positively correlated with rumination and worry. SPP was positively associated with worry but not rumination
Flett, Madorsky, Hewitt, & Heisel (2002)	Perfectionism cognitions, rumination, and psychological distress	HFMPS, PCI, Abbreviated Response Styles Questionnaire	Perfectionism cognitions, SOP, and SPP were all positively correlated with rumination
Harris, Pepper, & Maack (2008)	The relationship between maladaptive perfectionism and depressive symptoms: the mediating role of rumination	FMPS and Response Styles Questionnaire	Maladaptive perfectionism (COM and DAA was positively correlated with rumination, brooding, and reflective pondering. Adaptive perfectionism high PS and organization) was not linked with brooding

Table 6.2 (continued)

Author(s)	Title	Measures	Results: rumination and perfectionism
Hill, Huelsman, Furr, Kibler, Vicente, & Kennedy (2004)	A new measure of perfectionism: the perfectionism inventory	Perfectionism Inventory, FMPS, and HFMPS	The rumination subscale of the Perfectionism Inventory was positively correlated with all of the other subscales of this measure, as well as with the subscales of both the FMPS and HFMPS
Olson & Kwon (2008)	Brooding perfectionism: refining the roles of rumination and perfectionism in the etiology of depression	HFMPS and Response Styles Questionnaire	SOP and SPP were positively associated with ruminative brooding and reflection
O'Connor, O'Connor, & Marshall (2007)	Perfectionism and psychological distress: evidence of the mediating effects of rumination	HFMPS and Ruminative Responses Scale	Across three studies, SOP and SPP were positively linked with brooding, while OOP was positively correlated with brooding in one study
Randles, Flett, Nash, McGregor, & Hewitt (2010)	Dimensions of perfectionism, behavioral inhibition, and rumination	HFMPS and Rumination–Reflection Scale	SPP was positively linked with trait rumination
Rudolph, Flett, & Hewitt (2007)	Perfectionism and deficits in cognitive emotion regulation	HFMPS, PCI, and Cognitive Emotion Regulation Questionnaire	SPP and perfectionism cognitions were positively correlated with rumination from the CERQ
Short & Mazmanian (2013)	Perfectionism and negative repetitive thoughts: examining a multiple mediator model in relation to mindfulness	HFMPS, Ruminative–Responses Scale—brooding PSWQ	Both SOP and SPP were positively correlated with rumination as well as worry
Sirois, Monforton, & Simpson (2010)	"If only I had done better": perfectionism and the functionality of counterfactual thinking	Almost Perfect Scale—Revised and Ruminative–Response Scale	Maladaptive perfectionism was robustly associated with greater ruminative brooding, while maladaptive and PS perfectionism were positively linked with reflection
Wilson, Hunter, Rasmussen, & McGowan (in press)	They made you perfect: a test of the social reaction model of perfectionism	HFMPS Response Styles Questionnaire	Both SOP and SPP were positively correlated with brooding with the correlation with SPP being much stronger; only SPP was correlated positively with reflection

Another study did not test the association between rumination and perfectionism, as assessed by the FMPS, even though both types of measures were included. However, rumination and perfectionism were substantially elevated in those students who engaged in nonsuicidal self-injury when they were compared with the students who had not engaged in self-injury (Hoff & Muehlenkamp, 2009). In addition to rumination, self-injuring students had elevated COM and parental criticism, but lower scores on the FMPS organization factor.

In a study testing rumination as a potential mediator of the link between maladaptive perfectionism and depression (Harris, Pepper, & Maack, 2008), participants identified their most recent disappointing test score. Maladaptive perfectionism (COM and DAA) was positively correlated with rumination, brooding, reflective pondering, and depressive symptoms, whereas adaptive perfectionism (PS and organization) was correlated with brooding. Rumination also fully mediated the association between maladaptive perfectionism and depressive symptoms.

Rukmini, Sudhir, and Math (2014) examined the FMPS and rumination in 30 patients with social phobia and 30 community participants and found that brooding was associated with COM ($r=.40$) and with perceived criticism ($r=.47$) among the clinical participants. Group comparisons indicated that the clinical group was distinguished by having an exceptionally high level of COM. Similarly, one study showed that the maladaptive component of rumination was associated with COM and with DAA. It was not associated with PS perfectionism, and no support was found for the suggestion that a more adaptive form of rumination might be associated positively with PS perfectionism (Di Schiena, Luminet, Philippot, & Douilliez, 2012).

Studies Using the Hewitt Flett MPS (HFMPS)

Table 6.2 describes 12 studies that either used the HFMPS or a measure derived from it such as the Child–Adolescent Perfectionism Scale. The typical finding was that both SOP and SPP were associated significantly with ruminative brooding, with the link between rumination and SPP tending to be more robust. For example, Olson and Kwon (2008) examined perfectionism, brooding, and depression in a four-week longitudinal study and found that SOP and SPP were positively associated with brooding and reflection. Also, both SOP and SPP interacted with brooding and stress to predict depression.

O'Connor, O'Connor, and Marshall (2007) conducted three different studies assessing the mediating role of rumination in the perfectionism–distress link. Analyses indicated that across all three studies, SOP and SPP were positively linked with a brooding ruminative response style. Studies 1 and 2 demonstrated that cross-sectionally, brooding mediated the relations that SOP and SPP had with levels of depression and hopelessness. Study 3 showed that brooding mediated the links that SPP had with depression and hopelessness after a 2-month period. Taken together, these findings imply that rumination may be an important mechanism through which the aspects of perfectionism are linked with distress.

In another study on perfectionism, rumination, worry, distress, and dispositional mindfulness in students, both SOP and SPP were positively associated with worry and rumination (Short & Mazmanian, 2013). SPP, rumination, and worry were all linked with higher levels of negative affect. Rumination and worry mediated the link between SPP and negative affect. However, the mediating effect of rumination was not significant for those high in mindfulness. These findings point to dispositional mindfulness as a protective factor for perfectionistic students who engage in rumination.

A study by Blankstein and Lumley (2008) deserves special mention because their study focused specifically on examining possible sex differences, given the original emphasis by Nolen-Hoeksema (1991) on rumination and depression in women. Their results indicated that SPP was positively associated with brooding in response to distress among men and women, while SOP was only correlated with brooding in women. SOP, SPP, and brooding were also positively associated with current worry in men as well as women. A series of regression analyses showed that SOP, SPP, and brooding all uniquely predicted numerous forms of distress. The need for greater exploration of sex differences is a theme we revisit later in our chapter.

Other Research on Perfectionism and Rumination

Burns and Fedewa (2005) studied how aspects of perfectionism are associated with numerous cognitive styles, including rumination, and found that negative perfectionism, as assessed by the Positive and Negative Perfectionism Scale (Terry-Short, Owens, Slade, & Dewey, 1995), was positively correlated with rumination. This finding suggests that rumination is a response to coping with distress used by negative perfectionists. Negative perfectionists were also low on constructive thinking and had reported engaging in dangerous activities in response to distress.

Hill and colleagues (2004) created and tested a measure of perfectionism that has a rumination subscale. The other subscales are COM, high standards for others, need for approval, organization, parental pressure, planfulness, and striving for excellence. Across two studies, the rumination subscale was positively linked with all other subscales. In one study, they also found that the rumination subscale was positively correlated with all of the subscales from the FMPS and the HFMPS.

Summary

Collectively, the research described above and the studies found in Tables 6.1 and 6.2 highlight the links between various trait perfectionism dimensions and indices of worry and rumination. Attempts to interpret PS perfectionism and SOP as potentially adaptive are not supported by the existing correlational findings showing that rumination and worry are often linked with these dimensions, and PS perfectionism is substantially elevated among people with diagnosable GAD and people who are subthreshold for GAD, but who still have exceptionally high levels of worry. It could be argued that worry and rumination are seen by these people as beneficial, but our sense is that underlying this seemingly adaptive belief is a profound anticipatory fear about the consequences and costs that ensue if the need to be perfect is relaxed and perfection is no longer seen as an absolute imperative.

We now extend our analysis by introducing perfectionism cognition theory (PCT). Until now, the field of perfectionism and cognition has been devoid of any extensive theoretical accounts, and it can be argued that this lack of a conceptual perspective has limited the amount of empirical attention that this topic has received. Below, we take an initial step by providing an overview of the main tenets of PCT as a way of illustrating the many issues that merit further investigation.

Perfectionism Cognition Theory

The key guiding assumptions of our initial PCT are provided below. The PCT is a theoretical model that provides a conceptual framework to explicate and explore the cognitive mechanisms, processes, and outcomes that underscore and accompany perfectionism. It is a process model in that the cognitive aspects of perfectionism reflect the ongoing situational challenges and developing circumstances. But it also recognizes that cognitive tendencies such as rumination tend to be trait-like and our particular interest is in describing and understanding the perfectionist who habitually and chronically engages in types of rumination that are largely maladaptive.

Our initial version of PCT is an extension of the theoretical views outlined previously by Flett, Hewitt, Blankstein, and Gray (1998). The main tenets of PCT are as follows: (1) Perfectionism is associated with quicker onset and more frequent onset of rumination as well as a greater persistence of rumination; quicker onset and longer persistence of rumination are both implicated uniquely in risk for depression (Grafton & MacLeod, 2013); (2) Perfectionism is linked with a vast array of types of recurrent thoughts and forms of cognitive perseveration, including some types of overthinking that are quite unique to perfectionism and distinguish it from other personality vulnerabilities. These various types of thinking are described in more detail below; (3) The overthinking of perfectionists is associated with few benefits, but many predictable costs and consequences, such as deficits in attentional capacity and working memory during times of stress. Some costs and consequences are also described in more detail below; (4) Excessive cognitive activation and perseveration leads to an overdeveloped memory for mistakes, failures, and stressful experiences that highlight a sense of personal inadequacy. The high cognitive salience of past mistakes and failures among perseverating perfectionists is accompanied by a hypervigilance and cognitive bias toward related cues that signal the possibility of failure, mistakes, and negative social evaluations; (5) The ruminative thinking linked with perfectionism is a key contributor to health and mental health problems and amplified stress; (6) The impact of negative ruminations will be especially amplified among those perfectionists who engage in overgeneralization of the self (i.e., the belief that one flaw reflects the entire self) and who are focused on personally needing to be perfect (i.e., being the perfect person, having the perfect life, etc.) according to a fixed mindset that emphasizes a dispositional, entity view of the self. These perfectionists will have a chronically elevated level of self-focused attention that increases the intensity of emotional reactions such as shame and makes it more difficult to limit rumination and to have emotional self-control and cognitive and emotional self-regulation; and (7) The metacognitive aspects of perfectionism include the emphasis on emotional perfectionism that David Burns (1980) described in his early work. Because negative emotions signal falling short of the ideal of perfection, perfectionists are prone to becoming distressed about being distressed and this fuels their already-elevated level of rumination. This emotional perfectionism and associated metacognitive beliefs contribute to a strong desire to correct and improve the self and distract oneself so that negative emotions are avoided as much as possible.

Parenthetically, it should be noted that PCT is based largely on the contention that the ruminative tendencies of perfectionists reflect the type of thinking that people have when they have not achieved an important goal, as described by scholars such as Martin and Tesser (1989); however, this tendency to ruminate is a byproduct of several other contributing factors, including an unresolved need for social approval and acceptance and related concerns about negative social evaluation in keeping with recent evidence of the role of social evaluation threats in rumination (Zoccola, Dickerson, & Lam, 2012). This rumination is largely self-focused, and it highlights the discrepancy between the self (actual and unwanted/undesirable self) and the ideal, perfect self.

While our focus is largely on perfectionism, it is also important to note that work on perfectionism and rumination has clear implications in terms of advancing understanding of the nature of rumination as seen within the framework of Nolen-Hoeksema's (1991) response styles theory. For instance, the analyses that focus on the role of goal discrepancies in rumination (e.g., Watkins & Nolen-Hoeksema, 2014) should be qualified by recognizing the precipitating role of factors, such as perfectionism, that are likely to generate the goal discrepancies that ultimately elicit rumination about the goals or standards. The goals themselves and discrepancies from goals set the stage for ruminative brooding.

As for our proposed PCT, we will limit our focus to two key themes. First, we explore our contention that perfectionists are at risk for mental and physical health problems because they have many cognitive perseveration tendencies that are related to, but distinguishable from, cognitive worry and rumination. Table 6.3 lists several different types of automatic thoughts and rumination that have been linked with perfectionism, including procrastination-related automatic thoughts and negative automatic thoughts about the self. David Burns was among the first to discuss these negative self-thoughts (see Burns & Beck, 1978; Burns, 1980). Burns and Beck (1978) illustrated this by describing the depressed perfectionistic student who refused to take credit for her straight A's because she saw herself as lazy and incompetent according to all-or-none evaluative criteria. Burns (1980) suggested that these various negative thoughts involuntarily flood the mind of the perfectionist and

Table 6.3 Various types of cognition and recurrent thinking among perfectionists

Cognition category	Empirical examples
Anticipatory thinking	
Generalized worry	Buhr and Dugas (2006)
Hopelessness/negative future thinking	O'Connor, O'Connor, O'Connor, Smallwood, and Miles (2004)
Types of rumination	
Depressive and anxious rumination	Blankstein and Lumley (2008)
Mistake rumination	Besser, Flett, and Hewitt (2004)
Failure rumination	Hewitt et al. (2001)
Repetitive negative thinking	Macedo et al. (2015)
Post-event stress-related rumination	Brown and Kocovski (2014)
Work-related rumination	Flaxman, Menard, Bond, and Kinman (2012)
Anger rumination	Besharat and Shahidi (2010)
Types of frequent automatic thoughts	
Perfectionistic automatic thoughts	Flett, Hewitt, Blankstein, and Gray (1998)
Self-critical, negative automatic thoughts	Arpin-Cribbie and Cribbie (2007)
Procrastinatory automatic thoughts	Flett, Stainton, Hewitt, Sherry, and Lay (2012)
Bulimic automatic thoughts	Flett, Newby, Hewitt, and Persaud (2011)

they seem quite plausible to the perfectionist despite being quite irrational to other people. Burns (1980) also suggested that once the perfectionistic child has adopted a perfectionistic mindset, this mindset perpetuates itself quite easily. We go a step further in our work by showing that perfectionists are prone to various types of rumination, including ruminating about the need to be perfect.

Cognitive Perseveration as Automatic Thoughts Reflecting the Need to be Perfect

Flett and associates (1998) developed the Perfectionism Cognitions Inventory (PCI) to assess automatic thoughts reflecting the need to be perfect, such as "I must be perfect." The PCI is based on the premise that perfectionists who sense a discrepancy between their actual self and their ideal self, or between their actual level of attainment and their exceptionally high goals, will tend to experience thoughts that reflect perfectionistic themes. This conceptualization fits with the notion that certain people have a strong and highly salient ideal self-schema that facilitates selective attention recall of stimuli and outcomes signaling perfection as well as failures to be perfect and personal imperfections (see Hewitt & Genest, 1990). The PCI assesses the frequency of perfectionistic thoughts from "…a unique cognitive perspective" (Enns & Cox, 2002, p. 50) and while these thoughts are considered to be state-like, in reality, it can be considered ruminative thought in that people with high PCI scores tend to be obsessive. Numerous studies have confirmed that perfectionistic automatic thoughts contribute to maladjustment in that they tend to account for unique variance in psychological distress that is not accounted for by existing trait measures of perfectionism (Flett et al., 1998; Flett, Hewitt, Whelan, & Martin, 2007). The PCI is also linked to deficits in cognitive-emotion regulation and associated cognitive self-management deficits (see Flett et al., 2007; Rudolph, Flett, & Hewitt, 2007). As alluded to earlier, research indicates that the PCI is associated with health symptoms and that negative affect and daily hassles mediate the link between perfectionistic automatic thoughts and psychosomatic symptoms (Flett et al., 2012).

Two studies conducted have confirmed that the PCI is associated significantly with rumination, but not to the degree that they are redundant with each other (Flett, Madorsky, Hewitt, & Heisel, 2002; Rudolph et al., 2007). Flett et al. (2002) found that perfectionism cognitions, SOP, and SPP were all positively associated with a ruminative response orientation. The strongest correlate of rumination was perfectionism cognitions (r=.48), followed by SPP (r=.43). Perfectionism cognitions, SPP, and rumination were also associated with depression; the association between perfectionism cognitions and depression remained significant after controlling for rumination.

The tendency to experience perfectionistic automatic thoughts is also linked with worry. Flett, Coulter, Hewitt, & Nepon (2011) found among early adolescents that elevated PCI scores were associated jointly with rumination (r=.37) and worry (r=.39), as assessed by the children's version of the PSWQ. Supplementary analyses indicated that rumination mediated the link between the PCI and depressive symptoms.

As part of the validation of the PCI, Flett et al. (1998) administered the Distressing Thoughts Questionnaire (DTQ; Clark & Hemsley, 1985) which taps distressing thoughts and images related to anxiety and depression. Respondents are provided with six depression items (e.g., "thoughts and images that I am a failure") and six anxiety items (e.g., "thoughts or images that something is, or may in the future be wrong with my health"), rated across six response dimensions: frequency, sadness, worry, removal, guilt, and belief. The analyses showed that the PCI had significant correlations across all six response dimensions for both anxiety and depression items. Thus, people who experience frequent rumination about the need to be perfect also tend to report experiencing thoughts and images typically associated with depression and anxiety, and these thoughts and images add to their overall worry.

Finally, Lakey and Tanner (2013) conducted two studies in which participants completed the PCI various times to assess their thinking about people in their lives (i.e., mother, father, and friend). The analyses from Study 1 indicated that PCI scores experienced in these interpersonal contexts were positively associated with pathological worry. Perfectionistic thoughts were also negatively correlated with positive affect, appearance self-esteem, and positively correlated with negative affect and dysfunctional attitudes. The second study replicated these findings and found that perfectionistic automatic thoughts were linked with lower levels of optimism and higher levels of hopelessness.

Perfectionism and Stress-Related Forms of Cognitive Perseveration

The development of the PCI and the subsequent creation of another multidimensional measure of perfectionistic thinking (Stoeber, Kobori, & Tanno, 2010) have understandably resulted in a tendency for perfectionism researchers to focus primarily on this type of ruminative thinking. However, our survey of clinical cases and our encounters with people struggling with their perfectionism points to several other types of overthinking that seem implicated in exacerbating and prolonging the stress and distress of perfectionists. We will briefly discuss other relevant types of cognitive perseveration.

Mistake Rumination

The defining feature of the sadness and demoralization experienced chronically by some perfectionists is their inability to stop thinking about a mistake that they have made. Their sadness is fuelled by a sense of shame and incompetence about being exposed publicly in a way that cannot be recovered from and their remorse is often out of proportion to the importance of the mistake. This was the case for one perfectionist, referred to as Mr. C, receiving treatment from the third author. Mr. C lost his job primarily by his inability to stop ruminating about a mistake he made in a published work; this began a chain of events that resulted in a near fatal suicide attempt (see Hewitt & Flett, 2007). This emphasis on ruminating about a mistake that one is personally responsible for is a common theme among perfectionistic people suffering from post-traumatic stress, but it occurs in more benign situations as well. For instance, the perfectionistic student described by Burns and Beck (1978) presented earlier had a tendency to ruminate about her mistakes on a test after the test was over even when she did exceptionally well overall.

At present, there is only a limited degree of published empirical research on perfectionism and cognitive rumination over mistakes. A key study was conducted by Frost and Henderson (1991) in which a sample of female athletes provided structured reports of their thoughts in the 24 h prior to competition. The authors found that perfectionists had a greater propensity to experience such cognitive reactions as "Images of me making a mistake clog my mind." A subsequent daily diary investigation by Frost, Trepanier, Brown, & Heimberg (1997) focused on rumination about mistakes found evidence suggesting that the perceived importance of a mistake is a catalyst for cognitive perseveration. That is, participants with a high level of COM reported more thoughts about an important mistake, not about less important mistakes. Subsequent experimental research also established an association between trait perfectionism and rumination about mistakes (Besser, Flett, & Hewitt, 2004). In light of these findings, one team of investigators included a subscale tapping rumination about past mistakes, past performance outcomes, and possible future mistakes as part of their scale called the Perfectionism Inventory (see Hill et al., 2004).

Currently, we are in the process of supplementing our research with the PCI by developing an inventory that requires people to reflect on an important personal mistake and report their ongoing degree of cognitive perseveration about this mistake. Respondents are asked to indicate the extent to which they have had thoughts such as "Why can't I stop making mistakes like this?" and to indicate the extent to which they still think about their mistake and wish it had gone better. Work on this measure is still in its early phases, but the initial results are in keeping with expectations. Mistake rumination is associated significantly with SOP and SPP, as well as various indices of distress, and is associated with higher scores on the PCI and a measure of procrastination-related automatic thoughts. Importantly, initial results confirm that our new measure of mistake rumination accounts uniquely for psychological distress beyond the variance attributable to the PCI.

Rumination and Post-Event Thinking

One way to interpret mistake rumination is that it is a form of post-event cognitive perseveration. A growing number of studies indicate that this tendency to engage in ruminative thinking and other cognitive activity is not limited to making mistakes. Earlier, we alluded to the research linking perfectionism with a tendency to experience frequent counterfactual thoughts about "what might have been" (see Sirois et al., 2010). This research was conducted with a focus on the concept of falling short of perfectionistic standards and being discrepant. A link between perfectionism and counterfactual thinking was posited originally by Flett et al. (1998) as part of their discussion of perfectionistic automatic thoughts, and it is likely that future research using the PCI will establish a more robust link between perfectionism and counterfactual thinking than is currently recognized.

Other research by Nepon, Flett, Hewitt, & Molnar (2011) highlights the tendency of people high in social perfectionism to ruminate about stressful interpersonal events involving the people in their lives. Specifically, they investigated the associations among trait perfectionism, perfectionistic self-presentation, negative social feedback, interpersonal rumination, depressive symptoms, and social anxiety in a sample of students. The results confirmed that SPP and perfectionistic self-presentation were associated significantly with rumination following interpersonal events (i.e., being hurt, humiliated, and mistreated) as well as a reported history of negative social feedback. In addition, depressive symptoms and social anxiety were associated with negative social feedback, interpersonal rumination, trait perfectionism, and perfectionistic self-presentation. Additional analyses indicated that interpersonal rumination mediated the links between aspects of social perfectionism and distress. Overall, the results indicated clearly that self-reported receipt of frequent negative feedback from others and engaging in rumination about an interpersonal event play important roles in the distress experienced by individuals with high levels of perfectionism.

Another study points to the tendency to ruminate after being engaged in performance situations involving the possibility of negative evaluation. Brown and Kocovski (2014) examined the roles of both trait and state perfectionism on post-event rumination in a longitudinal study of students with elevated social anxiety. Students completed measures of rumination and distress, trait perfectionism (COM, DAA, and SPP), and modified versions to assess state perfectionism during an anxiety-inducing speech task. Two days later, post-event rumination was assessed. Both state and trait perfectionism dimensions were positively correlated with trait rumination. These state and trait perfectionism facets also predicted post-event rumination after 2 days, while controlling for initial levels of social anxiety, state anxiety, and depression.

Similarly, a study showed that after being required to give a brief speech, perfectionism predicted post-event rumination 24 h later (Cox & Chen, 2014). Post-event rumination was tapped by such thoughts as "I looked stupid." Perfectionism in this study was assessed with DAA and SPP, and both of these factors were also linked robustly with social anxiety.

Social Comparison Rumination

Another line of investigation in our laboratory is focusing on individual differences in rumination about how one compares with others. To our knowledge, our focus on individual differences in social comparison rumination is unique. The possibility of individual differences in social comparison rumination is supported by test anxiety research from Irwin Sarason. In their classic work on worry and cognitive interference, Sarason and colleagues incorporated a focus on thoughts related to social comparison as part of their class work on worry and cognitive interference. Indeed, the Cognitive Interference Questionnaire includes an item about thinking about how other students are doing during a test situation (see Sarason, 1978).

Our work in this area was inspired by a key observation made earlier by Nolen-Hoeksema and her colleagues. Treynor, Gonzalez, and Nolen-Hoeksema (2003) conducted a content analysis of what students were brooding about and they noted explicitly that "…social comparison was a key aspect of the brooding factor in this study" (pp. 257–258). This emphasis on social comparison thoughts is also reflected in the brooding scale item "Why do I have problems other people don't have?" Nolen-Hoeksema (2003) also emphasized this theme in her book *Women Who Think Too Much*.

We believe that there is a strong cognitive element to social comparison, and this element is highly relevant to an understanding of perfectionists who are constantly ruminating about the performance and stature of colleagues and competitors who are standard setters. The original classic work by Albert Bandura and his colleagues had much to say about the self-reward and self-evaluative tendencies of people with perfectionistic standards; Bandura and his colleagues showed convincingly that children will learn to imitate the exacting standards for self-reward displayed by an adult model (Bandura, Grusec, & Menlove, 1967; Bandura & Kupers, 1964; Bandura & Whelan, 1966). In addition, Bandura (1971) astutely described the dangers of social comparison for people with exacting standards. He observed that, "Many of the people who seek psychotherapy are behaviorally competent and free of debilitating anxiety, but they experience a great deal of personal distress stemming from excessively high standards of self-evaluation often supported by unfavorable comparisons with models noted for their extraordinary achievements." (p. 31). Similarly, Burns (1980) emphasized the profound upset of high-achieving perfectionists used to being "number one" who could not cope with being in the middle of the pack when competing with very talented students.

It is our contention that these unfavorable comparisons often include an obsessive cognitive preoccupation with one's standing relative to others who are or appear to be doing exceptionally well; for many perfectionists, their cognitive preoccupation with social comparison goes well beyond performance situations to include life comparisons across various life domains and personal attributes (e.g., physical appearance). This cognitive preoccupation with social comparison information adds to the distress and dissatisfaction of perfectionists.

We are now in the process of conducting research to evaluate the usefulness of a newly created brief self-report measure of social comparison rumination. Respondents indicate the extent of their agreement with items, such as "When someone does better than me, I spend a lot of time wondering why" and "I have been thinking a lot about how other students are doing versus how I am doing." Our initial work suggests that meaningful individual differences in social comparison rumination can be detected among children, adolescents, and emerging adults. For instance, in one study, social comparison rumination was associated significantly with SOP, SPP, and various facets of perfectionistic self-presentation (r's ranging from .30 to .54). Social comparison rumination was also associated significantly with a self-report depression measure ($r=.30$). We believe that this cognitive preoccupation with social comparison information is fuelled by the self-doubt and self-uncertainty of perfectionists, but it is just as likely that social comparison is contributing to this self-doubt and self-uncertainty.

The potential relevance of social comparison rumination was illustrated by the results of a new study. Specifically, we explored the associations among trait and self-presentational perfectionism, social comparison rumination, and both physical and mental health. The results revealed that SPP and all facets of perfectionistic self-presentation were positively linked with social comparison rumination and poorer mental health, while SPP and two facets of perfectionistic self-presentation were associated with poorer physical health (see Table 6.4). Social comparison rumination was also linked with poorer mental and physical health.

A related study explored the links among dimensions of trait and self-presentational perfectionism, mistake rumination, social comparison, depression, and student burnout. As can be seen in the lower portion of Table 6.4, SOP, SPP, and the three facets of perfectionistic self-presentation were positively correlated with mistake rumination, social comparison rumination, and depression. All dimensions of trait and self-presentational perfectionism were positively associated with the exhaustion subscale of student burnout, while SPP and perfectionistic self-presentation were positively linked with the cynicism subscale of student burnout. In addition, both mistake rumination and social comparison rumination were linked with higher levels of depression, exhaustion, and cynicism.

Table 6.4 Correlations between trait and self-presentational perfectionism and key rumination and well-being variables—Studies 1 and 2

Measures	SOP	OOP	SPP	Promote	Nondisplay	Nondisclose
Study 1						
SC rumination	.07	.01	.49**	.41**	.65**	.50**
Physical health	.03	.008	−.30**	−.12	−.22**	−.40**
Mental health	.03	.05	−.42**	−.22**	−.44**	−.40**
Study 2						
Mistake rumination	.34**	−.02	.39**	.39**	.50**	.36**
SC rumination	.35**	−.06	.51**	.51**	.58**	.44**
Depression	.26**	−.02	.48**	.35**	.38**	.36**
Burnout-exhaustion	.28**	.17*	.35**	.31**	.39**	.26**
Burnout-cynicism	.13	.12	.36**	.31**	.36**	.32**

SOP self-oriented perfectionism, *OOP* other-oriented perfectionism, *SPP* socially prescribed perfectionism, *Promote* perfectionistic self-promotion, *Nondisplay* nondisplay of imperfection, *Nondisclose* nondisclosure of imperfection, and *SC Rumination* social comparison rumination
$N=233$ for Study 1; $N=227$ for Study 2. * $p<.05$, ** $p<.01$, two-tailed

What are some of the costs and consequences of chronic cognitive perseveration for perfectionists such as Mike and Tom? Some of the possible costs and consequences for "perseverating perfectionists" are now briefly outlined. It should be noted from the outset that these costs and consequences have not been studied extensively by researchers, and these various themes reflect key directions for additional research.

The Costs and Consequences of Cognitive Perfectionism

Our analysis of the cognitive aspects of perfectionism is based on the presumption that this cognitive perfectionism contributes to the vulnerability of certain perfectionists and this translates into health and mental health problems. We conclude our chapter by exploring these costs in more detail and outlining key directions for future research. We begin by exploring the potential cost in terms of cognitive functioning.

Diminished Attention and Cognitive Capacity

When emotional events activate obsessive thinking, especially events that evoke strong feelings of negative arousal, perseverating perfectionists will be more likely to lack the attentional capacity to attend to other stimuli, especially when thoughts about being imperfect are predominant. Indeed, a new conceptual model details the limitations in attentional processing that accompany chronic rumination (see

Whitmer & Gotlib, 2013), and some data indicate that rumination is linked with reductions in elements of executive functioning (e.g., Connolly et al., 2014). This link with attentional problems has troubling implications for perfectionists at school or work who characteristically brood, but must learn and remember new material.

Some empirical support for the diminished cognitive capacity of ruminating perfectionists was provided by Flett et al. (1998) in their description of the correlates of the PCI. High PCI scorers reported performance difficulty as well as attentional control problems and mind wandering. These cognitive difficulties would be exacerbated among perseverating perfectionists who are engaging in various forms of overthinking and who have contemporary experiences (e.g., key mistakes) that are distracting them.

Longer Lasting Negative Emotions and Stress Reactions

Rumination should also contribute to more intense and longer lasting negative emotions and stress reactions. Implicit in our earlier description of the emotional preoccupation found among perfectionists with chronic health problems is the notion that ruminating perfectionists will tend to have negative emotions that persist. This proposed set of costs is in keeping with indications that trait perfectionism is associated with both state depression and chronic depression (Hewitt, Flett, Ediger, Norton, & Flynn, 1998). The study conducted with cardiac patients found that both trait perfectionism and perfectionistic self-presentation were correlated significantly with the component of the Type D distress prone personality that involves chronic negative emotionality (see Shanmugasegaram et al., 2014). An important point to underscore here is that the perfectionism measures were associated with chronic negative emotionality and with the social inhibition component of the Type D style; this is quite alarming given the link between Type D and risk of death.

Research examining the features and experiences of 27 emotions clearly indicates that rumination has its strongest link with persistent sadness (Verduyn & Lavrijsen, 2015). This finding has clear implications for perseverating perfectionists given the evidence we have presented thus far; distressed and stressed vulnerable perfectionists should have prolonged negative emotionality in ways that can protract and exacerbate the existing emotional distress, stress, and negative arousal, which help set the stage for experiencing health problems.

The extended diathesis-stress perfectionism model presented by Hewitt and Flett (2002) outlined several mechanisms implicated in the psychological distress of perfectionists, including stress anticipation, stress generation, stress perpetuation, and stress reactivity. This model can easily be extended to include vulnerability to health problems. Most importantly, a tendency to engage in worry, rumination, and other forms of cognitive perseveration is relevant to at least three mechanisms—stress anticipation, stress perpetuation, and stress reactivity. Thus, perseverating perfectionists can be at risk simply because of their ruminative ways, but they can also be at risk indirectly via these stress mechanisms.

Emotional and Physical Exhaustion

Emotional and physical exhaustion are likely byproducts of the tendency for stress reactive perfectionists to brood and worry. A third negative consequence for perseverating perfectionists is that they are likely prone to mental and physical exhaustion, and other forms of burnout due to the mental toll that accompanies cognitive perseveration and the constant pressure to be perfect. Exhaustion, burnout, and a sense of depletion are also likely when perfectionism gets translated into excessive and relentless striving. These proposed associations are in keeping with established links among obsessive passion, an inability to stop engaging in work-related rumination, and emotional exhaustion (see Donahue et al., 2012).

A link between perfectionistic overthinking and exhaustion has been documented in research which showed that the PCI was linked with burnout in terms of physical and emotional exhaustion (Hill & Appleton, 2011). A susceptibility to exhaustion was also demonstrated by Flaxman, Menard, Bond, & Kinman (2012) in a prospective study of academic employees on a holiday respite. A key finding that emerged was that the mood state and well-being of the more perfectionistic employees, relative to the less-perfectionistic employees, deteriorated to a greater extent upon returning to work, and this was mediated by their elevated levels of cognitive perseveration. A work-related rumination scale was created by adapting individual items from measures of worry, rumination, and the PCI (e.g., "I was worried about mistakes I have made or might make at work"). This measure was linked significantly with perfectionism ($r=.29$), and weekly measures of exhaustion and fatigue (r's ranging from .34 to .63) in a manner suggesting that workaholic perfectionists maintain a cognitive focus on work-related matters in ways that deplete them, both emotionally and physically.

Our discussion focused on only three negative consequences, but there are several other costs and consequences that likely follow from perfectionists' tendency to habitually engage in worry, rumination, and other forms of overthinking. For instance, we have not discussed the potential social consequences that follow from being highly ruminative and self-focused; it is quite plausible that the tendencies described in the current chapter can alienate other people and contribute to the social disconnection and loneliness that tends to be experienced by people with a pressure to be perfect. Indeed, Lyubomirsky et al. (2015) have summarized evidence suggesting that ruminators are less likely than nonruminators to elicit social support.

We also maintain that the chronic rumination experienced by many perfectionists is antithetical to a more protective cognitive orientation involving mindfulness. There are clear advantages to experiencing life in the here and now; but, for perseverating perfectionists, rather than experiencing life as it unfolds, they are very busy as they actively and tenaciously strive to meet impossible goals. We have illustrated throughout our chapter that this "busyness" is clearly evident at the cognitive level.

Summary and Future Directions

The current chapter introduced the framework of perfectionism cognition theory and illustrated three central themes: (1) both SOP and SPP and other dimensions reflecting evaluative concerns perfectionism (e.g., COM) are associated consistently with worry and rumination; (2) perfectionists are prone to several interrelated forms of cognitive perseveration (i.e., failure and mistake rumination, social comparison rumination, post-event rumination); and (3) in keeping with an expanded diathesis-stress perspective, the tendency to worry and ruminate contributes jointly to emotional distress and physical health problems.

One reason to "shine a light" on the cognitive aspects of perfectionism and to propose this initial version of perfectionism cognition theory is that there are several potentially important directions for future research, including the need for cross-sectional and longitudinal research on perfectionism, rumination, and physical illness. It is also important to identify factors that contribute to and underscore the link between perfectionism and rumination so that interventions can target these factors. Other key issues for further investigation can be extrapolated from a key review paper by Watkins (2008) who raised the possibility that there can be a constructive side to rumination. Is there an aspect that is actually constructive? Or is the constructive aspect perceived rather than actual? Many perfectionists believe that they will fall apart if they abandon their perfectionism—does this extend to their views of worry and rumination? Watkins (2008) also illustrated the need to consider the external and intrapersonal contexts when examining the association between rumination and psychological distress. What roles do these factors play in perfectionism and rumination and worry? Clearly, the level and types of stressors being experienced merit an extensive consideration. A person-focused approach that considers other cognitive-based personality styles such as the tendency to experience frequent thoughts involving procrastination and avoidance should also be considered.

As we noted in a commentary paper on the nature of perfectionistic automatic thoughts (see Flett & Hewitt, 2014b), research and clinical assessments have reinforced our sense that the cognitive perseveration inherent in dysfunctional perfectionism is largely about the issues involving the self and personal identity. That is, worry, rumination, and associated thoughts and images can be traced back to the fact that many people have a core need to be flawless in all aspects of their lives to compensate for feelings of unworthiness and self-doubt. We noted in this commentary that the type of overthinking should perhaps be conceptualized as "perfectionistic self-rumination." This emphasis on the self is important to keep in mind when trying to gain a better understanding of how and when cognitive perseveration will translate into health problems. Perfectionists who feel ashamed, inadequate, and perhaps humiliated will be highly stressed, and this stress will be amplified if they respond to coping challenges by constantly ruminating and worrying. Viewed from this perspective, the prolonged distress that comes from ruminating is a salient reminder to these vulnerable people that they are far from perfect, and they are imperfect in ways that are not easily remedied by people who tend to stringently apply all-or-none standards when evaluating their performance, their capabilities, and their longstanding and deeply ingrained personality attributes.

References

Aldao, A., Nolen-Hoeksema, S., & Schweizer, S. (2010). Emotion-regulation strategies across psychopathology: A meta-analytic review. *Clinical Psychology Review, 30,* 217–237.

Arpin-Cribbie, C. A., & Cribbie, R. A. (2007). Psychological correlates of fatigue: Examining depression, perfectionism, and automatic negative thoughts. *Personality and Individual Differences, 43,* 1310–1320.

Bandura, A. (1971). *Social learning theory*. New York: General Learning Press.

Bandura, A., & Kupers, C. J. (1964). Transmission of patterns of self-reinforcement through modeling. *Journal of Abnormal and Social Psychology, 69,* 1–9.

Bandura, A., Grusec, J. E., & Menlove, F. L. (1967). Some social determinants of self-monitoring reinforcement systems. *Journal of Personality and Social Psychology, 5,* 449–455.

Bandura, A., & Whelan, C. K. (1966). The influence of antecedent reinforcement and divergent modeling cues on patterns of self-reward. *Journal of Personality and Social Psychology, 3,* 373–382.

Besharat, M. A., & Shahidi, S. (2010). Perfectionism, anger, and anger rumination. *International Journal of Psychology, 45,* 427–434.

Besharat, M. A., Issazadegan, A., Etemadinia, M., Golssanamlou, S., & Abdolmanafi, A. (2014). Risk factors associated with depressive symptoms among undergraduate students. *Asian Journal of Psychiatry, 10,* 21–26.

Besser, A., Flett, G. L., & Hewitt, P. L. (2004). Perfectionism, cognition, and affect in response to performance failure vs. success. *Journal of Rational-Emotive and Cognitive Behavior Therapy, 22,* 301–328.

Blankstein, K. R., & Lumley, C. H. (2008). Multidimensional perfectionism and ruminative brooding in current dysphoria, anxiety, worry and anger. *Journal of Rational- Emotive and Cognitive-Behavior Therapy, 26,* 168–193.

Blankstein, K. R., Flett, G. L., Hewitt, P. L., & Eng, A. (1993). Dimensions of perfectionism and irrational fears: An examination with the fear survey schedule. *Personality and Individual Differences, 15,* 323–328.

Borkovec, T. D., Metzger, R. L., & Pruzinsky, T. (1986). Anxiety, worry, and the self. In L. M. Hartman & K. R. Blankstein (Eds.), *Perception of self in emotional disorder and psychotherapy* (pp. 219–260). New York: Plenum Press.

Borkovec, T. D., Alcaine, O., & Behar, E. (2004). Avoidance theory of worry and generalized anxiety disorder. In R. G. Heimberg, C. L. Turk, & D. S. Mennin (Eds.), *Generalized anxiety disorder: Advances in research and practice* (pp. 77–108). New York: Guilford Press.

Brosschot, J. F, Gerin, W., & Thayer, J. F. (2006). The preservative cognition hypothesis: A review of worry, prolonged stress-related physiological activation, and health. *Journal of Psychosomatic Research, 60,* 113–124.

Brown, J. R., & Kocovski, N. L. (2014). Perfectionism as a predictor of post-event rumination in a socially anxious sample. *Journal of Rational-Emotive and Cognitive-Behavior Therapy, 32,* 150–163.

Buhr, K., & Dugas, M. J. (2006). Investigating the construct validity of intolerance of uncertainty and its unique relationship with worry. *Journal of Anxiety Disorders, 20,* 222–236.

Burns, D. D. (1980). *Feeling good: The new mood therapy*. New York: New American Library.

Burns, D. D., & Beck, A. T. (1978). *Cognitive behavior modification of mood disorders* (pp. 109–134). London; Plenum Press.

Burns, L. R., & Fedewa, B. A. (2005). Cognitive styles: Links with perfectionistic thinking. *Personality and Individual Differences, 38,* 103–113.

Chang, E. C. (2006). Conceptualization and measurement of adaptive and maladaptive aspects of performance perfectionism: Relations to personality, psychological functioning, and academic achievement. *Cognitive Therapy and Research, 30,* 677–697.

Chang, E. C., Zumberg, K. M., Sanna, L. J., Girz, L. P., Kade, A. M., et al. (2007). Relationship between perfectionism and domains of worry in a college student population: Considering the role of BIS/BAS motives. *Personality and Individual Differences, 43,* 925–936.

Ciesla, J. A., & Roberts, J. E. (2007). Rumination, negative cognition, and their interactive effects on depressed mood. *Emotion, 7,* 555–565.

Clark, D. A., & Hemsley, D. R. (1985). Individual differences in the experience of depressive and anxious, intrusive thoughts. *Behaviour Research and Therapy, 23,* 625–633.

Connolly, S. L., Wagner, C. A., Shapero, B. G., Pendergast, L. L., Abramson, L. Y., et al. (2014). Rumination prospectively predicts executive functioning impairments in adolescents. *Journal of Behavior Therapy and Experimental Psychiatry, 45,* 46–56.

Costello, E., & Borkovec, T. D. (1992). Generalized anxiety disorder. In A. Freeman & F. M. Datillo (Eds.), *Casebook of cognitive therapy* (pp. 53–60). New York: Springer.

Cox, S. L., & Chen, J. (2014). Perfectionism: A contributor to social anxiety and its cognitive processes. *Australian Journal of Psychology.*

Di Schiena, R., Luminet, O., Philippot, P., & Douilliez, C. (2012). Adaptive and maladaptive perfectionism in depression: Preliminary evidence of the role of adaptive and maladaptive rumination. *Personality and Individual Differences, 53,* 774–778.

Donahue, E. G., Forest, J., Vallerand, R. J., Lemyre, P. N., Crevier-Braud, L., & Bergeron, E. (2012). Passion for work and emotional exhaustion: The mediating role of rumination and recovery. *Applied Psychology Health and Well-Being, 4,* 341–368.

Egan, S. J., Hattaway, M., & Kane, R. T. (2014). The relationship between perfectionism and rumination in post traumatic stress disorder. *Behvavioural and Cognitive Psychotherapy, 42,* 211–223.

Endler, N. S., Edwards, J. M., & Vitelli, R. (1991). *Endler multidimensional anxiety scales (EMAS): manual.* Los Angeles: Western Psychological Services.

Enns, M. W., & Cox, B. J. (2002). The nature and assessment of perfectionism. In G. Flett & P. Hewitt (Eds.), *Perfectionism: Theory, research, and treatment* (pp. 33–62). Washington, DC: American Psychological Association.

Essau, C. A., Leung, P. W. L., Conradt, J., Cheng, H., & Wong, T. (2008). Anxiety symptoms in Chinese and German adolescents: Their relationship with early learning experiences, perfectionism, and learning motivation. *Depression and Anxiety, 25,* 801–810.

Flaxman, P. E., Menard, J., Bond, F.W., & Kinman, G. (2012). Academics' experiences of a respite from work: Effects of self-critical perfectionism and perseverative cognition on postrespite well-being. *Journal of Applied Psychology, 97,* 854–865.

Flett, G. L. & Hewitt, P. L. (2014a). The assessment of perfectionism. In G. J. Boyle, D. H. Saklofske, & G. Matthews (Eds.), *Measures of personality and social psychological constructs* (Vol. 2, pp. 595–618). London: Elsevier.

Flett, G. L. & Hewitt, P. L. (2014b). The multidimensional assessment of perfectionistic automatic thoughts: A commentary on "Examining mutual suppression effects in the assessment of perfectionism cognitions: Evidence supporting multidimensional assessment." *Assessment, 21,* 661–665.

Flett, G. L., Hewitt, P. L., Endler, N. S., & Tassone, C. (1994/1995). Perfectionism and components of state and trait anxiety. *Current Psychology, 13,* 326–350.

Flett, G. L., Hewitt, P. L., Blankstein, K. R., & Gray, L. (1998). Psychological distress and the frequency of perfectionistic thinking. *Journal of Personality and Social Psychology, 75,* 1363–1381.

Flett, G. L., Madorsky, D., Hewitt, P. L., & Heisel, M. J. (2002). Perfectionism cognitions, rumination, and psychological distress. *Journal of Rational-Emotive and Cognitive-Behavior Therapy, 20,* 33–47.

Flett, G. L., Hewitt, P. L., Oliver, J. M., & Macdonald, S. (2002). Perfectionism in children and their parents: A developmental analysis. In G. Flett & P. Hewitt (Eds.), *Perfectionism: Theory, research, and treatment* (pp. 89–132). Washington, DC: American Psychological Association.

Flett, G. L., Hewitt, P. L., Whelan, T., & Martin, T. R. (2007). The Perfectionism Cognitions Inventory: Psychometric properties and associations with distress and deficits in cognitive self-management. *Journal of Rational-Emotive and Cognitive-Behavior Therapy, 25,* 255–277.

Flett, G. L., Newby, J., Hewitt, P. L., & Persaud, C. (2011). Perfectionistic automatic thoughts, trait perfectionism, and bulimic automatic thoughts in young women. *Journal of Rational-Emotive and Cognitive-Behavior Therapy, 29,* 192–206.

Flett, G. L., Baricza, C., Gupta, A., Hewitt, P. L., & Endler, N. S. (2011). Perfectionism, psychosocial impact and coping with irritable bowel disease: A study of patients with crohn's disease and ulcerative colitis. *Journal of Health Psychology, 16,* 561–571.

Flett, G. L., Coulter, L., Hewitt, P. L., & Nepon, T. (2011). Perfectionism, rumination, worry, and depressive symptoms in early adolescents. *Canadian Journal of School Psychology, 26,* 159–176.

Flett, G. L., Hewitt, P. L., Demerjian, A., Sturman, E. D., Sherry, S. B., & Cheng, W. (2012). Perfectionistic automatic thoughts and psychological distress in adolescents: An analysis of the perfectionism cognitions inventory. *Journal of Rational-Emotive and Cognitive-Behavior Therapy, 30,* 91–104.

Flett, G. L., Molnar, D. S., Nepon, T., & Hewitt, P. L. (2012). A mediational model of perfectionistic automatic thoughts and psychosomatic symptoms: The roles of negative affect and daily hassles. *Personality and Individual Differences, 52,* 565–570. doi:10.1016/j.paid.2011.09.010.

Flett, G. L., Stainton, M., Hewitt, P. L., Sherry, S. B., & Lay, C. (2012). Procrastination automatic thoughts as a personality construct: An analysis of the procrastinatory cognitions inventory. *Journal of Rational-Emotive and Cognitive-Behavior Therapy, 30,* 223–236.

Frost, R. O., & Henderson, K. J. (1991). Perfectionism and reactions to athletic competitions. *Journal of Sport and Exercise Psychology, 13,* 323–335.

Frost, R. O., Marten, P., Lahart, C., & Rosenblate, R. (1990). The dimensions of perfectionism. *Cognitive Therapy and Research, 14,* 449–468.

Frost, R. O., Trepanier, K. L., Brown, E. J., & Heimberg, R. G. (1997). Self-monitoring of mistakes among subjects high and low in perfectionistic concern over mistakes. *Cognitive Therapy and Research, 21,* 209–222.

Frost, R. O., Turcotte, T. A., Heimberg, R. G., Mattia, J. I., Holt, C. S., et al. (1995). Reactions to mistakes among subjects high and low in perfectionistic concern over mistakes. *Cognitive Therapy and Research, 19,* 195–205.

Gentes, E. L., & Ruscio, A. M. (2014). Perceptions of functioning in worry and generalized anxiety disorder. *Cognitive Therapy and Research, 38,* 518–529.

Grafton, B., & MacLeod, C. (2013). Don't start what you can't stop: Differentiating individual differences in ruminative onset and ruminative persistence, and their contributions to dysphoria. *Emotion, 13,* 1080–1085.

Gray, J. A. (1991). *The neuropsychology of temperament.* New York: Plenum Press.

Handley, A. K., Egan, S. J., Kane, R. T., & Rees, C. S. (2014). The relationships between perfectionism, pathological worry and generalised anxiety disorder. *BMC Psychiatry, 14,* 98–105.

Harris, P. W., Pepper, C. M., & Maack, D. J. (2008). The relationship between maladaptive perfectionism and depressive symptoms: The mediating role of rumination. *Personality and Individual Differences, 44,* 150–160.

Hewitt, P. L., Caelian, C. F., Flett, G. L., Sherry, S. B., Collins, L., et al. (2002). Perfectionism in children: Associations with depression, anxiety, and anger. *Personality and Individual Differences, 32,* 1049–1061.

Hewitt, P. L., & Flett, G. L. (1991). Perfectionism in the self and social contexts: Conceptualization, assessment, and association with psychopathology. *Journal of Personality and Social Psychology, 60,* 456–470.

Hewitt, P. L., & Flett, G. L. (2002). Perfectionism and stress processes in psychopathology. In G. L. Flett & P.L. Hewitt (Eds.), *Perfectionism: Theory, research, and treatment* (pp. 255–284). Washington, DC: American Psychological Association.

Hewitt, P. L., & Flett, G. L. (2004). *Multidimensional perfectionism scale: Technical manual*. Toronto: Multi-Health Systems Inc.
Hewitt, P. L., & Flett, G. L. (2007). When does conscientiousness become perfectionism? *Current Psychiatry, 6,* 49–60.
Hewitt, P. L., Flett, G. L., Turnbull-Donovan, W., & Mikail, S. F. (1991). The multidimensional perfectionism scale: Reliability, validity, and psychometric properties in psychiatric samples. *Psychological Assessment, 3,* 464–468.
Hewitt, P. L., Flett, G. L., Ediger, E., Norton, G. R., & Flynn, C. (1998). Dimensions of perfectionism and chronic symptoms of unipolar and bipolar depression. *Canadian Journal of Behavioural Science, 30,* 234–242.
Hewitt, P. L., & Genest, M. (1990). The ideal self: Schematic processing of perfectionistic content in dysphoric university students. *Journal of Personality and Social Psychology, 59,* 802–808.
Hill, A. P., & Appleton, P. R. (2011). The predictive ability of the frequency of perfectionistic cognitions, self-oriented perfectionism, and socially prescribed perfectionism in relation to symptoms of burnout in youth rugby players. *Journal of Sports Sciences, 29,* 695–703.
Hill, R. W., Huelsman, T. J., Furr, M., Kibler, J., Vicente, B. B., & Kennedy, C. (2004). A new measure of perfectionism: The Perfectionism Inventory. *Journal of Personality Assessment, 82,* 80–91.
Hoff, E. R., & Muehlenkamp, J. J. (2009). Nonsuicidal self-injury in college students: The role of perfectionism and rumination. *Suicide and Life-Threatening Behavior, 39,* 576–587.
Johnson, J. A., Key, B. L., Routledge, F. S., Gerin, W., & Campbell, T. S. (2014). High trait rumination is associated with blunted nighttime diastolic blood pressure dipping. *Annals of Behavioral Medicine, 48,* 384–391.
Kawamura, K. Y., Hunt, S. L., Frost, R. O., & Marten DiBartolo, P. (2001). Perfectionism, anxiety, and depression: Are the relationships independent? *Cognitive Therapy and Research, 25,* 291–301.
Key, B. L., Campbell, T. S., Bacon, S. L, & Gerin, W. (2008). The influence of trait and state rumination on cardiovascular recovery from a negative emotional stressor. *Journal of Behavioral Medicine, 31,* 237–248.
Khawaja, N.G., & Armstrong, K.A. (2005). Factor structure and psychometric properties of the frost multidimensional perfectionism scale: Developing shorter versions using an Australian sample. *Australian Journal of Psychology, 57,* 129–138.
Lakey, B., & Tanner, S. M. (2013). Social influences in negative thinking and affect. *Cognitive Therapy and Research, 37,* 160–172.
Leahy, R. (2002). Improving homework compliance in the treatment of generalized anxiety disorder. *Journal of Clinical Psychology, 58,* 499–511.
Lemaire, M., El-Hage, W., & Frangou, S. (2014). Reappraising suppression: Subjective and physiological correlates of experiential suppression in healthy adults. *Frontiers in Psychology, 5*(571), 1–9.
Lyubomirsky, S., Layous, K., Chancellor, J., & Nelson, K. S. (2015). The scholarly contributions and intellectual legacy of Susan Nolen-Hoeksema. *Annual Review of Clinical Psychology, 11,* 4.1–4.22.
Macedo, A., Marques, M., & Pereira, A.T. (2014). Perfectionism and psychological distress: A review of the cognitive factors. *Clinical Neurosciences and Mental Health, 1,* 6.
Macedo, A., Soares, M. J., Amaral, A. P., Nogueira, V., Madeira, N., Roque, C., … Pereira, A. T. (2015). Repetitive negative thinking mediates the association between perfectionism and psychological distress. *Personality and Individual Differences, 72,* 220–224.
Martin, L. L., & Tesser, A. (1989). Toward a motivational and structural theory of ruminative thought. In J. S. Vlema & J. A. Bargh (Eds.), *Unintended thought* (pp. 306–326). New York: Guilford Press.
McCullough, M. E., Orsulak, P., Brandon, A., & Akers, L. (2007). Rumination, fear, and cortisol: An in vivo study of interpersonal transgressions. *Health Psychology, 26,* 126–132.
Meyer, T. J., Miller, M. L., Metzger, R. L., & Borkovec, T. D. (1990). Development and validation of the Penn State Worry questionnaire. *Behaviour Research and Therapy, 28,* 487–495.

Nepon, T., Flett, G. L., Hewitt, P. L., & Molnar, D. S. (2011). Perfectionism, negative social feedback, and interpersonal rumination in depression and social anxiety. *Canadian Journal of Behavioral Science, 43,* 297–308.
Nolen-Hoeksema, S. (1991). Responses to depression and their effects on the duration of depressive episodes. *Journal of Abnormal Psychology, 100,* 569–582.
Nolen-Hoeksema, S. (2003). *Women who think too much.* New York: St. Martin's Griffin.
Nolen-Hoeksema, S., Morrow, J., & Fredrickson, B. L. (1993). Response styles and the duration of episodes of depressed mood. *Journal of Abnormal Psychology, 102,* 20–28.
Nolen-Hoeksema, S., Wisco, B. E., & Lyubomirsky, S. (2008). Rethinking rumination. *Perspectives on Psychological Science, 3,* 400–424.
O'Connor, D. B., O'Connor, R. C., & Marshall, R. (2007). Perfectionism and psychological distress: Evidence of the mediating effects of rumination. *European Journal of Personality, 21,* 429–452.
O'Connor, R. C., O'Connor, D. B., O'Connor, S. M., Smallwood, J., & Miles, J. (2004). Hopelessness, stress, and perfectionism: The moderating effects of future thinking. *Cognition and Emotion, 18,* 1099–1120.
Olson, M. L., & Kwon, P. (2008). Brooding perfectionism: Refining the roles of rumination and perfectionism in the etiology of depression. *Cognitive Therapy Research, 32,* 788–802.
Papadakis, A. A., Prince, R. P., Jones, N. P., & Strauman, T. J., (2006). Self-regulation, rumination, and vulnerability to depression in adolescent girls. *Development and Psychopathology, 18,* 815–829.
Randles, D., Flett, G. L., Nash, K. A., McGregor, I. D., & Hewitt, P. L. (2010). Dimensions of perfectionism, behavioral inhibition, and rumination. *Personality and Individual Differences, 49,* 83–87.
Roelofs, J., Papageorgiou, C., Gerber, R. D., Huibers, M., Peeters, F., & Arntz, A. (2007). On the links between self-discrepancies, rumination, metacognitions, and symptoms of depression in undergraduates. *Behaviour Research and Therapy, 45,* 1295–1305.
Rudolph, S. G., Flett, G. L., & Hewitt, P. L. (2007). Perfectionism and deficits in cognitive emotion regulation. *Journal of Rational-Emotive and Cognitive-Behavior Therapy, 25,* 343–357.
Rukmini, S., Sudhir, P. M., & Math, S. B. (2014). Perfectionism, emotion regulation and their relationship to negative affect in patients with social phobia. *Indian Journal of Psychological Medicine, 36,* 239–245.
Ruscio, A. M., Seitchik, A. E., Gentes, E. L., Jones, J. D., & Hallion, L. S. (2011). Perseverative thought: A robust predictor of response to emotional challenge in generalized anxiety disorder and major depressive disorder. *Behaviour Research and Therapy, 49,* 867–874.
Santanello, A. W., & Gardner, F. L. (2006). The role of experiential avoidance in the relationship between maladaptive perfectionism and worry. *Cognitive Therapy and Research, 30,* 319–332.
Sarason, I. G. (1978). The test anxiety scale: Concept and research. In C. D. Spielberger & I. G. Sarason (Eds.), *Stress and anxiety* (Vol. 5, pp. 193–216). Washington, DC: Hemisphere Publishing Corporation.
Shanmugasegaram, S., Flett, G. L., Madan, M., Oh, P., Marzolini, S., Reitav, J., Hewitt, P. L., & Sturman, E.C. (2014). Perfectionism, Type D personality, and illness-related coping styles in cardiac rehabilitation patients. *Journal of Health Psychology, 19,* 417–426.
Short, M. M., & Mazmanian, D. (2013). Perfectionism and negative repetitive thoughts: Examining a multiple mediator model in relation to mindfulness. *Personality and Individual Differences, 55,* 716–721. doi:10.1016/j.paid.2013.05.026.
Sirois, F. M., Monforton, J., & Simpson, M. (2010). "If only I had done better": Perfectionism and the functionality of counterfactual thinking. *Personality and Social Psychology Bulletin ,36,* 1675–1692.
Slaney, R. B., Rice, K. G., Mobley, M., Trippi, J., & Ashby, J. S. (2001). The almost perfect scale–revised. *Measurement and Evaluation in Counseling and Development, 34,* 130–145.
Smári, J., Olason, D. T., Eypórsdóttir, A., & Frölunde, M. B. (2007). Psychometric properties of the obsessive compulsive inventory-revised among Icelandic college students. *Scandinavian Journal of Psychology, 48,* 127–133.

Soo, H., Burney, S., & Basten, C. (2009). The role of rumination in affective distress in people with a chronic physical illness: A review of the literature and theoretical formulation. *Journal of Health Psychology, 14,* 956–966.

Spasojevic, J., & Alloy, L. B. (2001). Rumination as a common mechanism relating depressive risk factors to depression. *Emotion, 1,* 25–37.

Stöber, J., & Joormann, J. (2001). Worry, procrastination, and perfectionism: Differentiating amount of worry, pathological worry, anxiety, and depression. *Cognitive Therapy and Research, 25,* 49–60.

Stoeber, J., Kobori, O., & Tanno, Y. (2010). The multidimensional perfectionism cognitions inventory—english (MPCI-E): Reliability, validity, and relationships with positive and negative affect. *Journal of Personality Assessment, 92,* 16–25.

Tallis, F., Eysenck, M., & Mathews, A. (1992). A questionnaire for the measurement of nonpathological worry. *Personality and Individual Differences, 13,* 161–168.

Terry-Short, L. A., Owens, R. G., Slade, P. D., & Dewey, M. E. (1995). Positive and negative perfectionism. *Personality and Individual Differences, 18,* 663–668.

Thomsen, D. K., Mehlsen, M. Y., Hokland, M., Viidik, M., Olesen, F., et al. (2004). Negative thoughts and health: Associations among rumination, immunity, and health care utilization in a young and elderly sample. *Psychosomatic Medicine, 66,* 363–371.

Treynor, W., Gonzalez, R., & Nolen-Hoeksema, S. (2003). Rumination reconsidered: A psychometric analysis. *Cognitive Therapy and Research, 27,* 247–259.

Verduyn, P., & Lavrijsen, S. (2015). Which emotions last longest and why: The role of event importance and rumination. *Motivation and Emotion, 39,* 119–127.

Verduyn, P., & Lavrijsen, S. (in press). Which emotions last longest and why: The role of event importance and rumination. *Motivation and Emotion.*

Verkuil, B., Brosschot, J. F., Gebhardt, W. A., & Thayer, J. F. (2011). Perseverative cognition, psychopathology, and somatic health. In I. Nyklicek (Ed.), *Emotion regulation and well-being* (pp. 85–100). New York: Springer.

Watkins, E. R. (2008). Constructive and unconstructive repetitive thought. *Psychological Bulletin, 134,* 163–206.

Watkins, E. R., & Nolen-Hoeksma, S. (2014). A habit-goal framework of depressive rumination. *Journal of Abnormal Psychology, 123,* 24–34.

Whiting, S. E., Jenkins, W. S., May, A. C., Rudy, B. M., Davis, T. E., & Ruether, E. T. (2014). The role of intolerance of uncertainty in social anxiety subtypes. *Journal of Clinical Psychology, 70,* 260–272.

Whitmer, A. J., & Gotlib, I. H. (2013). An attentional scope model of rumination. *Psychological Bulletin, 139,* 1036–1061.

Wilson, C., Hunter, S. C., Rasmussen, S., & McGowan, A. (in press). They made you perfect: A test of the social reaction model of perfectionism. *Aggressive Behavior.*

Zoccola, P., Dickerson, S. S., & Lam, S. (2012). Eliciting and maintaining ruminative thought: The role of social-evaluative threat. *Emotion, 12,* 673–677.

Chapter 7
Personal Standards and Self-Critical Perfectionism and Distress: Stress, Coping, and Perceived Social Support as Mediators and Moderators

David M. Dunkley, Shauna Solomon-Krakus and Molly Moroz

Since 2007, an annual nationwide Stress in America survey has been commissioned by the American Psychological Association (e.g., 2014) that illustrates year after year a growing stress-induced public health crisis. Stress has been associated with the development of most major mental health problems, such as depression and anxiety disorders (e.g., Marin et al., 2011), and has been linked to all leading physical causes of death, including heart disease, cancer, and stroke (e.g., Cohen, Janicki-Deverts, & Miller, 2007). Furthermore, stress is indirectly related to increased physical health problems through negative health behaviors, such as smoking, alcohol and drug abuse, and lack of sleep (Ellis, Gehrman, Espie, Riemann, & Perlis, 2012; Herman, 2012; Kassel, Stroud, & Paronis, 2003).

Perfectionism has emerged as an important cognitive-personality factor that has a negative impact on the stress and coping process and heightens vulnerability to a variety of psychological problems, including depression, anxiety, and eating disorders (see Bardone-Cone et al., 2007; Egan, Wade, & Shafran, 2011; Flett & Hewitt, 2002b; Shafran & Mansell, 2001 for reviews). Perfectionism has also been associated with poorer physical health (Molnar, Sadava, Flett, & Colautti, 2012), lower health functioning in existing chronic conditions (Molnar, Flett, et al., 2012), and

D. M. Dunkley (✉)
Institute of Community and Family Psychiatry, Jewish General Hospital,
4333 Cote Ste. Catherine Road, Montreal, QC H3T 1E4, Canada
e-mail: david.dunkley@mcgill.ca

D. M. Dunkley · S. Solomon-Krakus · M. Moroz
Department of Psychiatry, Lady Davis Institute—Jewish General Hospital,
4333 Cote Ste. Catherine Road, Montreal, QC H3T 1E4, Canada

D. M. Dunkley · S. Solomon-Krakus
Department of Psychiatry, McGill University,
1033 Pine Avenue West, Montreal, QC H3A 1A1, Canada

D. M. Dunkley · M. Moroz
Department of Psychology, McGill University, 1205 Dr. Penfield Avenue,
H3A 1B1 Montreal, QC, Canada

F. M. Sirois, D. S. Molnar (eds.), *Perfectionism, Health, and Well-Being,*
DOI 10.1007/978-3-319-18582-8_7

early mortality (Fry & Debats, 2009). In addition, perfectionism has been found to have adverse effects on the therapeutic process and treatment outcomes (see Blatt & Zuroff, 2005; Kannan & Levitt, 2013). The general purpose of the present chapter is to examine the mediating and moderating roles of daily stress, coping, and perceived social support in the relation between self-critical and personal standards perfectionism dimensions and distress symptoms (i.e., depression, anxiety) in hopes of addressing what might constitute more effective prevention and intervention efforts for highly perfectionistic individuals.

Personal Standards and Self-Criticism Dimensions of Perfectionism: Differential Relations with Distress

Over the past two decades, the perfectionism construct has become viewed as a multidimensional construct and has been conceptualized and defined in many different ways (see Flett & Hewitt, 2002a). Three multidimensional conceptualizations have generated considerable interest, including those of Hewitt and Flett (1991), Frost and colleagues (Frost, Marten, Lahart, & Rosenblate,1990), and Slaney and colleagues (Slaney, Rice, Mobley, Trippi, & Ashby, 2001). Hewitt and Flett (1991) conceptualized the perfectionism construct as consisting of both intrapersonal (i.e., self-oriented perfectionism) and interpersonal (i.e., other-oriented perfectionism, socially prescribed perfectionism) dimensions. On the other hand, Frost and colleagues (1990) considered perfectionism to be comprised of several different aspects, including personal standards, concern over mistakes, doubts about actions, parental expectations, parental criticism, and organization. Finally, Slaney and colleagues (2001) conceptualized high standards and order as adaptive aspects of perfectionism and discrepancy (i.e., perceived inability to meet high standards set for the self) as the essential defining negative component of perfectionism.

Factor analytic studies have consistently identified two higher-order dimensions of perfectionism that underlie the many different perfectionism constructs and measures, with one dimension having both maladaptive and adaptive aspects and the other dimension being primarily maladaptive (see Dunkley, Blankstein, Masheb, & Grilo, 2006; Stoeber & Otto, 2006). These two higher-order dimensions have been referred to as *personal standards* (*PS*) *perfectionism* and *self-critical* (*SC*) *perfectionism*, respectively (e.g., Dunkley, Zuroff, & Blankstein, 2003). PS perfectionism involves the setting of and striving for high standards and goals for oneself. PS measures include the self-oriented perfectionism scale of the Hewitt and Flett (1991) Multidimensional Perfectionism Scale (HMPS), the personal standards scale of the Frost et al. (1990) Multidimensional Perfectionism Scale (FMPS), and the high standards scale of the Slaney et al. (2001) revised Almost Perfect Scale (APS-R). On the other hand, SC perfectionism involves constant and harsh self-scrutiny and overly critical self-evaluation tendencies that are closely linked with chronic concerns about others' criticism and disapproval (e.g., Dunkley et al., 2003). SC perfectionism measures include HMPS socially prescribed perfectionism, FMPS concern over mistakes, FMPS doubts about actions, APS-R discrepancy, as well as the self-criticism scores of the Depressive Experiences Questionnaire (DEQ; Blatt, D'Afflitti, & Quinlan, 1976) and the Dysfunctional Attitudes Scale (DAS; Weissman & Beck, 1978), respectively. In contrast to PS measures, SC perfectionism measures have been consistently related to depressive and anxious symptoms (see Dunkley, Blankstein, et al., 2006; Stoeber & Otto, 2006). Further, several studies have supported SC perfectionism as a prospective predictor of psychosocial maladjustment over periods ranging from several months (e.g., Rice, Leever, Christopher, & Porter, 2006; Sherry, Mackinnon, Macneil, & Fitzpatrick, 2013) to several years (Dunkley, Mandel, & Ma, 2014; Dunkley, Sanislow, et al., 2006, 2009).

Cognitive appraisals and coping are emphasized as critical explanatory processes in the relation between stressful person-environment relations and outcomes by the cognitive theory of psychological stress and coping developed by Lazarus and colleagues (e.g., Lazarus & Folkman, 1984). Both dispositional and situational factors play a role in the stress and coping process. Changes in stress, cognitive appraisals, and coping occur across situational contexts in perfectionistic individuals who can also be characterized as having stable traits of stress, cognitive appraisals, and coping (Dunkley, Mandel, et al., 2014; Dunkley et al., 2003). A growing body of literature has examined the dispositional and situational influences of perfectionism on the stress, appraisal, and coping process as an explanation for its relations with both negative and positive aspects of well-being. Three sections follow. First, we review several mediation studies that have tested theoretical models with stress, coping, and perceived social support as trait-like correlates of perfectionism that can explain how or why SC and PS dimensions are differentially associated with well-being outcomes. Second, we review several moderation studies that have examined certain types of stressors, appraisals, and coping strategies that determine when the relation between perfectionism dimensions and (mal)adjustment is maximized or minimized. Third, as stress has predominantly been assessed in previous studies using self-report measures, we examine emerging evidence that demonstrates the impact of perfectionism on physiological measures of stress (e.g., cortisol).

Structural Models of the Relation Between Perfectionism and Distress: Stress, Coping, and Perceived Social Support as Mediators

To understand the link between SC perfectionism and distress symptoms in depression and anxiety, it is necessary to examine the possible mediating mechanisms responsible for increased vulnerability to such negative outcomes, which, in turn, will inform prevention and intervention efforts. Several researchers have argued that SC perfectionism plays a role in the construction of a stressful environment (e.g., Blankstein & Dunkley, 2002; Hewitt & Flett, 2002; Zuroff, Mongrain, & Santor, 2004). Although there are many ways to group coping responses within the broad domain of coping, one of the oldest and most often used distinctions is between disengagement responses (e.g., avoidance), which are aimed at escaping the stressor and are emotionally negative, and engagement responses (e.g., problem-focused coping), which are aimed at dealing with the stressor and are emotionally positive (see Carver & Connor-Smith, 2010; Skinner, Edge, Altman, & Sherwood, 2003). Based on an integration of various theoretical perspectives, our conceptual model (Dunkley, Ma, Lee, Preacher, & Zuroff, 2014; Dunkley et al., 2003) considers in parallel disengagement and engagement tendencies that are organized around threats and challenges to competence and are differentially linked to negative affect and (lower) positive affect.

Several theorists have discussed how perfectionism develops in response to conditional parental approval that is conditional on attaining extremely high parental expectations of success and productivity (e.g., Blatt, 1995; Hamachek, 1978). Further, it has been theorized that the development of SC arises from exposure to a combination of excessive parental expectations as well as parental harshness and punitiveness (e.g., Blatt, 1995; Flett, Hewitt, Oliver, & Macdonald, 2002; Young, Klosko, & Weishaar, 2003). Individuals who possess higher levels of SC perfectionism are thought to instigate daily stress for themselves, as they tend to engage in harsh self-evaluations and magnify the negative aspects of events, thereby interpreting even mundane stressors as major threatening stressors (e.g., "I reviewed what I said in the meeting today, and I found so many things that I did not say or said mistakenly that I felt worse and worse"; see Dunkley et al., 2003; Hewitt & Flett, 2002). In addition, high-SC perfectionists fear interpersonal rejection and criticism from others, which is expressed through a defensive relational style that evokes more negative social interactions, and thus higher levels of daily stress (see Dunkley, Sanislow, et al., 2006; Flett, Hewitt, Garshowitz, & Martin, 1997; Zuroff et al., 2004). Individuals with higher SC perfectionism have a tendency to engage in avoidant coping resulting from their perceived inability to cope with stressful situations to their own and others' expectations and satisfaction (see Dunkley, Blankstein, Halsall, Williams, & Winkworth, 2000; Flett, Hewitt, Blankstein, Solnik, & Van Brunschot, 1996). An avoidant coping style, in turn, fails to address stressors directly, and thereby increases the severity and duration of stress, leading to a greater susceptibility to experience additional stressors (Carver & Connor-Smith, 2010; Dunkley et al., 2003). This tendency for individuals with higher SC perfectionism to engage in avoidant coping impedes their ability both to use other more adaptive coping strategies and to move past the distress related to stressful situations (e.g., "I stopped working and went home early. I kept thinking about the work I had not completed all evening and felt really sad and anxious"; see Carver & Connor-Smith, 2010; Dunkley et al., 2003).

In parallel, individuals with higher SC perfectionism often lack compensatory experiences of positive affect to provide a psychological respite because they typically do not utilize engagement resources and strategies (e.g., Dunkley, Ma, et al., 2014; Dunkley et al., 2003). Specifically, individuals with higher SC perfectionism often perceive that others are unwilling or unavailable to help them in times of stress (e.g., Dunkley et al., 2000). Subsequently, they lack an important resource (i.e., perceived social support) to encourage more adaptive coping strategies and make stressors seem less overwhelming. In contrast, individuals with higher PS have been theorized to internalize the high parental standards and actively strive to meet them (see Blatt, 1995; Hamachek, 1978). PS perfectionistic individuals may also experience higher levels of stress, but their tendency to engage in active and problem-focused coping appears to offset the potential negative outcomes of distress (see Dunkley et al., 2000).

Stress as a Mediator Several studies have examined stress as a single mediator between perfectionism and a wide range of outcomes, including depressive symptoms, positive and negative affect, satisfaction with life, and psychosocial functioning. For example, E. C. Chang (2000) demonstrated that total perfectionism, as measured by the FMPS, was related with negative affect, worry, and lower life satisfaction, respectively, through perceived stress in both younger and older adults. Similarly, perceived stress mediated the relation between SC perfectionism and lower psychological well-being in both Black and White female college students (Chang, Watkins, & Banks, 2004). Perceived stress also mediated the relations between SC perfectionism and three dimensions of psychological well-being (autonomy, environmental mastery, purpose of life) in college students (Chang, 2006). In other studies, the relationship between SC perfectionism and each of depressive symptoms and lower satisfaction with life was mediated by perceived stress in female undergraduate students (Ashby, Noble, & Gnilka, 2012). Further, stress mediated the relationship between SC perfectionism and depressive symptoms in bipolar patients (Corry et al., 2013), which demonstrates the generalizability of this model to a clinical sample. Finally, in a 16-week longitudinal study of Israeli adolescents, negative life events and lower positive life events mediated the effects of SC perfectionism on distress (Shahar & Priel, 2003).

Coping as a Mediator In addition to stress, coping has also been tested as an important mediator in the relation between SC perfectionism and various outcomes, including depressive symptoms, burnout, and anxiety. Several studies have looked at maladaptive coping (e.g., avoidant, emotion-focused) and problem-focused coping as potential mediators. In our initial study, we found that the relation between SC perfectionism and distress in undergraduate students was mediated by maladaptive (e.g., emotion-focused) coping (Dunkley & Blankstein, 2000). In another study of undergraduate students (Noble, Ashby, & Gnilka, 2014), the relation between PS perfectionism and lower depressive symptoms was mediated by higher problem-focused coping and lower avoidant coping, while the relation between SC perfectionism and depressive symptoms was mediated by avoidant coping. In another study of undergraduate students (Gnilka, Ashby, & Noble, 2012), ineffective coping processes (e.g., escape–avoidance) mediated the relationship between SC perfectionism and anxiety. In addition, Weiner and Carton (2012) demonstrated in a study of college participants that avoidant coping mediated the relation between SC perfectionism and test anxiety. In a study of junior elite athletes (Hill, Hall, & Appleton, 2010), the relation between PS perfectionism and lower athlete burnout was mediated by problem-focused coping and lower avoidant coping, whereas the relation between SC perfectionism and athlete burnout was mediated by avoidant coping. Similarly, emotion-focused coping mediated the relation between SC perfectionism and burnout in a sample of Taiwanese nurses (Chang, 2012).

Lower Perceived Social Support as a Mediator Perceived social support has also been established as a mediator between SC perfectionism and depressive symptoms. The relation between SC perfectionism and depressive symptoms was partially mediated by lower perceived social support in a study of undergraduate students (Sherry, Law, Hewitt, Flett, & Besser, 2008). Further, a test of a 3-wave mediational model in a sample of patients demonstrated that negative perceptions of social support at 3 years mediated the relation between Time 1 SC perfectionism and depression over 4 years (Dunkley et al., 2009).

Stress, Coping, and Lower Perceived Social Support as Simultaneous Mediators Studies have also examined stress, avoidant coping, and perceived social support simultaneously as three mediators in the relation between SC perfectionism and distress. In our first investigation of this model (Dunkley et al., 2000), we found that daily hassles, avoidant coping, and lower perceived social support were all unique mediators that fully explained the relationship with SC perfectionism and distress in university students. The generalizability of these findings has been examined in different populations. In a study of university professors, avoidant coping and hassles mediated the relation between SC perfectionism and distress, but perceived social support did not mediate this relationship (Dunn, Whelton, & Sharpe, 2006). In our study of patients over 3 years, the relation between Time 1 SC perfectionism and depressive symptoms 3 years later was explained by negative social interactions, avoidant coping, and lower perceived social support (Dunkley, Sanislow, et al., 2006).

Daily Diary Studies: Stress, Coping, and Lower Perceived Social Support as Maintenance Factors Whereas most of these previous mediation studies used retrospective summary assessments of stress, coping, and perceived social support, we included a major methodological enhancement by using a daily diary approach and aggregating daily reports across several stressors to empirically derive maintenance measures of daily stress, appraisals, coping, and affect (Dunkley et al., 2003). In our study of university students, the relation between SC perfectionism and negative affect maintenance over 7 days was mediated by daily avoidant coping and stress maintenance factors, whereas the relation between SC perfectionism and the maintenance of lower positive affect over 7 days was mediated by event stress and lower perceived social support. In our 6-month follow-up study of community adults (Dunkley, Ma, et al., 2014), we incorporated an additional methodological advance by using multilevel structural equation modeling to provide unbiased estimates of between-cluster (or between-persons) means of several daily stress, coping, and affect reports for each participant, which allowed a more rigorous test of the indirect effects of perfectionism dimensions on maintenance of daily affect through stress and coping than previous studies. As shown in Fig. 7.1, the relation between SC perfectionism and daily negative affect maintenance 6 months later was mediated by daily avoidant coping and event stress maintenance factors, with avoidant coping

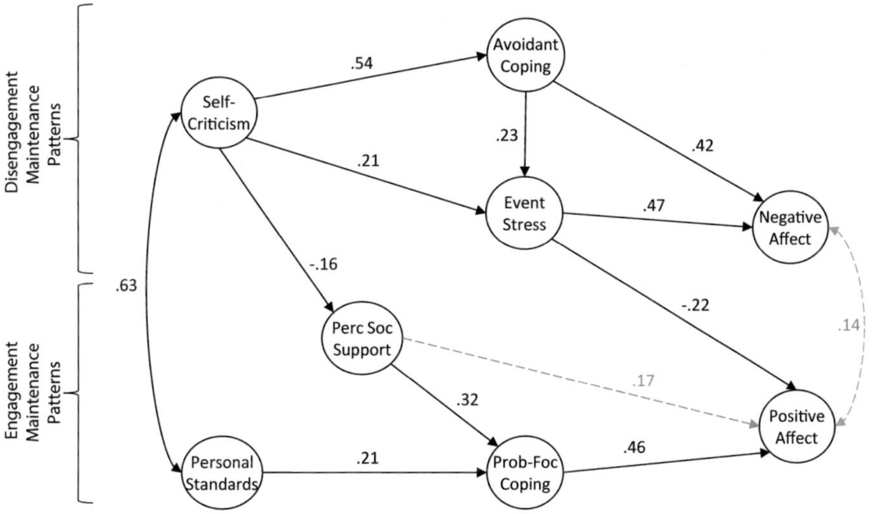

Figure 7.1 Standardized parameter estimates for the mediation model relating self-criticism and personal standards, avoidant and problem-focused coping, event stress, perceived social support, and negative and positive affect. Significant estimates are shown in *solid black* and nonsignificant estimates ($p > 0.05$) in *dashed grey*. *Perc Soc* Perceived Social, *Prob-Foc* Problem-focused. (Copyright © 2014 by the American Psychological Association. Reproduced with permission. The official citation that should be used in referencing this material is Reprinted from Dunkley et al., (2014). The use of APA information does not imply endorsement by APA.)

related to negative affect directly and negative and lower positive affect indirectly through its association with event stress. Our findings also indicated that SC perfectionism had an indirect association with the maintenance of lower positive affect 6 months later through lower perceived social support and problem-focused coping maintenance. Further, the adaptive potential of PS was exhibited by an indirect relation with positive affect through higher average daily problem-focused coping (Dunkley, Ma, et al., 2014).

In summary, the extant research consistently suggests that stress and avoidant coping are important characteristics associated with SC perfectionism that explains its association with different psychological problems that are often comorbid. Indeed, several studies indicate that SC perfectionism is not specific to depression and cuts across a wide variety of disorders, including social phobia, obsessive-compulsive disorder, and eating disorders (e.g., Bardone-Cone et al., 2007; Egan et al., 2011; Flett & Hewitt, 2002b). On the other hand, lower perceived social support might be specific to the experience of depression for individuals with higher SC perfectionism. In addition, a growing number of findings show that PS is indirectly associated with lower distress or higher positive affect through problem-focused tendencies, which illustrate secondary gains to having high personal standards that might make these individuals reluctant to lower their standards even a little bit (see Young et al., 2003).

Interactive Models of the Relation Between Perfectionism and Distress: Stress, Coping, and Perceived Social Support as Moderators

In addition to examining the associations between perfectionism, stress, coping, social support, and distress in structural models, several studies have tested the possibility that stress and coping moderate the link between PS and SC perfectionism and distress, respectively. This is particularly relevant to PS perfectionism because the often weak or negligible relation between PS perfectionism and distress calls for research to establish when the association between PS perfectionism and distress is amplified or diminished (see Dunkley et al., 2000). Indeed, a more complex association between self-oriented perfectionism and distress, in which other variables may moderate the relation (e.g., stress, coping), was initially proposed by Hewitt, Flett, and colleagues (Hewitt & Flett, 1993; Hewitt, Flett, & Endler, 1995).

Perfectionism General Vulnerability, Specific Vulnerability, and Stress-Regulation Models

General Vulnerability Model Several studies have supported a general perfectionism vulnerability model that maintains that individuals with higher levels of PS/SC perfectionism who are experiencing life stress will be especially vulnerable to psychological distress symptoms (e.g., Chang & Rand, 2000; Enns, Cox, & Clara, 1995; Flett, Hewitt, Blankstein, & Mosher, 1995). In a study of university students (Flett et al., 1995), both socially prescribed perfectionism and self-oriented perfectionism interacted with major life stress to predict higher levels of depressive symptoms in college students. As well, a relation was found between self-oriented perfectionism—but not socially prescribed perfectionism—and dysphoria 3 months later for students who had experienced a major life event. Similarly, for university students with higher SC perfectionism and for those with higher PS, we found daily hassles to be more strongly related to distress (Dunkley et al., 2000). On the other hand, several studies have found SC perfectionism measures, but not PS perfectionism measures, to interact with stress to predict distress outcomes. In a study of university students (Lynd-Stevenson & Hearne, 1999), SC perfectionism—but not PS perfectionism—moderated the relation between stressful life events and depressive symptoms. E. C. Chang and Rand (2000) found that socially prescribed perfectionism, but not self-oriented perfectionism, combined with self-appraised life stress to predict psychological symptoms and hopelessness 1 month later in university students. In a study of medical students, SC perfectionism measures (i.e., concern over mistakes, socially prescribed perfectionism), but not PS perfectionism measures, interacted with negative life events to predict increases in depression over 5 months (Enns et al., 2005).

In addition, there are some studies that have examined stress as a moderator of the association between SC perfectionism and suicidality. Psychiatric adolescents with higher socially prescribed perfectionism who had higher daily hassles were found to have an increased likelihood of concurrent suicide potential even after controlling for depression, hopelessness, and prior suicide attempt (Hewitt, Caelian, Chen, & Flett, 2014). Similarly, in a study of adolescent school children over a 6-month period (O'Connor, Rasmussen, & Hawton, 2010), PS perfectionism did not predict levels of self-harm, but SC perfectionism in combination with acute life stress predicted elevated levels of depression and self-harm 6 months later. In sum, although the general vulnerability model has been supported for both PS and SC perfectionism, research has more consistently demonstrated that individuals with higher SC perfectionism who are also experiencing higher stress have higher levels of distress symptoms.

Specific Vulnerability Model A large body of research has examined a specific vulnerability model: individuals with higher PS/SC perfectionism, who have contingent self-worth that is based on success and productivity (e.g., Sturman, Flett, Hewitt, & Rudolph, 2009), are theorized to be specifically vulnerable to achievement-related stressors that reflect personal failure and loss of control (see Blatt & Zuroff, 1992; Dunkley et al., 2003; Hewitt & Flett, 1993). Relatedly, because individuals with higher SC perfectionism have heightened sensitivity to criticism and disapproval from others, these individuals might experience more distress in response to negative social exchanges with others (see Dunkley et al., 2003; Hewitt & Flett, 1993). In a cross-sectional study, Hewitt and Flett (1993) found PS perfectionism combined with only achievement stressors to predict depression in depressed patients and general psychiatric patients. On the other hand, socially prescribed perfectionism interacted with interpersonal stressors in depressed patients and with achievement stressors in general psychiatric patients to predict depression. Similarly, SC perfectionism measures have been found to interact with both achievement hassles and interpersonal hassles to predict depression in female university students (Sherry, Hewitt, & Flett, 2003).

Three longitudinal studies have supported the hypothesis that individuals with higher PS/SC perfectionism are vulnerable to psychological distress symptoms in the context of achievement-related major life events (Enns & Cox, 2005; Enns et al., 2005; Hewitt, Flett, & Ediger, 1996). In a study of patients, Hewitt et al. (1996) found that self-oriented perfectionism combined only with achievement-related stress to predict depression 4 months later, whereas socially prescribed perfectionism did not interact with stress to predict depression over time. Similarly, Enns and Cox (2005) found that self-oriented perfectionism in conjunction with achievement life events predicted nonremission of depression symptoms over 1 year in a sample of depressed patients, whereas socially prescribed perfectionism did not interact with life events to predict nonremission of depressive symptoms. On the other hand, Enns et al. (2005) found that socially prescribed perfectionism—not self-oriented perfectionism—interacted with achievement-related stressors to predict greater hopelessness 5 months later in medical students. In sum, although there is some evidence to suggest that the relation between SC perfectionism and distress symptoms is even stronger for those who are also experiencing achievement and/or interpersonal stress, the findings are mixed. On the other hand, several studies have demonstrated that individuals with higher PS perfectionism who are also experiencing greater achievement-related stress have elevated levels of depressive symptoms.

Stress-Regulation Models Given that perfectionistic individuals have a heightened vulnerability to stress, it is important to discern whether certain coping strategies commonly exacerbate the negative impact of stressors or can serve a buffering role. A few studies have tested self-regulation models (e.g., Baumeister, 1990), which posit that individuals with perfectionistic standards who typically make use of maladaptive coping responses will be especially prone to maladjustment. For instance, in a sample of psychiatric patients, Hewitt and colleagues (1995) found that self-oriented perfectionism combined with higher levels of emotion-focused coping was associated with higher levels of depressive symptoms. Avoidant coping may be especially detrimental for individuals with higher PS/SC perfectionism in that it might add to the perception that they are failing or have failed to meet high expectations of success and productivity (O'Connor & O'Connor, 2003; Shafran, Cooper, & Fairburn, 2002). In a longitudinal study, individuals with higher SC perfectionism who reported greater use of avoidant coping had higher distress symptoms four to five weeks later (O'Connor & O'Connor, 2003). On the other hand, in our cross-sectional study, PS or SC perfectionism did not interact with avoidant coping to predict distress symptoms (Dunkley et al., 2000).

Perceived Social Support as a Buffer Given that perfectionism is considered to be a stress-generating mechanism, perfectionistic individuals with higher levels of perceived social support may be less prone to experience maladjustment than those with lower levels of perceived support. Two studies have supported the suggestion that perceived social support may buffer the impact of perfectionism on distress. We found that the relation between PS and SC perfectionism and distress was stronger for individuals who had more negative perceptions of social support than for those who had more positive perceptions of support (Dunkley et al., 2000). Similarly, Zhou, Zhu, Zhang, and Cai (2013) demonstrated that the relation between negative perfectionism and depressive and anxious symptoms is weaker for individuals with higher perceived social support than for those with lower perceived social support. On the other hand, Sherry et al. (2008) did not find evidence that the relation between self-oriented or socially prescribed perfectionism and depressive symptoms was moderated by perceived social support.

Although the mixed findings observed across studies might be interpreted as failure to fully support the moderator hypotheses, it is important to keep in mind that detecting moderator effects in designs and analyses such as these is difficult (see McClelland & Judd, 1993). Further, as the number of statistically significant interaction effects in theorized directions increases, the possibility that the effects are false-positive becomes unlikely (see Murayama, Pekrun, & Fiedler, 2014).

Differential Stress Reactivity and Coping Effectiveness Models: Within-Person Analyses

An important shortcoming of most research examining these moderator hypotheses is that between-persons designs and analyses were used, which address whether SC perfectionism in conjunction with individual differences in certain variables (e.g., stress) predicts individual differences in maladjustment. Moreover, these studies were based on single, one-occasion measures of the moderators and outcomes, which do not illuminate the common precipitants or triggers of an individual's distress. Conversely, in evidence-based interventions such as cognitive-behavior therapy (CBT), therapists focus on the present in collecting numerous specific instances of clients' thoughts, feelings, and behaviors for several cross sections of daily life (e.g., "I thought that I will never be able to write a good proposal and that my supervisor would think I am stupid, and I felt sad," "I procrastinated and had less time to do the report, and I felt really nervous and afraid about not doing the report to the standard that I would like"). Therapists then look for themes and patterns across several situations when clients' presenting problems are activated to ascertain common triggers (see Kuyken, Padesky, & Dudley, 2009).

Two of our studies of university students (Dunkley et al., 2003) and community adults (Dunkley, Mandel, et al., 2014) have addressed some of the limitations of previous research by using a daily diary approach to gather simultaneous measures of daily appraisals, coping, and affect for each individual across different stressors in their natural day-to-day lives. Consistent with CBT, within-person analyses examined whether within-person variations in appraisals and coping across many different stressors were linked to within-person fluctuations in daily affect, with participants serving as their own control across all the stressors that they reported.

Stress Reactivity We found support for the specific vulnerability hypothesis in that students with higher SC perfectionism, relative to students with lower SC perfectionism, exhibited greater increases in daily negative affect when they experienced more academic hassles and perceived criticism from others than usual, and less perceived control than usual (Dunkley et al., 2003). Further, we have examined the differential stress reactivity of individuals with higher perfectionism across the short and long term (Dunkley, Mandel, et al., 2014). Community adults completed daily diaries for 14 consecutive days repeatedly at 6-month and 3-year follow-ups. We found that for both adults higher on SC perfectionism and those higher on PS, compared to individuals lower on these dimensions, more event stress than usual was associated with greater increases in negative affect and sadness and greater decreases in positive affect at Month 6 and Year 3. We also found some support for the specific reactivity hypothesis in that adults with higher SC/PS perfectionism experienced greater increases in negative affect and sadness and greater decreases in positive affect at Year 3 when they perceived less control than usual. However, this finding was not replicated at Month 6. In addition, daily increases in depressive affect were connected to more negative social interactions than usual for SC perfectionists only at Month 6 and Year 3. Finally, our findings also highlighted conditions under which individuals with higher PS perfectionism feel more resilient than those with lower PS perfectionism. Specifically, adults with higher PS perfectionism had higher daily positive affect than adults with lower PS on days when they perceived less event stress (at Month 6 and Year 3), more control over their most bothersome event (at Year 3), and experienced fewer negative social interactions (at Year 3) than usual (Dunkley, Mandel, et al., 2014).

Coping (In)Effectiveness Three studies have examined whether certain coping strategies with most bothersome daily events may be especially (in)effective for perfectionistic individuals. We found that, across many different daily stressors, engaging in more self-blame than usual was coupled with greater increases in daily negative affect for university students higher on SC perfectionism than for those lower on SC perfectionism (Dunkley et al., 2003). In addition, using more problem-focused coping and less avoidant coping than usual was coupled with greater increases in daily positive affect for students with lower—but not higher—SC perfectionism, which indicates that problem-focused coping might be ineffective for those with higher SC perfectionism. On the other hand, across many different daily stressful situations, using more positive reinterpretation than usual was coupled with greater increases in daily positive affect for students with higher SC perfectionism (Dunkley et al., 2003). Stoeber and Janssen (2011) replicated this latter finding in showing that the more students with higher SC perfectionism used positive reinterpretation to deal with the day's most bothersome failures, the more satisfied they felt at the end of the day. Thus, cognitive reframing might work especially well for SC perfectionistic individuals.

As we found that community adults with higher levels of perfectionism have heightened reactivity to stress as they get older (Dunkley, Mandel, et al., 2014), it is important to examine the (in)effectiveness of coping strategies in adult populations because the cumulative burden of daily stressors may diminish their coping resources. We found more avoidant coping than usual was connected with greater increases in negative affect and sadness at Month 6 and Year 3 in adults who have higher levels of SC/PS perfectionism (Dunkley, Mandel, et al., 2014). Also, engaging in more problem-focused coping than usual was associated with greater decreases in sadness at Month 6 for adults with higher SC/PS perfectionism and with greater increases in positive affect at Month 6 for those with higher SC perfectionism. Previous theory and findings (e.g., O'Connor & O'Connor, 2003; Sturman et al., 2009) can help explain these findings. Individuals with higher perfectionism possess conditional self-worth that is contingent on success and productivity. When goals are not being met as expected, perfectionists believe that they are failing and feel heightened anxiety, irritability, and guilt (e.g., Blatt, 1995; Shafran et al., 2002; Young et al., 2003). On the other hand, we found that engaging in more positive reinterpretation than usual was associated with greater decreases in sadness for adults with higher SC perfectionism at Month 6 and Year 3 (Dunkley, Mandel, et al., 2014), which bolsters emerging evidence that perfectionistic individuals respond well to perceiving stressors as challenges rather than as threats (Dunkley et al., 2003; Stoeber & Janssen, 2011).

Overall, the extant literature suggests that perfectionism is an important moderator in the stress and coping process at both between-persons and within-person levels of analysis. At the between-persons level, perfectionism dimensions in combination with individuals differences in general stress, specific stressors (e.g., achievement, interpersonal), and maladaptive coping tendencies are associated with higher levels of distress symptoms. At the within-person level, individuals with higher perfectionism have heightened affective reactivity to changes in various stress appraisals and the use of certain coping strategies. These results can be explained by previous theory that proposes that conditional self-worth that is contingent on success and productivity is integral to different kinds of perfectionistic vulnerability, regardless of whether the emphasis is on unrelenting personal standards or overly self-critical evaluative tendencies (e.g., Blatt, 1995; Flett et al., 2002; Young et al., 2003).

The Impact of Perfectionism on Physiological Responses to Stress

One important shortcoming in the literature is that stress has typically been assessed using self-report measures, which does not allow for objective situation-specific aspects to be separated from subjective aspects of the individual stress response. A few studies have used a well-established paradigm, the Trier Social Stress Test (TSST; Kirschbaum, Pirke, & Hellhammer, 1993), to induce achievement-related stress. The TSST involves participants completing a simulated job interview and a highly demanding arithmetic task in front of a two-person committee. The TSST has been found to be effective at activating two major physiological systems activated during the stress response, the hypothalamic pituitary–adrenal (HPA) axis and the sympathetic nervous system.

Middle-aged men with higher SC perfectionism (as assessed by the FMPS concern over mistakes and doubts about actions subscales), in contrast to those with higher PS, were found to exhibit heightened HPA axis activation in response to the TSST (Wirtz et al., 2007). Specifically, an association between SC perfectionism scores and salivary cortisol stress reactivity, an indicator of HPA axis activity, was supported. In another study of adults (McGirr & Turecki, 2009), SC perfectionism (assessed by DEQ self-criticism) was not associated with increases in salivary cortisol, but SC perfectionism was associated with increases in salivary α-amylase, which is an indicator of sympathetic activity. On the other hand, a study of undergraduate students (Richardson, Rice, & Devine, 2014) found that the combination of SC and PS perfectionism was associated with a lower or blunted cortisol response to the TSST. The authors suggested that individuals with higher scores on both perfectionism dimensions experience chronic stress, which, in turn, leads to blunted cortisol stress responses because overactivation of the HPA axis eventually results in a hypoactive HPA axis (Richardson et al., 2014). Finally, in another study of university students (Zureck, Altstötter-Gleich, Wolf, & Brand, 2004), the combination of high levels of PS and high levels of SC perfectionism was associated with heightened affective arousal in response to the TSST. However, there were no main or interaction effects of PS and SC perfectionism for the HPA stress response.

In sum, there is emerging evidence to suggest that perfectionism plays an important role in modifying psychophysiological responses to psychosocial stress.

Clinical Implications

In considering the role of clients' perfectionism in the maintenance of distress, the findings reviewed in the present chapter further indicate that more clinical attention should be focused on self-critical evaluative tendencies than on high personal standards (e.g., Dunkley, Blankstein, et al., 2006). As SC perfectionism has exhibited an adverse impact on psychotherapeutic processes and outcomes (see Blatt & Zuroff, 2005; Egan et al., 2011; Kannan & Levitt, 2013), it is important to consider what might constitute more effective prevention/intervention for these individuals.

The mediational roles of stress and ineffective (e.g., avoidant) coping demonstrated in the extant literature suggest that interventions that target maintenance processes of ongoing stress and avoidant coping may be critical for alleviating the chronic distress of individuals with higher SC perfectionism (Dunkley et al., 2000; 2003). Deriving from empirical evidence (e.g., Dunkley et al., 2003) and the treatment literature (see Kannan & Levitt, 2013; Kelly & Zuroff, 2013), the heightened stress and avoidant coping tendencies of individuals with higher SC perfectionism might be addressed by helping these individuals diminish their tendency to destructively blame themselves across many stressors and increase their propensity to adopt more constructive approaches of habitually relating to themselves (e.g., from self-denigration to self-encouragement). The development of a more compassionate view by individuals with higher SC perfectionism might also decrease their perceptions of criticism from others and increase their perceptions of social support. Perceived social support might also be increased by helping individuals with higher SC perfectionism reconceptualize relationships with their family of origin, curb negative distortions in interpreting social interactions, and improve interpersonal communication skills (see Brand, Lakey, & Berman, 1995; Dunkley et al., 2000). This, in turn, might help change the tendency of individuals with higher SC perfectionism to engage in avoidant coping to a more habitual focus on problem-focused coping to bolster resilience (see Dunkley, Ma, et al., 2014; Dunkley et al., 2003).

The findings demonstrating the moderating role of stress and coping on the relation between perfectionism and distress suggest that the heightened vulnerability of perfectionistic individuals might be addressed in three ways. First, cognitive approaches can help individuals with higher SC/PS perfectionism reconceptualize their intensified vulnerability to stressors as a result, in part, of excessively controlling and/or harsh significant figures in childhood (see Young et al., 2003). This reattribution can be used to nurture more self-compassionate ways of relating to the self that are more adaptive (e.g., "When I make mistakes, it does not make me any less worthwhile as a person"; see Kannan & Levitt, 2013; Kuyken et al., 2009). Second, behavioral activation techniques can be adopted to specifically lessen avoidant coping and facilitate problem-focused coping to boost resilience for individuals when stressors occur (see Kuyken et al., 2009). Further, several findings suggest additional choice points for intervention of increasing perceptions of social support, perceived control, and positive reinterpretation, which can help decrease distress and foster resilience (e.g., Dunkley, Ma, et al., 2014; Dunkley, Mandel, et al., 2014). Finally, the findings reviewed in the present chapter suggest that individuals with higher SC perfectionism should be aided to transition from a reactive mode of responding habitually to stress (e.g., avoidance) to a response mode, in which they respond mindfully to stressors with awareness of consequences while working toward goals that are derived from their values (see Kuyken et al., 2009).

Future Directions

There are a number of limitations in the extant literature that should be addressed in future research. First, daily diary studies have assessed stress, coping, and affect only once a day. Future research should assess these variables multiple times throughout the day to better capture the dynamics of stress and coping processes as they unfold. This would also help ascertain the direction of causality among variables. Second, stress appraisals are very rapid and require more frequent measures than are possible using daily diaries. Future cognitive priming studies that expose individuals to experimental stimuli and examine subsequent cognitive reactions would be useful to better examine how stress and coping processes evolve. Third, as the majority of studies have relied on self-report measures, future studies might also want to supplement self-report measures with informant reports or assessments of observable behaviors (e.g., coping). Fourth, the majority of the research presented in this chapter focused on perfectionists' appraisals of and reactions to minor or daily stressors. It would be important to examine the role of stress appraisals and coping in response to major life events from different domains (e.g., interpersonal, achievement) because more severe negative events may have a greater effect on the onset of certain problems, such as depression (see Hammen, 2005). Fifth, the generalizability of these findings must be examined in various clinical and nonclinical populations, and in different age or sociocultural groups. It will be important to replicate and extend these findings in various psychopathologies (e.g., depression, anxiety disorders, eating disorders) as well as chronic illness populations (e.g., functional somatic syndromes). Finally, it will be important to develop and evaluate interventions integrating the various strategies outlined above to see whether treatment outcomes can be improved for individuals with higher perfectionism.

Conclusions

The present review underscores the importance of distinguishing between personal standards and self-critical dimensions in considering the role of perfectionism in the stress, coping, and adjustment process. A considerable amount of research has accumulated that confirms that the direct associations between self-critical perfectionism and various distress symptoms (e.g., depression, anxiety, negative affect, low positive affect) can be explained by its association with a number of maladaptive tendencies such as daily event stress, avoidant coping, and negative perceptions of social support. On the other hand, personal standards appears to be primarily linked to active, problem-focused coping, which might help protect these individuals to some degree from the negative impact of stress and negative mood. Interestingly, although PS and SC perfectionism exhibit very different associations with stress, coping, and perceived social support, both dimensions similarly interact with stress and coping to predict heightened levels of distress. Given the developing stress-induced public health crisis (e.g., American Psychological Association, 2014), continued research efforts are needed to better understand the contribution of perfectionism to this escalating problem to improve prevention and intervention efforts.

References

American Psychological Association. (2014). Stress in America: Are teens adopting adults' stress habits? http://stressinamerica.org. Accessed 25 March 2014.

Ashby, J. S., Noble, C. L., & Gnilka, P. B. (2012). Multidimensional perfectionism, depression, and satisfaction with life: Differences among perfectionists and tests of a stress-mediation model. *Journal of College Counseling, 15,* 130–143. doi:10.1002/j.2161-1882.2012.00011.x.

Bardone-Cone, A. M., Wonderlich, S. A., Frost, R. O., Bulik, C. M., Mitchell, J. E., Uppala, S., & Simonich, H. (2007). Perfectionism and eating disorders: Current status and future directions. *Clinical Psychology Review, 27,* 384–405. doi: 10.1016/j.cpr.2006.12.005.

Baumeister, R. F. (1990). Suicide as escape from self. *Psychological Review, 97*(1), 90–113.

Blankstein, K. R., & Dunkley, D. M. (2002). Evaluative concerns, self-critical, and personal standards perfectionism, hassles, coping, social support, and distress: A structural equation modeling strategy. In G. L. Flett & P. L. Hewitt (Eds.), *Perfectionism: Theory, research, and treatment* (pp. 285–315). Washington, DC: American Psychological Association.

Blatt, S. J. (1995). The destructiveness of perfectionism: Implications for the treatment of depression. *American Psychologist, 50,* 1003–1020. doi:10.1037/0003-066x.50.12.1003.

Blatt, S. J., & Zuroff, D. C. (1992). Interpersonal relatedness and self-definition: Two prototypes for depression. *Clinical Psychology Review, 12,* 527–562. doi: 10.1016/0272-7358(92)90070-o.

Blatt, S. J., & Zuroff, D. C. (2005). Empirical evaluation of the assumptions in identifying evidence based treatments in mental health. *Clinical Psychology Review, 25,* 459–486. doi:10.1016/j.cpr.2005.03.001.

Blatt, S. J., D'Afflitti, J. P., & Quinlan, D. M. (1976). Experiences of depression in normal young adults. *Journal of Abnormal Psychology, 85,* 383–389. doi:10.1037/0021-843X.85.4.383.

Brand, E. F., Lakey, B., & Berman, S. (1995). A preventive, psychoeducational approach to increase perceived social support. *American Journal of Community Psychology, 23,* 117–135. doi:10.1007/BF02506925.

Carver, C. S., & Connor-Smith, J. (2010). Personality and coping. *Annual Review of Psychology, 61,* 679–704. doi:10.1146/annurev.psych.093008.100352.

Chang, E. C. (2000). Perfectionism as a predictor of positive and negative psychological outcomes: Examining a mediation model in younger and older adults. *Journal of Counseling Psychology, 47,* 18–26. doi:10.1037/0022-0167.47.1.18.

Chang, E. C. (2006). Perfectionism and dimensions of psychological well-being in a college student sample: A test of a stress-mediation model. *Journal of Social and Clinical Psychology, 25,* 1001–1022. doi:10.1521/jscp.2006.25.9.1001.

Chang, Y. (2012). The relationship between maladaptive perfectionism with burnout: Testing mediating effect of emotion-focused coping. *Personality and Individual Differences, 53,* 635–639. doi: 10.1016/j.paid.2012.05.002.

Chang, E. C., & Rand, K. L. (2000). Perfectionism as a predictor of subsequent adjustment: Evidence for a specific diathesis-stress mechanism among college students. *Journal of Counseling Psychology, 47,* 129–137. doi:10.1037/0022-0167.47.1.129.

Chang, E. C., Watkins, A., & Banks, K. H. (2004). How adaptive and maladaptive perfectionism relate to positive and negative psychological functioning: Testing a stress-mediation model in black and white female college students. *Journal of Counseling Psychology, 51,* 93–102. doi:10.1037/0022-0167.51.1.93.

Cohen, S., Janicki-Deverts, D., & Miller, G. E. (2007). Psychological stress and disease. *Journal of the American Medical Association, 298,* 1685–1687. doi:10.1001/jama.298.14.1685.

Corry, J., Green, M., Roberts, G., Frankland, A., Wright, A., Lau, P., Mitchell, P. B. (2013). Anxiety, stress and perfectionism in bipolar disorder. *Journal of Affective Disorders, 151,* 1016–1024. doi:10.1016/j.jad.2013.08.029.

Dunkley, D. M., & Blankstein, K. R. (2000). Self-critical perfectionism, coping, hassles, and current distress: A structural equation modeling approach. *Cognitive Therapy and Research, 24,* 713–730. doi:10.1023/a:1005543529245.

Dunkley, D. M., Blankstein, K. R., Halsall, J., Williams, M., & Winkworth, G. (2000). The relation between perfectionism and distress: Hassles, coping, and perceived social support as mediators and moderators. *Journal of Counseling Psychology, 47,* 437–453. doi:10.1037/0022-0167.47.4.437.

Dunkley, D. M., Zuroff, D. C., & Blankstein, K. R. (2003). Self-critical perfectionism and daily affect: Dispositional and situational influences on stress and coping. *Journal of Personality and Social Psychology, 84,* 234–252. doi:10.1037/0022-3514.84.1.234.

Dunkley, D. M., Blankstein, K. R., Masheb, R. M., & Grilo, C. M. (2006). Personal standards and evaluative concerns dimensions of "clinical" perfectionism: A reply to Shafran et al. (2002, 2003) and Hewitt et al. (2003). *Behaviour Research and Therapy, 44,* 63–84. doi:10.1016/j.brat.2004.12.004.

Dunkley, D. M., Sanislow, C. A., Grilo, C. M., & McGlashan, T. H. (2006). Perfectionism and depressive symptoms 3 years later: Negative social interactions, avoidant coping, and perceived social support as mediators. *Comprehensive Psychiatry, 47,* 106–115. doi:10.1016/j.comppsych.2005.06.003.

Dunkley, D. M., Sanislow, C. A., Grilo, C. M., & McGlashan, T. H. (2009). Self-criticism versus neuroticism in predicting depression and psychosocial impairment for 4 years in a clinical sample. *Comprehensive Psychiatry, 50,* 335–346. doi:10.1016/j.comppsych.2008.09.004.

Dunkley, D. M., Ma, D., Lee, I. A., Preacher, K. J., & Zuroff, D. C. (2014). Advancing complex explanatory conceptualizations of daily negative and positive affect: Trigger and maintenance coping action patterns. *Journal of Counseling Psychology, 61,* 93–109. doi: 10.1037/a0034673.

Dunkley, D. M., Mandel, T., & Ma, D. (2014). Perfectionism, neuroticism, and daily stress reactivity and coping effectiveness 6 months and 3 years later. *Journal of Counseling Psychology, 61,* 616–633. doi:10.1037/cou0000036.

Dunn, J. C., Whelton, W. J., & Sharpe, D. (2006). Maladaptive perfectionism, hassles, coping, and psychological distress in university professors. *Journal of Counseling Psychology, 53,* 511–523. doi:10.1037/0022-0167.53.4.511.

Egan, S. J., Wade, T. D., & Shafran, R. (2011). Perfectionism as a transdiagnostic process: A clinical review. *Clinical Psychology Review, 31,* 203–212. doi:10.1016/j.cpr.2010.04.009.

Ellis, J. G., Gehrman, P., Espie, C. A., Riemann, D., & Perlis, M. L. (2012). Acute insomnia: Current conceptualizations and future directions. *Sleep Medicine Reviews, 16,* 5–14. doi:10.1016/j.smrv.2011.02.002.

Enns, M. W., & Cox, B. J. (2005). Perfectionism, stressful life events, and the 1-year outcome of depression. *Cognitive Therapy and Research, 29*, 541–553. doi:10.1007/s10608-005-2414-8.

Enns, M. W., Cox, B. J., & Clara, I. P. (2005). Perfectionism and neuroticism: A longitudinal study of specific vulnerability and diathesis-stress models. *Cognitive Therapy and Research, 29,* 463–478. doi:10.1007/s10608-005-2843-04.

Flett, G. L., & Hewitt, P. L. (2002a). Perfectionism and maladjustment: An overview of theoretical, definitional, and treatment issues. In G. L. Flett & P. L. Hewitt (Eds.), *Perfectionism: Theory, research, and treatment* (pp. 5–31): Washington, DC: American Psychological Association.

Flett, G. L., & Hewitt, P. L. (Eds.). (2002b). *Perfectionism: Theory, research, and treatment*. Washington, DC: American Psychological Association.

Flett, G. L., Hewitt, P. L., Blankstein, K. R., & Mosher, S. (1995). Perfectionism, life events, and depressive symptoms: A test of a diathesis-stress model. *Current Psychology, 14,* 112–137. doi:10.1007/bf02686885.

Flett, G. L., Hewitt, P. L., Blankstein, K. R., Solnik, M., & Van Brunschot, M. (1996). Perfectionism, social problem-solving ability, and psychological distress. *Journal of Rational—Emotive and Cognitive—Behavior Therapy, 14,* 245–274.

Flett, G. L., Hewitt, P. L., Garshowitz, M., & Martin, T. R. (1997). Personality, negative social interactions, and depressive symptoms. *Canadian Journal of Behavioural Science, 29,* 28–37. doi:10.1037/0008-400x.29.1.28.

Flett, G. L., Hewitt, P. L., Oliver, J. M., & Macdonald, S. M. (2002). Perfectionism in children and their parents: A developmental analysis. In G. L. Flett & P. L. Hewitt (Eds.), *Perfectionism: Theory, research, and treatment* (pp. 89–132). Washington, DC: American Psychological Association.

Frost, R. O., Marten, P., Lahart, C., & Rosenblate, R. (1990). The dimensions of perfectionism. *Cognitive Therapy and Research, 14,* 449–468. doi:10.1007/bf01172967.

Fry, P. S., & Debats, D. L. (2009). Perfectionism and the five-factor personality traits as predictors of mortality in older adults. *Journal of Health Psychology, 14,* 513–524. doi:10.1177/1359105309103571.

Gnilka, P. B., Ashby, J. S., & Noble, C. M. (2012). Multidimensional perfectionism and anxiety: Differences among individuals with perfectionism and tests of a coping-mediation model. *Journal of Counseling and Development*, *90*(4), 427–436. doi:10.1002/j.1556-6676.2012.00054.x.

Hamachek, D. E. (1978). Psychodynamics of normal and neurotic perfectionism. *Psychology, 15,* 27–33.

Hammen, C. (2005). Stress and depression. *Annual Review of Clinical Psychology,* 293–319. doi:10.1146/annurev.clinpsy.1.102803.143938.

Herman, J. P. (2012). Neural pathways of stress integration relevance to alcohol abuse. *Alcohol Research: Current Reviews, 34,* 441–447.

Hewitt, P. L., & Flett, G. L. (1991). Perfectionism in the self and social contexts: Conceptualization, assessment, and association with psychopathology. *Journal of Personality and Social Psychology, 60,* 456–470. doi:10.1037/0022-3514.60.3.456.

Hewitt, P. L., & Flett, G. L. (1993). Dimensions of perfectionism, daily stress, and depression: A test of the specific vulnerability hypothesis. *Journal of Abnormal Psychology, 102,* 58–65. doi:10.1037/0021-843x.102.1.58.

Hewitt, P. L., & Flett, G. L. (2002). Perfectionism and stress processes in psychopathology. In G. L. Flett & P. L. Hewitt (Eds.), *Perfectionism: Theory, research, and treatment* (pp. 255–284): Washington, DC: American Psychological Association.

Hewitt, P. L., Flett, G. L., & Endler, N. S. (1995). Perfectionism, coping, and depression symptomatology in a clinical sample. *Clinical Psychology and Psychotherapy, 2,* 47–58. doi:10.1002/cpp.5640020105.

Hewitt, P. L., Flett, G. L., & Ediger, E. (1996). Perfectionism and depression: Longitudinal assessment of a specific vulnerability hypothesis. *Journal of Abnormal Psychology*, *105*, 276–280. doi:10.1037/0021-843x.105.2.276.

Hewitt, P. L., Caelian, C. F., Chen, C., & Flett, G. L. (2014). Perfectionism, stress, daily hassles, hopelessness, and suicide potential in depressed psychiatric adolescents. *Journal of Psychopathology and Behavioral Assessment*. doi:10.1007/s10862-014-9427-0.

Hill, A. P., Hall, H. K., & Appleton, P. R. (2010). Perfectionism and athlete burnout in junior elite athletes: The mediating role of coping tendencies. *Anxiety, Stress, & Coping, 23,* 415–430. doi:10.1080/10615800903330966.

Kannan, D., & Levitt, H. M. (2013). A review of client self-criticism in psychotherapy. *Journal of Psychotherapy Integration, 23,* 166–178. doi:10.1037/a0032355.
Kassel, J. D., Stroud, L. R., & Paronis, C. A. (2003). Smoking, stress, and negative affect: Correlation, causation, and context across stages of smoking. *Psychological Bulletin, 129,* 270–304. doi:10.1037/0033-2909.129.2.270.
Kelly, A. C., & Zuroff, D. C. (2013). Treating perfectionism. In L. Grossman & S. Walfish (Eds.), *Translating psychological research into practice* (pp. 265–270). New York: Springer.
Kirschbaum, C., Pirke, K. M., & Hellhammer, D. H. (1993). The 'Trier social stress test'—A tool for investigating psychobiological stress responses in a laboratory setting. *Neuropsychobiology, 28,* 76–81. doi:10.1159/000119004.
Kuyken, W., Padesky, C. A., & Dudley, R. (2009). *Collaborative case conceptualization: Working effectively with clients in cognitive-behavioral therapy*. New York: Guilford Press.
Lazarus, R. S., & Folkman, S. (1984). *Stress, appraisal, and coping*. New York: Springer.
Lynd-Stevenson, R. M., & Hearne, C. M. (1999). Perfectionism and depressive affect: The pros and cons of being a perfectionist. *Personality and Individual Differences, 26,* 549–562. doi:10.1016/s0191-8869(98)00170-6.
Marin, M. F., Lord, C., Andrews, J., Juster, R. P., Sindi, S., Arsenault-Lapierre, G., Lupien, S. J. (2011). Chronic stress, cognitive functioning and mental health. *Neurobiology of Learning and Memory, 96,* 583–595. doi:10.1016/j.nlm.2011.02.016.
McClelland, G. H., & Judd, C. M. (1993). Statistical difficulties of detecting interactions and moderator effects. *Psychological Bulletin, 114,* 376–390.
McGirr, A., & Turecki, G. (2009). Self-critical perfectionism is associated with increases in sympathetic indicators in a controlled laboratory stress paradigm. *Psychosomatic Medicine, 71,* 588. doi:10.1097/PSY.0b013e3181a99b64.
Molnar, D. S., Flett, G. L., Sadava, S. W., & Colautti, J. (2012). Perfectionism and health functioning in women with fibromyalgia. *Journal of Psychosomatic Research, 73,* 295–300. doi:10.1016/j.jpsychores.2012.08.001.
Molnar, D. S., Sadava, S. W., Flett, G. L., & Colautti, J. (2012). Perfectionism and health: A mediational analysis of the roles of stress, social support and health-related behaviours. *Psychology and Health, 27,* 846–864. doi:10.1080/08870446.2011.630466.
Murayama, K., Pekrun, R., & Fiedler, K. (2014). Research practices that can prevent an inflation of false-positive rates. *Personality and Social Psychology Review, 18,* 107–118. doi:10.1177/1088868313496330.
Noble, C. L., Ashby, J. S., & Gnilka, P. B. (2014). Multidimensional perfectionism, coping, and depression: Differential prediction of depression symptoms by perfectionism type. *Journal of College Counseling, 17,* 80–94. doi:10.1002/j.2161-1882.2014.00049.x.
O'Connor, R. C., & O'Connor, D. B. (2003). Predicting hopelessness and psychological distress: The role of perfectionism and coping. *Journal of Counseling Psychology, 50,* 362–372. doi:10.1037/0022-0167.50.3.362.
O'Connor, R. C., Rasmussen, S., & Hawton, K. (2010). Predicting depression, anxiety and self-harm in adolescents: The role of perfectionism and acute life stress. *Behaviour Research and Therapy*, *48*, 52–59. doi:10.1016/j.brat.2009.09.008.
Rice, K. G., Leever, B. A., Christopher, J., & Porter, J. D. (2006). Perfectionism, stress, and social (dis)connection: A short-term study of hopelessness, depression, and academic adjustment among honors students. *Journal of Counseling Psychology, 53,* 524–534. doi:10.1037/0022-0167.53.4.524.
Richardson, C. M. E., Rice, K. G., & Devine, D. P. (2014). Perfectionism, emotion regulation, and the cortisol stress response. *Journal of Counseling Psychology, 61,* 110–118. doi:10.1037/a0034446.
Shafran, R., & Mansell, W. (2001). Perfectionism and psychopathology: A review of research and treatment. *Clinical Psychology Review, 21,* 879–906. doi:10.1016/s0272-7358(00)00072-6.
Shafran, R., Cooper, Z., & Fairburn, C. G. (2002). Clinical perfectionism: A cognitive-behavioural analysis. *Behaviour Research and Therapy, 40,* 773–791. doi:10.1016/s0005-7967(01)00059-6.

Shahar, G., & Priel, B. (2003). Active vulnerability, adolescent distress, and the mediating/suppressing role of life events. *Personality and Individual Differences, 35,* 199–218. doi:10.1016/s0191-8869(02)00185-x.

Sherry, S. B., Hewitt, P. L., & Flett, G. L. (2003). Perfectionism dimensions, perfectionistic attitudes, dependent attitudes, and depression in psychiatric patients and university students. *Journal of Counseling Psychology, 50,* 373–386. doi:10.1037/0022-0167.50.3.373.

Sherry, S. B., Law, A., Hewitt, P. L., Flett, G. L., & Besser, A. (2008). Social support as a mediator of the relationship between perfectionism and depression: A preliminary test of the social disconnection model. *Personality and Individual Differences, 45,* 339–344. doi:10.1016/j.paid.2008.05.001.

Sherry, S. B., Mackinnon, S. P., Macneil, M. A., & Fitzpatrick, S. (2013). Discrepancies confer vulnerability to depressive symptoms: A three-wave longitudinal study. *Journal of Counseling Psychology, 60,* 112–126. doi:10.1037/a0030439.

Skinner, E. A., Edge, K., Altman, J., & Sherwood, H. (2003). Searching for the structure of coping: A review and critique of category systems for classifying ways of coping. *Psychological Bulletin, 129,* 216–269. doi:10.1037/0033-2909.129.2.216.

Slaney, R. B., Rice, K. G., Mobley, M., Trippi, J., & Ashby, J. S. (2001). The revised almost perfect scale. *Measurement and Evaluation in Counseling and Development, 34,* 130–145.

Stoeber, J., & Janssen, D. P. (2011). Perfectionism and coping with daily failures: Positive reframing helps achieve satisfaction at the end of the day. *Anxiety, Stress, & Coping, 24,* 477–497. doi:10.1080/10615806.2011.562977.

Stoeber, J., & Otto, K. (2006). Positive conceptions of perfectionism: Approaches, evidence, challenges. *Personality and Social Psychology Review, 10,* 295–319. doi:10.1207/s15327957pspr1004_2.

Sturman, E. D., Flett, G. L., Hewitt, P. L., & Rudolph, S. G. (2009). Dimensions of perfectionism and self-worth contingencies in depression. *Journal of Rational—Emotive and Cognitive—Behavior Therapy, 27,* 213–231. doi:10.1007/s10942-007-0079-9.

Weiner, B. A., & Carton, J. S. (2012). Avoidant coping: A mediator of maladaptive perfectionism and test anxiety. *Personality and Individual Differences*, *52*, 632–636. doi:10.1016/j.paid.2011.12.009.

Weissman, A. N., & Beck, A. T. (1978). *Development and validation of the Dysfunctional Attitude Scale: A preliminary investigation.* Paper presented at the 62nd Annual Meeting of the American Educational Research Association, Toronto, Ontario, Canada.

Wirtz, P. H., Elsenbruch, S., Emini, L., Rüdisüli, K., Groessbauer, S., & Ehlert, U. (2007). Perfectionism and the cortisol response to psychosocial stress in men. *Psychosomatic Medicine, 69,* 249–255. doi:10.1097/PSY.0b013e318042589e.

Young, J. E., Klosko, J. S., & Weishaar, M. E. (2003). *Schema therapy: A practitioner's guide.* New York: Guilford Press.

Zhou, X., Zhu, H., Zhang, B., & Cai, T. (2013). Perceived social support as moderator of perfectionism, depression, and anxiety in college students. *Social Behavior and Personality, 41,* 1141–1152. doi:10.2224/sbp.2013.41.7.1141.

Zureck, E., Altstötter-Gleich, C., Wolf, O. T., & Brand, M. (2014). It depends: Perfectionism as a moderator of experimentally induced stress. *Personality and Individual Differences, 63,* 30–35. doi:10.1016/j.paid.2014.01.038.

Zuroff, D. C., Mongrain, M., & Santor, D. A. (2004). Conceptualizing and measuring personality vulnerability to depression: Comment on Coyne and Whiffen (1995). *Psychological Bulletin, 130,* 489–511. doi:10.1037/0033-2909.130.3.489.

Chapter 8
Anxiety and Perfectionism: Relationships, Mechanisms, and Conditions

Alexandra M. Burgess and Patricia Marten DiBartolo

Anxiety and Perfectionism: Relationships

Responses from a qualitative interview investigation on the meaning of perfectionism indicate that people often associate their understanding of the construct with an increased psychological distress (Rice, Bair, Castro, Cohen, & Hood, 2003). Indeed, as the current volume makes clear, a burgeoning research literature finds robust relationships between perfectionism and many forms of psychopathology. The following chapter offers a brief review of the well-established and robust relationship between perfectionism and anxiety and delves into the literature regarding potential mechanisms underlying this relationship while highlighting their clinical implications. The chapter concludes with methodological recommendations for the direction of future research on causal mechanisms that can help us to understand and address the perfectionism–anxiety link.

Perfectionism is a combination of setting excessively high standards and having an overly critical evaluative style (Hamachek, 1978). Although universal consensus has yet to be fully reached regarding the essential structure of perfectionism (Frost, Marten, Lahart, & Rosenblate, 1990; Hewitt & Flett, 1991; Hewitt, Flett, Besser, Sherry, & McGee, 2003; Shafran, Cooper, & Fairburn, 2002), most researchers share a bidimensional approach to measuring and understanding perfectionism that includes the two broad categories of achievement striving and evaluative concerns (for a detailed review, see Chap. 1). In the following chapter, "achievement striving" will be used to describe dimensions of perfectionism that reflect the setting of rigorous standards (also referred to as positive, adaptive, or standards perfectionism), and "evaluative concerns" will be used to describe dimensions of perfectionism relating to fears of failure and negative evaluation (also referred to as negative, maladaptive, or clinical perfectionism). Indeed, this bidimensional model of perfectionism indicated by the initial factor analytic study by Frost and colleagues (1993)

A. M. Burgess (✉) · P. M. DiBartolo
Department of Psychology, Smith College, Northampton, MA 01063, USA
e-mail: aburgess@smith.edu

F. M. Sirois, D. S. Molnar (eds.), *Perfectionism, Health, and Well-Being,*
DOI 10.1007/978-3-319-18582-8_8

has now been replicated by subsequent research (Frost, Heimberg, Holt, Mattia, & Neubauer, 1993; Pearson & Gleaves, 2006).

Evidence suggests that evaluative concerns correlates with negative mental health outcomes, whereas the data are mixed regarding achievement striving and other-oriented perfectionism (cf. Antony, Purdon, Huta, & Swinson, 1998; Frost et al., 1993; Brown et al., 1999). Among other adverse outcomes, evaluative concerns maintains relationships with a wide variety of anxiety symptomology, including social anxiety, general state or trait anxiety, and obsessive-compulsive disorder (OCD). The association of evaluative concerns dimensions with these other forms of psychopathology (e.g., depression, eating disorders) suggests that evaluative concerns may function as a transdiagnostic risk factor (Egan, Wade, & Shafran, 2011). Although there is also some evidence to suggest that dimensions of perfectionism are associated with both post-traumatic stress disorder (e.g., Kawamura, Hunt, Frost, & DiBartolo, 2001) and panic disorder (e.g., Antony et al., 1998), the literature in these areas remains comparatively underdeveloped and therefore will not be discussed in the present chapter.

Trait Anxiety

Evaluative concern consistently maintains a robust positive association with general trait or state anxiety (cf., Flett, Hewitt, Endler, & Tassone, 1994–1995; Frost et al., 1990; Hewitt & Flett, 1991; Kawamura et al., 2001). The mechanisms for this association are likely numerous, transactional, and range across a variety of intra- and interpersonal domains such as patterns of cognitions, behaviors, and social interactions. Unlike evaluative concerns, achievement striving demonstrates a varied relationship with trait anxiety, sometimes being positively correlated (cf., Stöber, 1998) and sometimes being uncorrelated (cf., Flett, Hewitt, Endler, & Tassone, 1994–1995). The inconsistency in findings suggests that this association may only exist under certain conditions. Additionally, the quality of the relationship between achievement striving and trait anxiety sometimes changes once evaluative concerns is accounted for; specifically, a positive or absent relationship often becomes an absent or negative relationship (cf., Wu & Wei, 2008). The focus of later sections of this chapter will be the exploration of possible mechanisms through which and circumstances under, which dimensions of perfectionism relate to trait anxiety.

Social Anxiety

Social anxiety and evaluative concerns are consistently, positively correlated among community samples (DiBartolo et al., 2007; Nepon, Flett, Hewitt, & Molnar, 2011) and individuals diagnosed with social phobia (Antony et al., 1998; Juster, Heimberg, Frost, & Holt, 1996; Wheeler, Blankstein, Antony, McCabe, & Bieling, 2011). Furthermore, when individuals diagnosed with social phobia were compared to those with other anxiety disorders (i.e., OCD and panic disorder), individuals with social phobia reported the highest levels of socially prescribed perfectionism and maladaptive evaluative concerns (Wheeler et al., 2011). Antony and colleagues (1998) also found that individuals with social phobia had higher levels of evaluative concerns than anxiety-disordered clinical comparison groups and nonclinical controls (Antony et al., 1998). Similar to trait anxiety, the processes that give rise to this association are not fully understood, are likely numerous and interrelated, and will be explored in subsequent sections. In contrast, achievement striving is most often unrelated to social anxiety symptoms (cf. Levinson et al., 2013; Nepon, Flett, Hewitt, & Molnar, 2011; Santanello & Gardner, 2007; Xie, Leong, & Feng, 2008), but very occasionally, researchers discover a significant positive relationship (cf., Saboonchi & Lundh, 1997). This pattern of associations indicates that there may be certain circumstances under which these constructs are related, but these conditions are not presently well understood.

Obsessive-Compulsive Disorder

OCD is characterized by obsessions (e.g., intrusive thoughts, images, and impulses), and compulsions, which are voluntary, repetitive behaviors that an individual feels compelled to perform (e.g., counting, washing); these features are collectively termed OC symptoms. Researchers have considered perfectionism both a risk factor for the development of OC symptoms (Rasmussen & Eisen, 1989) and one of the six belief structures inherent to OCD (Obsessive Compulsive Cognitions Working Group, 1997). A body of empirical literature links evaluative concerns, especially features related to doubts about actions and concern over mistakes, with OC symptoms in both community (cf. Rhéaume, Freeston, Dugas, Letarte, & Ladouceur, 1995) and clinical samples (cf. Antony et al., 1998; Frost & Steketee, 1997). Unlike trait and social anxiety, a few studies have demonstrated that achievement striving is associated with specific OC symptoms, such as not just right experiences (e.g., the uncomfortable sensation that something is not *just right*), subclinical compulsive symptoms that do not meet the criteria for a formal diagnosis of OCD (Frost, Steketee, Cohn, & Griess, 1994), and hoarding (Lee et al., 2009; Frost & Gross, 1993; Yorulmaz, Karanci, & Tekok-Kilic, 2006). The complex and varied mechanisms that give rise to this association are unknown; however, some of the theorized mediators will be discussed in later sections of this chapter.

Anxiety and Perfectionism: Mechanisms and Conditions

As reviewed, evaluative concerns maintains a consistently strong, positive relationship with features of anxiety such as social anxiety, trait and state anxiety, and OC symptoms across research studies. Given these high rates of co-occurrence for anxiety and evaluative concerns, researchers have appropriately focused on research investigating the mechanisms that underlie these relationships (Frazier, Tix, & Barron, 2004; Rose, Holmbeck, Coakley, & Franks, 2004). Mediational research clarifies the processes or mechanisms through which a relationship exists. Therefore, this type of analysis is appropriate to the study of evaluative concerns and anxiety. However, mediational research is difficult to interpret when no consistent relationship exists between a set of variables, as is the case with dimensions of achievement striving and anxiety (Frazier et al., 2004). In contrast to mediational analyses, moderational research identifies the circumstances or conditions under which two constructs are related; these analyses are most appropriate for investigating the association between variables that are inconsistently related in the literature, such as achievement striving and anxiety (Frazier et al., 2004; Rose, Holmbeck, Coakley, & Franks, 2004).

Using mediational and moderational analyses to clarify the conditions and processes through which perfectionism and anxiety are associated is useful for deepening our understanding of these phenomena and has the potential to inform the treatment literature. Despite the value of this type of research, the current literature is not consistently and clearly theoretically grounded. Ideally, mediational and moderational research designs are driven by theory (Frazier et al., 2004); however, no unifying theory accounting for the relationship between the two dimensions of perfectionism and the development of the full range of anxiety symptoms has been proposed. Thus, researchers often test mechanisms posited by broader theories of psychopathology (e.g., Barlow's model of anxious apprehension; Barlow, 2000) and contextualize their empirical findings within these frameworks.

The mechanisms presented in this chapter's review are broadly categorized into three groups informed by a variety of theoretical models related to the development of anxious symptomology. Each section explores a set of potential mechanisms explaining the anxiety–perfectionism connection—stress/emotion regulation, social factors, and cognitions—and begins with a brief review of theories relevant to the mechanism and continues with a description of related empirical literature (see Table 8.1). Reflecting the multidimensional nature of perfectionism, findings for evaluative concerns and achievement striving are presented separately within each section, as the two dimensions typically demonstrate a different pattern of associations in each study. At the chapter's end, we consolidate the current understanding of potential mechanisms for this relationship, suggest a preliminary model for the connection between evaluative concerns and anxious psychopathology, and illuminate potential avenues for future investigations.

Table 8.1 Mediational and moderational research evaluating the relationship of dimensions of perfectionism and anxiety

Study	Sample: *N*	Perfectionism dimension (instrument)	Mediator (instrument)	Anxiety dimension (instrument)	Analysis type	Results
Stress and emotion regulation						
Dunkley et al., (2000)	443	EC/PS (MPS and FMPS)	Hassles (GASHSS) avoidant coping (COPE), perceived social support (SPS)	Distress (MASQ)	Mediation: SEM	Full mediation of EC to distress with the three mediators; PS had no relationship to distress after EC was included in the model
					Moderation: regression	Hassles and perceived social support both moderated for EC/PS to distress
Gnilka et al., (2012)	350	Standards/discrepancy (APS-R)	Coping (WCC-R)	Trait anxiety (STAI)	Mediation: multiple bootstrapping	Four coping methods (distancing, self-controlling, accepting responsibility, and escape-avoidance) fully mediated between discrepancy and trait anxiety; standards had no relationship with trait anxiety
Santanello & Gardner, (2007)	125	MP/PS (FMPS)	Experiential avoidance (AAQ)	Worry (PSWQ)	Mediation: regression	Partial mediation of MP to worry; PS had no relationship with experiential avoidance or worry
Klibert et al., (2014)	413	SPP/SOP/OOP (MPS)	Resilience (DRS-LF)	Anxiety (BSI)	Mediation: path analysis *and* multiple bootstrapping	Partial mediation effect of SSP to anxiety; SOP and OOP had no relationship with resilience
Moretz & McKay, (2009)	188	MEC (FMPS)	Trait anxiety (STAI)	OC symptoms (VOCI, just right and checking subscales)	Mediation: SEM	Full mediation of MEC to OC symptoms

Table 8.1 (continued)

Study	Sample: N	Perfectionism dimension (instrument)	Mediator (instrument)	Anxiety dimension (instrument)	Analysis type	Results
Social factors						
Chang et al., (2008)	383	SSP/SOP/OOP (MPS)	Loneliness (R-UCLA)	Anxiety (BAI)	Moderation: regression	Moderation of SPP and OOP to anxiety; SOP had no relationship with anxiety
Wu & Wei, (2008)	295	EC/PS (FMPS, APS-R)	Validation from self/others (brief FNE, RMLAM, FSRQ)	Anxiety (DASS-A short form, SRAS)	Mediation: SEM *and* multiple bootstrapping	Full mediation of EC to anxiety with the two mediators; partial mediation of PS to anxiety
DiBartolo et al., (2008)	274	MEC/PPS (FMPS)	Self-concealment, contingent self-worth (SCS, CSWS/PSW)	Fear of negative evaluation (brief FNE)	Mediation: multiple bootstrapping	CSW and SC partially mediated MEC to FNE; CSW fully mediated PPS to FNE
Nepon et al., (2011)	155	SPP/SOP/OOP (MPS)	Negative social feedback (SFQ)	Social anxiety (LSAS)	Mediation: regression *and* multiple bootstrapping	Partial mediation of SPP to social anxiety; SOP and OOP had no relationship with anxiety
Cognitions						
DiBartolo et al., (2007)	342	MEC/PPS (FMPS)	Perceived probability and cost of negative events (CONSE-Q, PCQ)	Social phobia (SPAI-SP), state anxiety (DASS-A)	Multiple bootstrapping	Partial mediation of MEC to social and state anxiety with the two mediators; full mediation of PPS to state anxiety with the two mediators; PPS had no relationship with social anxiety
Wimberley & Stashio, (2013)	113	EC/PS (FMPS)	Perfectionistic cognitions (PCI)	Anxiety (POMS T-A)	Mediation: multiple bootstrapping	Partial mediation of EC to anxiety; PS had no relationship with anxiety
					Moderation: regression	No moderation effects were found

Table 8.1 (continued)

Study	Sample: *N*	Perfectionism dimension (instrument)	Mediator (instrument)	Anxiety dimension (instrument)	Analysis type	Results
Pirbaglou et al., (2013)	992	Perfectionistic cognitions (PCI)	Anxiety sensitivity (ASI), automatic negative thoughts (ATQ)	Anxiety (BAI)	Mediation: SEM *and* multiple bootstrapping	Mediation of perfectionistic cognitions to anxiety with the two mediators (full or partial not specified)
Yorulmaz et al., (2006)	408	SSP/SOP/OOP (MPS)	Sense of responsibility (RAS)	OC symptoms: cleaning and checking (MOCI)	Mediation: regression	Full mediation of SPP to OC symptoms; full mediation of SOP to checking; partial mediation of SOP to cleaning; OOP had no relationship to OC symptoms
Reuther et al., (2013)	475	Perfectionism (FMPS)	Intolerance for uncertainty (IUS)	OC symptoms and severity (FOCI)	Mediation: SEM *and* multiple bootstrapping	Full mediation of perfectionism to both OC symptoms and severity
Pleva & Wade, (2006)	303	Concern over mistakes (FMPS)	Misinterpretation of thoughts (RIQ-B)	OC symptoms (MOCI total)	Mediation: regression	Partial mediation of concern over mistakes to OC symptoms

All samples consisted of undergraduate students

EC evaluative concerns, *PS* personal standards, *MPS* Multidimensional Perfectionism Scale, *FMPS* Frost Multidimensional Perfectionism Scale, *GASHSS* General, Academic, and Social Hassle Scale for Students, *COPE* COPE Inventory, *SPS* Social Provisions Scale, *MASQ* Mood and Anxiety Symptom Questionnaire, *SEM* structural equation modeling, *APS-R* Almost Perfect Scale—Revised, *WOC-R* Ways of Coping Inventory—Revised, *STAI* State-Trait Anxiety Inventory, *OC* obsessive-compulsive, *MP* maladaptive perfectionism, *AAQ* Acceptance and Action Questionnaire, *PSWQ* Penn State Worry Questionnaire, *SPP* socially prescribed perfectionism, *SOP* self-oriented perfectionism, *OOP* other-oriented perfectionism, *DRS-LF* Dispositional Resilience Scale—Long Form, *BSI* Brief Symptom Inventory, *MEC* maladaptive evaluation concerns, *VOCI* Vancouver Obsessional Compulsive Inventory, *R-UCLA* Revised UCLA Loneliness Scale, *BAI* Beck Anxiety Inventory, *Brief FNE* Fear of Negative Evaluation—Brief Version, *RMLAM* Revised Martin–Larsen Approval Motivation, *FSRQ* Frequency of Self-reinforcement Questionnaire, *DASS-A* Depression, Anxiety, and Stress Scale—Anxiety, *SRAS* Self-Rating Anxiety Scale, *PPS* pure personal standards, *SCS* Self-Concealment Scale, *CSWS* Contingent Self-Worth Scale, *PSW* Perfectionistic Self-Worth Scale, *SFQ* Social Feedback Questionnaire, *LSAS* Liebowitz Social Anxiety Scale, *CONSE-Q* Consequences of Negative Social Events Questionnaire, *PCQ* Subjective Probability and Cost Questionnaire, *SPAI-SP* Social Phobia and Anxiety Inventory—Social Phobia, *PCI* Perfectionistic Cognitions Inventory, *POMS T-A* Profile of Mood States Tension–Anxiety, *ASI* Anxiety Sensitivity Index, *ATQ* Automatic Thoughts Questionnaire, *RAS* Responsibility Attitude Scale, *MOCI* Maudsley Obsessive-Compulsive Inventory, *IUS* Intolerance for Uncertainty Scale, *FOCI* Florida Obsessive-Compulsive Inventory, *RIQ-B* Responsibility Interpretation Questionnaire—Beliefs

Stress and Emotion Regulation

Theoretical Underpinnings

Stress is best defined by a person–environment interaction in which (a) an individual perceives a challenging situation to be threatening, and (b) the demand or response required from the individual may exceed their available resources (Lazarus & Folkman, 1984). Lazarus and Folkman's (1984) cognitive theory of psychological stress and coping provides one means of understanding the relationship between stress, perfectionism, and anxiety pathology. The theory's two stages of cognitive appraisal describe the ways in which potentially harmful situations lead to varying levels of stress across individuals depending on their interpretations and reactions to the event. During primary cognitive appraisal of a stressful event, individuals determine the personal relevance and importance of the potentially threatening situation which influences the emotional response they will experience in reaction to the event. Perfectionists are more likely to interpret challenging situations as relevant to their well-being and as having high stakes (Flett & Hewitt, 2002; Flett et al., 1994–1995). Further, perfectionists experience more situations as stressors because they experience more distress following perceived mistakes and experience a high level of interpersonal sensitivity following social interactions (Frost et al., 1997; Hewitt & Flett, 1993). Perfectionism therefore acts as an underlying vulnerability within a diathesis-stress model to increase the likelihood of anxious symptomology when an individual is faced with challenging life events or hassles (Flett, Hewitt, Blankstein, & Mosher, 1991).

An individual's coping response following a stressor may also relate dimensions of perfectionism to the development of psychopathology. According to Lazarus and Folkman's cognitive model, during secondary appraisal an individual inventories his/her personal and social resources to determine an adaptive response to a stressor. At this point, perfectionists may approach threatening situations with hopelessness and a lack of self-efficacy in their ability to cope well (Flett, Hewitt, Blankstein, Solnik, & Brunschot, 1996). This sense of hopelessness may develop out of a learning history of failing to meet excessively high standards. Perfectionistic standards for behavior that are imposed by an individual, or perceived to be imposed by others, are extremely difficult to reach. Even if these standards are momentarily met, the expectation for behavior increases such that the previously acceptable behavior becomes substandard. Furthermore, clinical interviews with perfectionists reveal that they often set higher standards for themselves following a failed attempt to meet a goal (Egan, Piek, Dyck, Rees, & Hagger, 2013). Through repeated experiences with falling short of high standards, perfectionists may develop a sense of hopelessness that leads to poor coping strategies such as avoidance.

Avoidance is known to maintain and intensify future anxiety about similar situations (Barlow, 2000); thus, avoidant coping in response to perfectionistic evaluative concerns may serve to maintain and intensify anxious symptomology over time. Further, Slade and Owens (1998) posited a related model in which individuals high in achievement striving aim to receive positive reinforcement, whereas those high in evaluative concerns are motivated by the avoidance of criticism. The threat of negative evaluation may be so powerful that an individual becomes immobilized and procrastinates (Flett, Blankstein, Hewitt, & Koledin, 1992; Frost et al., 1990). Similarly, Hamachek (1978) suggested that the fear of performance evaluation related to evaluative concerns creates trepidation and avoidance in response to new tasks. Perfectionism has also been associated with both a lack of self-acceptance of stressful situations and a desire to keep signs of distress hidden (Flett & Hewitt, 2002; Flett, Russo, & Hewitt, 1994). These factors may inhibit healthy coping as an individual denies the problem and/or is reticent to take healthy, although potentially exposing, steps towards handling a difficult situation effectively.

Closely associated with coping style, resilience is a set of flexible attitudes that facilitates problem-solving and assists in adjustment to stress through positive coping (Neenan, 2009). Individuals who are high in evaluative concerns are less likely to engage in resilience-building activities, which may lead to an increase in their experience of anxiety. For example, they tend to have a poor problem-solving orientation due to a stance of helplessness and decreased engagement in social support networks, possibly as a result of defensiveness (Besser, Flett, & Hewitt, 2010). In sum, resilience, coping styles, and the experience of stress may be related to the way in which perfectionism leads to anxious symptomology. The following section will discuss literature investigating these potential mechanisms.

Mediational and Moderational Research

To date, a handful of studies have evaluated stress and emotion regulation as mechanisms underlying the association between dimensions of perfectionism and anxiety (see Table 8.1). This literature suggests that evaluative concerns is related to anxiety through stress and coping style via mediation and/or moderation. For example, research investigating the impact of daily hassles and avoidant coping indicates that both variables serve as mediators. Dunkley and colleagues (2000) tested a mediational model in which evaluative concerns (along with personal standards) predicted distress, which included items assessing anxiety and depression (Dunkley, Blankstein, Halsall, Williams, & Winkworth, 2000). Mediators in their model included hassles, comprising general, academic, and social hassles, and avoidant coping, including denial, behavioral disengagement, and mental disengagement. Both daily hassles and avoidant coping were found to be mediators of the evaluative concerns–distress relationship. Although not derived from a longitudinal study, the results provided support for the notion of the diathesis-stress model for evaluative concerns and anxiety, and suggested that coping style is important to the development of distress following life challenges for perfectionists. In additional exploratory analyses of the perfectionism–distress relationship, hassles was also evaluated as a moderator (Dunkley et al., 2000). Perhaps not surprisingly, hassles served as a moderator for the relationship between evaluative concerns and distress, which captured both anxiety and depression, wherein the highest levels of distress were found when individuals high in evaluative concerns were also experiencing daily hassles.

In another study, the frequency of avoidant coping style use was significantly related to evaluative concerns and functioned as a mediator for predicting trait anxiety (Gnilka, Ashby, & Noble, 2012). Frequent use of alternative coping styles including distancing, self-controlling, and accepting responsibility was also significantly related to evaluative concerns and functioned as a mediator. The only healthy coping style (as classified by the Ways of Coping—Revised; Folkman & Lazarus, 1985) that was a significant mediator of the anxiety–evaluative concerns relationship was a self-controlling style; seeking social support, planful problem-solving, or positive reappraisal were not significant mediators. The self-controlling subscale items relate to concealing one's emotions (e.g., "Kept others from knowing how bad things were") and trying to calmly and thoughtfully plan behavior rather than impulsively react out of emotion (e.g., "I tried to keep my feelings from interfering with other things too much" and "I tried to see things from the other person's point of view"). Hewitt and colleagues (2003) argue that perfectionism and self-concealment are related, which may help to explain why using a self-controlling style was significantly, positively related to evaluative concerns. These results suggest that perfectionists tend to use particular types of coping strategies and that these methods, especially when unhealthy, can serve as mechanisms through which evaluative concerns give rise to anxious pathology.

Relatedly, Santanello and Gardner (2007) investigated experiential avoidance as a mediator between dimensions of perfectionism and worry, the hallmark characteristic of generalized anxiety disorder (Santanello & Gardner, 2007). The authors hypothesized that intense aversion to negative evaluation leads to increased experiential avoidance, or the tendency to avoid unpleasant internal thoughts, emotions, and sensations. The authors suggested that experiential avoidance and worry would then be cyclically related as perfectionistic individuals worried to avoid evaluative threat by distracting themselves from the distressing topic. Results indicated that experiential avoidance was indeed a partial mediator of the relationship between evaluative concerns and worry.

Klibert and colleagues (2014) examined a different aspect of emotional response to distress: resilience, or the ability to successfully adapt to stressful situations (Klibert et al., 2014). The authors used Hewitt and Flett's conceptualization of self-oriented, other-oriented, and socially prescribed perfectionism to evaluate whether resilience functioned as a mediator for perfectionism's relationship with state anxiety. Although all three aspects of perfectionism were positively and significantly related to psychopathology, resilience correlated only with socially prescribed perfectionism, in a negative direction. Resilience partially mediated socially prescribed perfectionism's relationship with state levels of anxiety, reducing the strength of the relationship between these two constructs. The results further support the mediational role of coping response in the relationship between perfectionism and anxiety.

Studies presented up to this point have investigated the mechanisms underlying the relationship between perfectionism and general feelings of anxiety. Contrastingly, Moretz and McKay (2009) investigated trait anxiety as a mediator for the relationships between perfectionism and a specific type of anxious symptomology,

OC symptoms. The authors tested two structural equation models that predicted checking symptoms and not just right experiences separately with maladaptive evaluative concerns being mediated by trait anxiety. Both models demonstrated significant indirect effects for evaluative concerns through trait anxiety, indicating a mediation effect. These results suggest that trait anxiety may function as a mechanism through which perfectionism leads to other forms of anxious pathology.

Unlike evaluative concerns, which evidenced a consistent association with anxiety mediated by stress and coping factors, achievement striving demonstrated varied patterns of association within the five studies presented. Mediational analyses were not conducted for the achievement striving dimension in any of these studies because (a) achievement striving and anxiety were unrelated in the study sample (Dunkley et al., 2000; Gnilka, Ashby, & Noble, 2012; Santanello & Gardner, 2007), (b) achievement striving and anxious symptomology are not as consistently related in the broader literature (Moretz & McKay, 2009), or (c) achievement striving was unrelated to the study mediator (Klibert et al., 2014). Regarding moderational analyses, one study examined potential moderators of the relationship between achievement striving and distress. Dunkley and colleagues (2000) found that individuals with high levels of achievement striving, in comparison with those with low levels, experienced a larger increase in distress in the presence of hassles (Dunkley et al., 2000). The authors suggested that high stress levels reduced the ability to pursue positive coping strategies, and added that general and social hassles, not just academic hassles, appear to relate to the experience of distress for individuals high in achievement striving.

In sum, research to date demonstrates that evaluative concerns has a consistently positive relationship with anxiety that is mediated by hassles, resilience, and coping strategies. Importantly, avoidant coping is indicated as a pathway between perfectionism and psychopathology. These results suggest that meaningful treatment strategies may include the use of exposure therapy for the fear of performance evaluation and coaching in alternative, positive coping strategies. Achievement striving is most often unrelated to anxiety and/or coping, and thus, no mediation was tested. Results from these studies support the notion of distinguishing the different patterns of results for the evaluative concerns and achievement striving dimensions of perfectionism. Further, the inconsistent relationship between achievement striving and psychopathology indicates that moderational analyses (as one by Dunkley et al., 2000), rather than mediational, may be the most suitable for evaluating these constructs. Moderational analyses may provide insight into the conditions under which dimensions of achievement striving relate to negative psychological outcomes.

Social Factors

Theoretical Underpinnings

Hewitt and colleagues (2006) developed a model illuminating perfectionism's relationship with social factors and distress (Hewitt, Flett, Sherry, & Caelian, 2006) that was initially created to describe the relationship between evaluative concerns and suicidality but has relevance to understanding the association between evaluative concerns and anxiety. The Perfectionism Social Disconnection Model suggests that socially prescribed perfectionists often experience objective and subjective social isolation, which in turn predicts psychopathology (see also Chap. 9). Related to objective social isolation, Hewitt and colleagues (2006) argue that the socially prescribed dimension of perfectionism increases the likelihood of objective social isolation by generating interpersonal hostility (e.g., anger and suspiciousness) that often leads to negative social interactions. Socially prescribed perfectionists may develop these feelings because they perceive others to be overly critical while simultaneously expecting impossibly high standards. Perfectionistic self-presentation might also play a role in objective social isolation for those with high evaluative concerns. Perfectionists tend to lack social support and resources due to their desire to present a flawless image (Hewitt et al., 2003). In this way, individuals high in evaluative concerns further isolate themselves from social support that might otherwise be available to them. As Nepon and colleagues (2011) observe, this type of interpersonal style may also seem distant and inauthentic to others, thereby decreasing even further the frequency of positive and supportive social contact (Nepon et al., 2011).

Within the Perfectionism Social Disconnection Model, socially prescribed perfectionists experience subjective social isolation as well. These individuals are often highly interpersonally sensitive due to their need for acceptance and reliance on others' approval as a basis for self-worth (Hewitt et al., 2006; Nepon et al., 2011). This hypersensitivity can lead to the interpretation of neutral or ambiguous social feedback as negative and to the experience of distress following perceived failures or humiliations. Individuals high in evaluative concerns may therefore experience a higher level of negative social feedback both through objectively poor social interactions and through their overly sensitive perception of social feedback. Over time, accumulated negative interactions may lead these individuals to socially isolate themselves and feel lonely.

Compounding this difficulty, evaluative concerns is related to the use of social reinforcement, rather than self-reinforcement, to modulate feelings of efficacy, self-esteem, and self-worth. Hamachek (1978) proposed a difference in motivation for individuals high in achievement striving compared to evaluative concerns. He hypothesized that the former group strives to fulfill high personal standards to achieve self-satisfaction, whereas the latter group pursues rigorous standards to avoid negative evaluation from others. Wu and Wei (2008) suggested that evaluative concerns is associated with a relative deficit in the ability to self-reinforce and a high need for validation from others. Wu and Wei (2008) noted that individuals who rely on external reinforcement are likely to experience increased levels of anxiety depending on the availability of reassurance from others. Treatment evidence supporting this notion suggests that lessening reliance on reinforcement from others and increasing the ability to self-reinforce decreases symptoms of anxiety (Rehm & Marston, 1968). Given that perfectionists may foster negative social interactions and are hypersensitive to negative social feedback, a reliance on validation from others is especially problematic. As previously noted, although initially developed to explain the relationship between perfectionism and suicidality, the Perfectionism Social Disconnection Model may also accurately describe factors related to the development of anxiety for perfectionists. The following section will discuss literature pertaining to the role of social factors in the relationship between dimensions of perfectionism and anxious psychopathology.

Mediational and Moderational Research

Research evidence suggests that social factors are related, through mediation and moderation, to the experience of psychopathology for individuals high in evaluative concerns (see Table 8.1). Dunkley and colleagues (2000) evaluated the role of social support as both a mediator and moderator for the relationship between evaluative concerns and distress, which included components of anxiety and depression (Dunkley et al., 2000). Evaluative concerns maintained a significant negative relationship with social support, which suggests that these individuals feel others do not value them and cannot be counted on in times of need. Social support, in combination with hassles and avoidant coping (see Stress and Emotion Regulation for a discussion of these results), fully mediated the relationship between evaluative concerns and distress. Concerning a moderation effect, high levels of social support reduced distress for all groups of participants regardless of their level of perfectionism. However, for those individuals high in maladaptive evaluative concerns, social support had a much more powerful effect in reducing distress, indicating that it may serve as an important protective factor for mitigating the impact of evaluative concerns on distress.

Perfectionists may often be lonely due to their experience of both objective and subjective social isolation. Chang and colleagues (2008) were interested in whether perfectionists who were experiencing loneliness had higher levels of anxiety than those with a low level of loneliness. In this study, moderational analyses were conducted to see whether self-oriented, other-oriented, and socially prescribed perfectionism predicted anxiety at high and low levels of loneliness. Although the self-oriented and other-oriented dimensions of perfectionism are not consistently related to negative outcomes in the broader literature and thus are often not investigated in studies predicting psychopathology (See Anxiety and Perfectionism above), Chang et al. (2008) found that other-oriented perfectionism as well as socially prescribed perfectionism maintained relationships with trait anxiety, with loneliness acting as a significant moderator. In comparison with individuals low in these dimensions of perfectionism, participants with elevated scores for other-oriented or socially prescribed perfectionism experienced disproportionate increases in anxiety symptoms when they felt alone. These results again suggest a protective role for social contact against the development of psychopathology for individuals with high levels of perfectionism.

Beyond mere social contact, the need for reassurance from others may also impact the perfectionist's experience of anxiety. Wu and Wei (2008) investigated the need for reassurance from others ("Other-Validation") and the capacity to self-reinforce ("Self-Validation") as mediators for the relationship between evaluative concerns and anxiety (Wu & Wei, 2008). Evaluative concerns was shown to have a positive relationship with Other-Validation and a negative relationship with Self-Validation. Self-Validation maintained a strong negative correlation with anxiety, whereas Other-Validation demonstrated a moderate positive correlation with anxiety. In a structural equation model, the relationship of evaluative concerns with anxiety was fully mediated by Self- and Other-Validation together. Although not explicitly empirically tested in this study, the authors suggested a potential common developmental pathway leading to evaluative concerns, an overreliance on Other-Validation, and the underutilization of Self-Validation: Children with critical, demanding caregivers strive to receive love and approval through perfection, focusing so much on their own critical evaluation of their performance that they are insensitive to their internal cues for reward. What is unclear given the cross-sectional design of this study is which of these traits precedes the other, whether they causally relate to one another, and whether their relationship is truly one of mediation.

Related to validation from others, another group of researchers investigated contingent self-worth and self-concealment as potential mediators for the relationship between maladaptive evaluative concerns and fear of negative evaluation, a central component of social anxiety (DiBartolo, Li, & Frost, 2008). Contingent self-worth represented the extent to which self-esteem was based on others' approval, physical appearance, success and competition, academic competence, and participation in activities, whereas self-concealment referred to the tendency to hide one's negative qualities or mistakes. The predictor, maladaptive evaluative concerns, mediators, self-concealment and contingent self-worth, and criterion variable, fear of negative evaluation, all maintained significant and positive correlations with one another. Mediational analyses suggested partial mediation for self-concealment and contingent self-worth together. Findings indicated that individuals with perfectionistic qualities have lower unconditional self-acceptance, which is associated with a fear of negative social feedback. Results of this investigation are also consistent with Hewitt and colleagues' (2003) concept of perfectionistic self-presentation and suggest that individuals high in evaluative concerns may be reticent to expose their mistakes, and that this self-concealment contributes to fear of negative evaluation from others.

Negative social feedback is another potential mediator for the relationship between evaluative concerns and anxiety. A study by Nepon and colleagues (2011) evaluated the impact of this potential mechanism on socially prescribed perfectionism specifically and social anxiety (Nepon et al., 2011). Negative social feedback was measured using a self-report form in which respondents were asked to rate how often they received certain messages from others (e.g., "You should be really disappointed in yourself"). Negative social feedback partially mediated social anxiety levels for socially prescribed perfectionism, indicating that socially prescribed perfectionism may lead to elevated levels of social anxiety through a perception of receiving negative social feedback.

Although evaluative concerns was consistently associated with social factors and anxiety in these five studies, achievement striving was significantly related to distress in only three of them. When modeled without maladaptive evaluative concerns, Wu and Wei (2008) found that personal standards had no relationship with Other-Validation, or the need to seek approval from others, and a significant negative relationship with Self-Validation, or the ability to provide self-reinforcement and anxiety (Wu & Wei, 2008). However, when maladaptive evaluative concerns was considered in the model, achievement striving maintained a negative relationship with Other-Validation and anxiety, and a positive relationship with Self-Validation. These results suggest the contamination of personal standards measurement with elements of maladaptive evaluative concerns. In other words, measures that purport to assess achievement striving may also be tapping evaluative concerns. The findings also support the notion of personal standards perfectionism as an adaptive dimension unless it is paired with high levels of evaluative concerns. The authors further found a partial mediation effect for both Self- and Other-Validation for the personal standards–anxiety relationship. The lower levels of anxiety found for individuals with high achievement striving may be explained by their higher levels of Self-Validation and lower need for reassurance from others. Similarly, DiBartolo and colleagues (2008) found that pure personal standards was unrelated to self-concealment. However, personal standards was significantly and positively related to both fear of negative evaluation and contingent self-worth, and mediational analyses revealed that contingent self-worth fully mediated the relationship between pure personal standards and fear of negative evaluation.

Dunkley and colleagues (2000) found that achievement striving was not significantly correlated with either distress or social support, and thus, mediational analyses were not pursued. Social support was then considered as a moderator for the relationship between personal standards perfectionism and distress (Dunkley et al., 2000). When social support was low, individuals high in personal standards perfectionism experienced a larger increase in distress than those without strong personal standards perfectionism. The authors note that low social support is a condition under which achievement striving may be related to negative health outcomes because a lack of social support may overwhelm the individual's ability to cope with the distress that accompanies the pursuit of rigorous standards. As noted in the previous section, the findings from Dunkley et al. (2000) suggest that moderational research may be the most suited for identifying the ways in which high personal standards can lead to psychopathology.

Overall, these studies suggest that social support and positive social feedback are protective factors against the development of anxiety for individuals high in both achievement striving and evaluative concerns. Evaluative concerns appears to be uniformly related to negative psychological outcomes, and this relationship is consistently mediated in part by social factors. Interviews with perfectionists with high levels of negative perfectionism revealed that they recognize the interpersonal consequences of perfectionism, including annoying or putting pressure on others because of their exacting standards, although they also indicated that one perceived advantage of perfectionism is to gain respect from others (Egan et al., 2013). Clinically, these findings suggest that improvement in interpersonal skills, especially ways to appropriately garner affection from and connection to others, may be an important treatment target for individuals who have high levels of evaluative concerns. The findings for achievement striving are more complex. Whereas Wu and Wei (2008) found that achievement striving was negatively related to anxiety and positively related to the healthy ability to self-reinforce (when controlling for evaluative concerns), Dunkley and colleagues (2000) observed a relationship between achievement striving and anxiety in conditions of low social support. Additionally, DiBartolo and colleagues (2008) found a positive relationship between achievement striving and fear of negative evaluation mediated by contingent self-worth. Taken together, these three studies indicate that achievement striving may relate to anxiety in particular circumstances, but is not consistently a predictor of psychopathology (DiBartolo et al., 2008; Dunkley et al., 2000; Wu & Wei, 2008).

Cognitions

Theoretical Underpinnings

The literature relating evaluative concerns to anxiety through cognitive mechanisms is perhaps the most theoretically and methodologically disjointed. Most cognitive theories assert that attitudes and belief structures are often established early in life (cf. Chorpita & Barlow, 1998), and may interact to produce both evaluative concerns and anxiety. A difficulty then arises in building models that accurately represent when cognitive variables, including perfectionism's dimensions, serve as predictors, mediators, and outcome variables in investigating these relationships. However, evaluating the relationship between these cognitive variables is of particular relevance to treatment, especially in identifying treatment targets for cognitive behavioral therapy.

Barlow (2000) provides a comprehensive model for the development of anxiety which includes at its core a feeling that future events are unpredictable, uncontrollable, and potentially dangerous. Cognitive biases, including memory biases, interpretive biases, enhanced recognition of threat, and attention narrowing on sources of threat, interfere with healthy coping and generate avoidance and worry. This "anxious apprehension" increases autonomic arousal and negative affect, thereby cyclically worsening anxiety. Hewitt and Flett (2002) hypothesized that individuals high in evaluative concerns have similar cognitive characteristics that generate anxiety (Flett & Hewitt, 2002). For example, perfectionists are more likely to experience intrusive and automatic negative thoughts about their performance during stressful events, anticipate failure in the future, and ruminate about past failures (Flett et al., 1991; Flett, Madorsky, Hewitt, & Heisel, 2002; Fry, 1995). These attentional and memory biases lead perfectionists to overestimate the probability of future failure and inflate the cost of failure. As Pirbaglou and colleagues (2013) note, the presence of, and attention to, these negative thoughts, termed "perfectionistic cognitions," may distinguish perfectionists characterized by achievement striving from those characterized by evaluative concerns (Pirbaglou et al., 2013).

OCD The theoretical foundation underlying the relationship of evaluative concerns with OC symptoms through cognitive factors is somewhat of a special case. Perfectionism has at times been considered a risk factor for OCD as well as an integral part of the disorder (OCCWG, 1997). As they are currently understood, perfectionism and OCD share several common belief structures. For both perfectionists and individuals with OCD, a need for certainty and belief in the possibility of perfect performance may enhance personal responsibility about avoiding negative outcomes (Bouchard, Rheaume, & Ladouceur, 1999; OCCWG, 1997). Whereas perfectionists are more likely to be concerned over personal failures and negative evaluation, an individual with OCD may fear a wide variety of consequences as a result of their imperfection (e.g., contamination, harm to self or loved ones, unknown catastrophic outcome). The individual's belief that s/he is responsible for consequences that are both likely and serious without perfect performance fuels perfectionistic striving (e.g., high achievements) and OC symptoms (e.g., checking, ordering; Bouchard, et al., 1999; Rasmussen & Eisen, 1989).

The relationship between perfectionism and OCD is particularly complex due to these common cognitive structures, and perfectionism's current status as a definitional belief domain of OCD (OCCWG, 1997). However, both inflated responsibility and intolerance of uncertainty have been investigated as potential mediators for the relationship between evaluative concerns and OC symptoms. Further, Pleva and Wade (2006) proposed that misinterpretation of intrusive thoughts might serve as a mechanism between maladaptive evaluative concerns and OC symptoms. As per Salkovskis's theory of OCD, OC symptoms develop because normative intrusive thoughts (e.g., "there are harmful germs in my house") are misinterpreted as accurate and meaningful (Salkovskis, 1985). These intrusions become especially problematic when the individual assumes personal responsibility for avoiding the catastrophic consequences that might arise based on the intrusions (e.g., cleaning excessively and repeatedly to avoid getting themselves or loved ones sick). Bouchard and colleagues (1999) suggested that perfectionistic beliefs may lead to unhelpful interpretation of intrusions because unacceptable thoughts could be considered a mark of imperfection (Bouchard et al., 1999).

Mediational Research

Empirical research supports theoretical models indicating cognitive processes as a mediating factor of the evaluative concerns–anxiety relationship. DiBartolo and colleagues (2007) were interested in two cognitive biases common among both anxious and perfectionistic individuals (DiBartolo et al., 2007). The authors evaluated the perceived probability and negative impact of future stressful events as mediators of the relationship between dimensions of perfectionism and two types of anxiety, social phobia and state anxiety. Evaluative concerns was significantly correlated with measures of the two cognitive biases and with both measures of psychopathology. Regression analyses indicated that maladaptive evaluative concerns was a significant predictor for each cognitive bias while controlling for current levels of depression, anxiety, and stress. The perceived probability of negative events and the perceived consequences of future negative events together partially mediated the relationship between evaluative concerns and both forms of anxiety. When evaluated individually, perceived cost of negative events mediated the relationship with social anxiety only, whereas perceived probability mediated the relationship with both forms of anxiety. These results highlight the complex nature of these cognitive mechanisms while suggesting that interpretive biases may play a role in the relationship between evaluative concerns and the development of anxiety.

Wimberley and Stasio (2013) investigated perfectionistic cognitions as a mediator between maladaptive evaluative concerns and state anxiety (Wimberley & Stasio, 2013). Perfectionistic cognitions partially mediated the relationship between maladaptive evaluative concerns and anxiety. Results indicated that evaluative concerns may relate to anxiety through perfectionistic cognitions as a result of the activation of their ideal-self schema that perpetuates failure-related thoughts and worry (Flett et al., 2002).

Relational mechanisms between perfectionistic cognitions and anxiety were also evaluated by a separate group of researchers (Pirbaglou et al., 2013) who constructed a model in which perfectionistic cognitions predicted two indices of psychopathology, depression and anxiety. The model included two mediators, anxiety sensitivity and automatic negative thoughts, which each predicted depression and anxiety. The proposed model fit the data well, and significant indirect effects were found for both anxiety sensitivity and automatic negative thoughts, indicating the presence of mediation. These results indicate that individuals with high levels of evaluative concerns tend to experience frequent negative thoughts, including fears related to the consequences of anxiety (anxiety sensitivity; e.g., embarrassment, escalated anxiety), which lead to an increase in the experience of anxiety and depression. Pirbaglou and colleagues further speculate that the activation of negative thoughts serves as a boundary between perfectionistic strivings and evaluative concerns. The importance of perfectionistic cognitions and automatic negative thoughts suggests the potential utility of cognitive approaches (e.g., cognitive restructuring) in ameliorating the negative impact of perfectionism on mental health.

The literature presented suggests that cognitive factors may mediate the relationship between negative health outcomes and evaluative concerns (DiBartolo et al., 2007; Pirbaglou et al., 2013; Wimberley & Stasio, 2013). However, two of the studies described above also investigated the relationship of achievement striving with anxiety via cognitive mechanisms (DiBartolo et al., 2007; Wimberley & Stasio, 2013). DiBartolo and colleagues (2007) found that personal standards significantly and positively correlated with general state anxiety but not with social anxiety (DiBartolo et al., 2007). Perceived probability and cost of negative events together fully mediated the relationship between personal standards and anxiety, with perceived probability significantly contributing to the overall indirect effects. Wimberley and Stasio (2013) also investigated the mediating effect of perfectionistic cognitions on the association between personal standards and anxiety. Personal standards was not correlated with anxiety, but did maintain a positive relationship with perfectionistic cognitions, the mediator for the study. Mediational analyses indicated that personal standards was related to anxiety when accounting for the variance from perfectionistic cognitions; the authors concluded that perfectionistic cognitions mediated the relationship between personal standards and anxiety. However, the pattern of associations found within their data set suggests that analyses involving moderation, rather than mediation, may have been more appropriate given the lack of a significant correlation between personal standards and anxiety.

Evidence from these three studies suggests that evaluative concerns may be related to negative mental health outcomes through cognitive factors such as automatic negative thoughts, perfectionistic cognitions, and the perceived probability and cost of future negative events (DiBartolo et al., 2007; Pirbaglou et al., 2013; Wimberley & Stasio, 2013). Achievement striving may be related to the aspects of anxious symptomology through perfectionistic cognitions along with the perceived probability and consequences of negative events (DiBartolo et al., 2007; Wimberley & Stasio, 2013). Underscoring the difficulty of this area of study, researchers have conceptualized perfectionistic cognitions both as a specific domain of automatic negative thoughts (Flett et al., 2002) and as a mediator for perfectionism rather than an indicator of perfectionism (Wimberley & Stasio, 2013). Nonetheless, this research highlights the ways in which the distorted thinking typical of evaluative concerns likely fuels distress by rigidly imposing cognitive "absolutes and extremes" (Rice et al., 2003, p. 53). Despite these often-recognized costs, many individuals with clinical distress tied to their evaluative concerns reported worrying about catastrophic consequences if they were to relinquish their perfectionism, stating that "wheels would be falling off," or "I would sink" (Egan et al., 2013, p. 572). These data suggest that it is essential to address cognitive distortions and dysfunctional schema in clients with marked evaluative concerns, especially since they can serve to interfere with establishing motivation to change and therapeutic alliance (cf. Zuroff et al., 2000).

OCD Cognitive mechanisms have also been evaluated with regard to understanding the association between dimensions of perfectionism and a specific form of anxious symptomology, OC symptoms. Yorulmaz and colleagues (2006) investigated heightened personal responsibility as a potential mediator between Hewitt and Flett's conceptualization of perfectionism and OC symptoms (Yorulmaz et al., 2006). Socially prescribed perfectionism significantly correlated with measures of anxiety, responsibility, OC checking, and OC cleaning, whereas other-oriented perfectionism correlated only with cleaning symptoms. The authors controlled for variance related to depression and trait anxiety within the mediational regression analyses. Regression analyses including all three dimensions of perfectionism demonstrated no significant relationship between other-oriented perfectionism and cleaning; therefore, mediational analyses were not pursued with other-oriented perfectionism as a predictor. Results indicated that a sense of inflated responsibility fully mediated the relationship of socially prescribed perfectionism with both checking and cleaning. The authors hypothesized that in the presence of an imperfect state, high levels of evaluative concerns trigger the belief domain of over-responsibility for outcomes, and actions are taken to reduce threat.

Reuther and colleagues (2013) evaluated another potential cognitive mediator, intolerance for uncertainty, as a mechanism for the relationship between perfectionism and OC symptoms and severity, separately (Reuther et al., 2013). The authors measured perfectionism with the total FMPS score, a strategy that is not recommended given the distinct patterns of relationships seen for achievement striving and maladaptive evaluative concerns. Nonetheless, intolerance for uncertainty was found to mediate total perfectionism's relationship with both OCD indicators in one structural model. The authors also tested whether perfectionism was in fact a mediator between intolerance for uncertainty and OC symptoms and severity. This alternative model indicated that perfectionism did not function as a mediator. Despite these results, it is not clear whether intolerance for uncertainty is a mediator or a common vulnerability underlying both perfectionism and OC symptoms. As the authors suggest, an intolerance for uncertainty may in fact lead to the development of perfectionistic beliefs in order to ease the anxiety caused by uncertainty.

Lastly, another group of researchers investigated a third potential cognitive mechanism for understanding the association between dimensions of perfectionism and OC symptoms. Misinterpretation of intrusive thoughts was tested as a mediator between the Concern over Mistakes subscale of the FMPS and OC symptoms (Pleva & Wade, 2006). Inflated responsibility, but not depression, was controlled for in the regression analyses. When all variables were included in their model, Pleva and Wade (2006) found that heightened responsibility was a stronger predictor than Concern over Mistakes of both misinterpretation of intrusive thoughts and OC symptoms. However, the relationship between Concern over Mistakes and OC symptoms was partially mediated by misinterpretation of intrusive thoughts, even after controlling for responsibility. The results support Salkovskis's theory that intrusive thoughts become problematic when they are interpreted as accurate and meaningful; however, questions remain about the direction of the causal relationships.

Achievement striving was only evaluated in one of these three studies (Yorulmaz et al., 2006); the other two either did not distinguish the two dimensions of perfectionism (Reuther et al., 2013) or did not include a measure of achievement striving (Pleva & Wade, 2006). Yorulmaz and colleagues found that self-oriented perfectionism was significantly, positively correlated with anxiety, heightened responsibility, and both OC checking and cleaning (Yorulmaz et al., 2006). Mediational analyses for self-oriented perfectionism suggested that heightened personal responsibility fully mediated the association with checking and partially mediated the association with cleaning. The authors suggested that the association with cleaning may have been only partially mediated because of the difference between those wanting to reach a perfect state of cleanliness and those who are seeking to avoid contamination and sickness. Danger expectancy may play a larger role in cleaning compulsions for this later group.

The results of the three studies presented indicate that cognitive factors may be mediators through which dimensions of perfectionism relate to OC symptoms.

Specifically, authors suggested that: evaluative concerns relate to OC symptoms through heightened personal responsibility and misinterpretation of intrusive thoughts, total perfectionism is associated with OC symptoms via intolerance for uncertainty, and the relationships between achievement striving and OC symptoms are fully mediated by heightened personal responsibility (Pleva & Wade, 2006; Reuther et al., 2013; Yorulmaz et al., 2006). However, these cognitive mechanisms may also be epiphenomenon, or they may be causes of both perfectionism and OC symptoms. Regardless, the presented data further support the use of cognitive behavioral therapy in treating OC symptoms, an approach which is already considered by many to be the best practice (Frost & Steketee, 2002).

Summary

This literature demonstrates that evaluative concerns is consistently related to a variety of negative mental health outcomes, including worry, social anxiety, OC symptomology, and state and trait anxiety (see Fig. 8.1). A developing body of

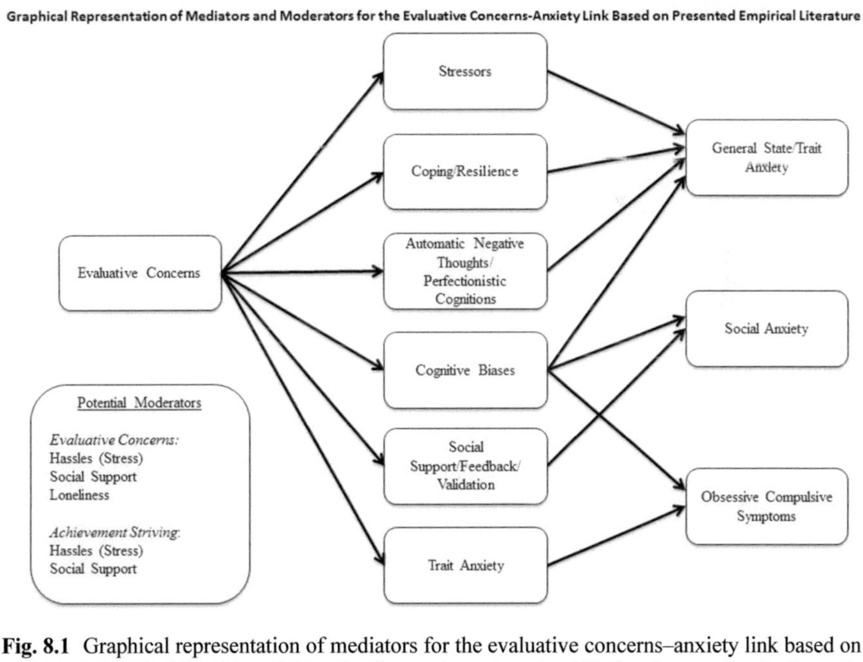

Fig. 8.1 Graphical representation of mediators for the evaluative concerns–anxiety link based on presented empirical literature. (Note: the figure above is a simplified and generalized schematic of the mediational themes arising within the describing literature. All constructs represented likely interact with one another in an iterative, reciprocal fashion at each level of the model. However, the status of the field at the present time does not allow for these fine distinctions to be made and represented. Moderators cannot be represented directly in the figure because it is unknown which of these mediational paths they impact)

research suggests that certain mechanisms mediate this relationship. In short, individuals high in evaluative concerns may be more likely to experience life stressors and subjective and objective social isolation to which they tend to respond by using unhelpful interpretive and attentional biases along with maladaptive coping strategies. Each of these mechanisms increases the likelihood of anxious symptomology. Additionally, these processes represent potential treatment targets for individuals with perfectionistic qualities who are suffering from anxious symptomology.

Of the 15 studies discussed, 6 reported significant findings for mediators of the achievement striving–anxious symptomology relationship. Individuals high in personal standards perfectionism tend to have increased contingent self-worth and perfectionistic cognitions, and may overestimate the probability and cost of negative events along with their personal responsibility. These characteristics may then contribute to an increase in anxiety symptoms, which may be further exacerbated by the moderators of life stress and low social support. However, some evidence reviewed suggested either a negative relationship or no relationship between achievement striving and anxiety. Recommendations provided below suggest ways in which research may clarify the associations between these constructs.

Recommendations

There is a growing body of research related to the mechanisms underlying the association between anxiety and perfectionism. Based on a review of the literature, a few recommendations are offered that may facilitate the advancement of this area of research. The field might consider moving towards the development of a comprehensive theory to describe the mechanisms through which and conditions under which dimensions of perfectionism relate to the development of anxiety. Currently, theoretical models of the relationship between perfectionism and psychopathology do not appear to be the driver behind the selection of study predictors, mediators, and criterion variables. Rather, researchers seem to couch empirical findings in broad theories of the development of psychopathology. Developing *a priori* hypotheses determined by theoretically specified causal relationships does not appear to be the norm, potentially due to the lack of a theoretical foundation underlying the relationship between evaluative concerns and anxiety. The development of this type of comprehensive foundation might allow for specific, theory-driven hypotheses to be tested regarding the nature of perfectionism and its impact on anxious symptomology.

Researchers may also wish to be more intentional when selecting methods of evaluating potential mediational relationships. Often, the rationale that significant correlations exist between an independent variable and a mediator, and the mediator and a dependent variable, is used to justify mediational analysis. Although this pattern of correlations is recommended for mediational analysis, it may not be sufficient to justify this procedure. Mediational analyses provide meaningful information when (a) the relationships under investigation are grounded theoretically and

(b) the predictor and criterion variables maintain a consistent relationship in the literature. The meaning of mediational analyses becomes unclear when predictor and criterion variables are unrelated (e.g., mediating a relationship that may not exist) either in past literature or the study at hand, or when the constructs under study have acted as predictors, mediators, and criterion variables in various investigations without a strong theoretical rationale. At times, moderational analyses may be more suitable. Because evaluative concerns and anxiety are robustly and consistently associated, it is appropriate to evaluate the mechanisms underlying this connection using mediational analysis. Contrastingly, achievement striving has an unstable pattern of associations with anxiety. These inconsistent results lead us to ask not why the constructs are related, but rather, under which circumstances they are related (Frazier, Tix, & Barron, 2004; Rose, Holmbeck, Coakley, & Franks, 2004). Moderational analyses may be best suited for clarifying the conditions through which positive achievement striving is related to anxiety.

Similarly, common developmental pathways that contribute to the co-occurrence of perfectionism and anxiety may contribute to some of the study findings. Within each of the studies presented, the question remains of whether the identified mechanism is truly a causal factor or an epiphenomenon of perfectionism. To understand the causal mechanisms underlying the associations between dimensions of perfectionism and anxiety, longitudinal and experimental designs are required. These types of studies can be challenging, but they effectively advance our understanding of causal relationships and have the potential to foster advances in the prevention and treatment of psychopathology. The literature presented here suggests potential efficacy for treatment approaches that address the development of positive coping mechanisms, improvement in social support, and cognitive restructuring (such as cognitive behavioral therapy). Identifying the processes that contribute to negative mental health outcomes for individuals high in dimensions of perfectionism may further clarify appropriate treatment targets for this population.

References

Antony, M. M., Purdon, C. L., Huta, V., & Swinson, R. P. (1998). Dimensions of perfectionism across the anxiety disorders. *Behaviour Research and Therapy, 36,* 1143–1154. doi:10.1016/S0005-7967(98)00083–7.

Barlow, D. H. (2000). Unraveling the mysteries of anxiety and its disorders from the perspective of emotion theory. *American Psychologist, 55,* 1247–1263. doi:10.1037/0003-066X.55.11.1247.

Besser, A., Flett, G. L., & Hewitt, P. L. (2010). Perfectionistic self-presentation and trait perfectionism in social problem-solving ability and depressive symptoms. *Journal of Applied Social Psychology, 40,* 2121–2154.

Bouchard, C., Rhéaume, J., & Ladouceur, R. (1999). Responsibility and perfectionism in OCD: An experimental study. *Behaviour Research and Therapy, 37,* 239–248. doi:10.1016/S0005-7967(98)00141-7.

Brown, E. J., Heimberg, R. G., Frost, R. O., Makris, G. S., Juster, H. R., & Leung, A. W. (1999). Relationship of perfectionism to affect, expectations, attributions and performance in the classroom. *Journal of Social and Clinical Psychology, 18,* 98–120. doi:10.1521/jscp.1999.18.1.98.

Chang, E. C., Sanna, L. J., Chang, R., & Bodem, M. R. (2008). A preliminary look at loneliness as a moderator of the link between perfectionism and depressive and anxious symptoms in college students: Does being lonely make perfectionistic strivings more distressing? *Behaviour Research and Therapy, 46,* 877–886. doi:10.1016/j.brat.2008.03.012.

Chorpita, B. F., & Barlow, D. H. (1998). The development of anxiety: The role of control in the early environment. *Psychological Bulletin, 124,* 3–21. doi:10.1037/0033-2909.124.1.3.

DiBartolo, P., Frost, R. O., Chang, P., LaSota, M., & Grills, A. E. (2004). Shedding light on the relationship between personal standards and psychopathology: The case for contingent self-worth. *Journal of Rational-Emotive and Cognitive-Behavior Therapy, 22,* 237–250. doi:10.1023/B:JORE.0000047310.94044.ac.

DiBartolo, P., Li, C., Averett, S., Skotheim, S., Smith, L. M., Raney, C., & McMillen, C. (2007). The relationship of perfectionism to judgmental bias and psychopathology. *Cognitive Therapy and Research, 31,* 573–587. doi:10.1007/s10608-006-9112-z.

DiBartolo, P., Li, C., & Frost, R. O. (2008). How do the dimensions of perfectionism relate to mental health? *Cognitive Therapy and Research, 32,* 401–417. doi:10.1007/s10608-007-9157-7.

Dunkley, D. M., Blankstein, K. R., Halsall, J., Williams, M., & Winkworth, G. (2000). The relation between perfectionism and distress: Hassles, coping, and perceived social support as mediators and moderators. *Journal of Counseling Psychology, 47,* 437–453. doi:10.1037/0022-0167.47.4.437.

Egan, S. J., Wade, T. D., & Shafran, R. (2011). Perfectionism as a transdiagnostic process: A clinical review. *Clinical Psychology Review, 31*(2), 203–212. doi:10.1016/j.cpr.2010.04.009.

Egan, S. J., Piek, J. P., Dyck, M. J., Rees, C. S., & Hagger, M. S. (2013). A clinical investigation of motivation to change standards and cognitions about failure in perfectionism. *Behavioural and Cognitive Psychotherapy, 41,* 565–578. doi:10.1017/S135246581200063X.

Flett, G. L., & Hewitt, P. L. (2002). *Perfectionism: Theory, research, and treatment.* Washington, DC: American Psychological Association. doi:10.1037/10458-000.

Flett, G. L., Hewitt, P. L., Blankstein, K. R., & Mosher, S. W. (1991). Perfectionism, self-actualization, and personal adjustment. *Journal of Social Behavior and Personality, 6,* 147–160.

Flett, G. L., Blankstein, K. L., Hewitt, P. L., & Koledin, S. (1992). Components of perfectionism and procrastination in college students. *Social Behavior and Personality, 20,* 85–94.

Flett, G. L., Hewitt, P. L., Endler, N. S., & Tassone, C. (1994–1995). Perfectionism and components of state and trait anxiety. *Current Psychology: A Journal for Diverse Perspectives on Diverse Psychological Issues, 13,* 326–350. doi:10.1007/BF02686891.

Flett, G. L., Russo, F., & Hewitt, P. L. (1994). Dimensions of perfectionism and constructive thinking as a coping response. *Journal of Rational-Emotive and Cognitive-Behaviour Therapy, 12,* 163–179.

Flett, G. L., Hewitt, P. L., Blankstein, K. R., Solnik, M., & Brunschot, M. (1996). Perfectionism, social problem-solving ability, and psychological distress. *Journal of Rational-Emotive and Cognitive-Behavior Therapy, 14,* 245–275. doi:10.1007/BF02238139.

Flett, G. L., Madorsky, D., Hewitt, P. L., & Heisel, M. J. (2002). Perfectionism cognitions, rumination, and psychological distress. *Journal of Rational-Emotive and Cognitive-Behavior Therapy, 20,* 33–47.

Folkman, S., & Lazarus, R. (1985). If it changes it must be a process: Study of emotion and coping during three stages of a college examination. *Journal of Personality and Social Psychology, 48,* 150–170. doi:10.1037/0022-3514.48.1.150.

Frazier, P. A., Tix, A. P., & Barron, K. E. (2004). Testing moderator and mediator effects in counseling psychology research. *Journal of Counseling Psychology, 51,* 115–134. doi:10.1037/0022-0167.51.1.115.

Frost, R. O., & Gross, R. C. (1993). The hoarding of possessions. *Behaviour Research and Therapy, 31,* 367–381. doi:10.1016/0005-7967(93)90094-B.

Frost, R. O., & Steketee, G. (1997). Perfectionism in obsessive-compulsive disorder patients. *Behaviour Research and Therapy, 35,* 291–296. doi:10.1016/S0005-7967(96)00108-8.

Frost, R. O., & Steketee, G. (2002). *Cognitive approaches to obsessions and compulsions: Theory, assessment, and treatment.* Amsterdam: Pergamon/Elsevier Science Inc.

Frost, R. O., Marten, P., Lahart, C., & Rosenblate, R. (1990). The dimensions of perfectionism. *Cognitive Therapy and Research, 14,* 449–468. doi:10.1007/BF01172967.

Frost, R. O., Heimberg, R. G., Holt, C. S., Mattia, J. I., & Neubauer, A. L. (1993). A comparison of two measures of perfectionism. *Personality and Individual Differences, 14,* 119–126.

Frost, R. O., Steketee, G., Cohn, L., & Griess, K. (1994). Personality traits in subclinical and non-obsessive-compulsive volunteers and their parents. *Behaviour Research and Therapy, 32,* 47–56. doi:10.1016/0005-7967(94)90083-3.

Frost, R. O., Trepanier, K. L., Brown, E. J., Heimberg, R. G., Juster, H. R., & Makris, G. S. (1997). Selfmonitoring of mistakes among subjects high and low in concern over mistakes. *Cognitive Therapy and Research, 21,* 209–222.

Fry, P. S. (1995). Perfectionism, humor, and optimism as moderators of health outcomes and determinants of coping styles of women executives. *Genetics, Social, and General Psychology Monographs, 121,* 211–245.

Gnilka, P. B., Ashby, J. S., & Noble, C. M. (2012). Multidimensional perfectionism and anxiety: Differences among individuals with perfectionism and tests of a coping-mediation model. *Journal of Counseling and Development, 90,* 427–436. doi:10.1002/j.1556-6676.2012.00054.x.

Hamachek, D. E. (1978). Psychodynamics of normal and neurotic perfectionism. *Psychology, 15,* 27–33.

Hewitt, P. L., & Flett, G. L. (1991). Perfectionism in the self and social contexts: Conceptualization, assessment, and association with psychopathology. *Journal of Personality and Social Psychology, 60,* 456–470.

Hewitt, P. L., & Flett, G. L. (1993). Dimensions of perfectionism, daily stress, and depression: A test of the specific vulnerability hypothesis. *Journal of Abnormal Psychology, 102,* 58–65.

Hewitt, P. L., Flett, G. L., Sherry, S. B., Habke, M., Parkin, M., Lam, R. W., & Stein, M. B. (2003). The interpersonal expression of perfection: Perfectionistic self-presentation and psychological distress. *Journal of Personality and Social Psychology, 84,* 1303–1325. doi:10.1037/0022-3514.84.6.1303.

Hewitt, P. L., Flett, G. L., Besser, A. A., Sherry, S. B., & McGee, B. B. (2003). Perfectionism is multidimensional: A reply to Shafran, Cooper and Fairburn (2002). *Behaviour Research and Therapy, 41,* 1221–1236. doi:10.1016/S0005-7967(03)00021-4.

Hewitt, P. L., Flett, G. L., Sherry, S. B., & Caelian, C. (2006). Trait perfectionism dimensions and suicidal behavior. In T. E. Ellis (Ed.), *Cognition and suicide: Theory, research, and therapy* (pp. 215–235). Washington, DC: American Psychological Association. doi:10.1037/11377-010.

Juster, H. R., Heimberg, R. G., Frost, R. O., & Holt, C. S. (1996). Social phobia and perfectionism. *Personality and Individual Differences, 21,* 403–410. doi:10.1016/0191-8869(96)00075-X.

Kawamura, K. Y., Hunt, S. L., Frost, R. O., & DiBartolo, P. (2001). Perfectionism, anxiety, and depression: Are the relationships independent? *Cognitive Therapy and Research, 25,* 291–301. doi:10.1023/A:1010736529013.

Klibert, J., Lamis, D. A., Collins, W., Smalley, K., Warren, J. C., Yancey, C., & Winterowd, C. (2014). Resilience mediates the relations between perfectionism and college student distress. *Journal of Counseling and Development, 92,* 75–82. doi:10.1002/j.1556-6676.2014.00132.x.

Lazarus, R. S., & Folkman, S. (1984). *Stress, appraisal, and coping*. New York: Springer.

Lee, J. C., Prado, H. S., Diniz, J. B., Borcato, S., da Silva, C. B., Hounie, A. G., & do Rosário, M. C. (2009). Perfectionism and sensory phenomena: Phenotypic components of obsessive-compulsive disorder. *Comprehensive Psychiatry, 50,* 431–436. doi:10.1016/j.comppsych.2008.11.007.

Levinson, C. A., Rodebaugh, T. L., White, E. K., Menatti, A. R., Weeks, J. W., Iacovino, J. M., & Warren, C. S. (2013). Social appearance anxiety, perfectionism, and fear of negative evaluation: Distinct or shared risk factors for social anxiety and eating disorders? *Appetite, 67,* 125–133. doi:10.1016/j.appet.2013.04.002.

Moretz, M. W., & McKay, D. (2009). The role of perfectionism in obsessive-compulsive symptoms: "Not just right" experiences and checking compulsions. *Journal of Anxiety Disorders, 23,* 640–644. doi:10.1016/j.janxdis.2009.01.015.

Neenan, M. (2009). *Developing resilience: A cognitive-behavioural approach.* New York: Routledge/Taylor & Francis Group.

Nepon, T., Flett, G. L., Hewitt, P. L., & Molnar, D. S. (2011). Perfectionism, negative social feedback, and interpersonal rumination in depression and social anxiety. *Canadian Journal of Behavioural Science/Revue Canadienne Des Sciences Du Comportement, 43,* 297–308. doi:10.1037/a0025032.

Obsessive Compulsive Cognitions Working Group. (1997). Cognitive assessment of obsessive-compulsive disorder. *Behaviour Research and Therapy, 35,* 667–681.

Pearson, C. A., & Gleaves, D. H. (2006). The multiple dimensions of perfectionism and their relation with eating disorder features. *Personality and Individual Differences, 41,* 225–235. doi:10.1016/j.paid.2006.01.013.

Pirbaglou, M., Cribbie, R., Irvine, J., Radhu, N., Vora, K., & Ritvo, P. (2013). Perfectionism, anxiety, and depressive distress: Evidence for the mediating role of negative automatic thoughts and anxiety sensitivity. *Journal of American College Health, 61,* 477–483. doi:10.1080/07448481.2013.833932.

Pleva, J., & Wade, T. D. (2006). The mediating effects of misinterpretation of intrusive thoughts on obsessive-compulsive symptoms. *Behaviour Research and Therapy, 44,* 1471–1479. doi:10.1016/j.brat.2005.11.003.

Rasmussen, S. A., & Eisen, J. L. (1989). Clinical features and phenomenology of obsessive compulsive disorder. *Psychiatric Annals, 19,* 67–73.

Rehm, L. P., & Marston, A. R. (1968). Reduction of social anxiety through modification of self-reinforcement: An instigation therapy technique. *Journal of Consulting and Clinical Psychology, 32,* 565–574. doi:10.1037/h0026406.

Reuther, E. T., Davis, T., Rudy, B. M., Jenkins, W. S., Whiting, S. E., & May, A. C. (2013). Intolerance of uncertainty as a mediator of the relationship between perfectionism and obsessive-compulsive symptom severity. *Depression and Anxiety, 30,* 773–777.

Rhéaume, J., Freeston, M. H., Dugas, M. J., Letarte, H., & Ladouceur, R. (1995). Perfectionism, responsibility and obsessive-compulsive symptoms. *Behaviour Research and Therapy, 33,* 785–794. doi:10.1016/0005-7967(95)00017-R.

Rice, K. G., Bair, C. J., Castro, J. R., Cohen, B. N., & Hood, C. A. (2003). Meanings of perfectionism: A quantitative and qualitative analysis. *Journal of Cognitive Psychotherapy, 17,* 39–58. doi:10.1891/jcop.17.1.39.58266.

Rose, B. M., Holmbeck, G. N., Coakley, R., & Franks, E. A. (2004). Mediator and moderator effects in developmental and behavioral pediatric research. *Journal of Developmental and Behavioral Pediatrics, 25,* 58–67. doi:10.1097/00004703-200402000-00013.

Saboonchi, F., & Lundh, L. (1997). Perfectionism, self-consciousness and anxiety. *Personality and Individual Differences, 22,* 921–928. doi:10.1016/S0191-8869(96)00274-7.

Salkovskis, P. M. (1985). Obsessional-compulsive problems: A cognitive-behavioural analysis. *Behaviour Research and Therapy, 23,* 571–558.

Santanello, A. W., & Gardner, F. L. (2007). The role of experiential avoidance in the relationship between maladaptive perfectionism and worry. *Cognitive Therapy and Research, 31,* 319–332. doi:10.1007/s10608-006-9000-6.

Shafran, R., Cooper, Z., & Fairburn, C. G. (2002). Clinical perfectionism: A cognitive-behavioural analysis. *Behaviour Research and Therapy, 40,* 773–791. doi:10.1016/S0005-7967(01)00059–6.

Slade, P. D., & Owens, R. G. (1998). A dual process model of perfectionism based on reinforcement theory. *Behavior Modification, 22,* 372–390.

Stöber, J. (1998). The Frost multidimensional perfectionism scale revisited: More perfect with four (instead of six) dimensions. *Personality and Individual Differences, 24,* 481–491. doi:10.1016/S0191-8869(97)00207-9.

Wheeler, H. A., Blankstein, K. R., Antony, M. M., McCabe, R. E., & Bieling, P. J. (2011). Perfectionism in anxiety and depression: Comparisons across disorders, relations with symptom severity, and role of comorbidity. *International Journal of Cognitive Therapy, 4,* 66–91. doi:10.1521/ijct.2011.4.1.66.

Wimberley, T. E., & Stasio, M. J. (2013). Perfectionistic thoughts, personal standards, and evaluative concerns: Further investigating relationships to psychological distress. *Cognitive Therapy and Research, 37,* 277–283. doi:10.1007/s10608-012-9462-7.

Wu, T., & Wei, M. (2008). Perfectionism and negative mood: The mediating roles of validation from others versus self. *Journal of Counseling Psychology, 55,* 276–288. doi:10.1037/0022-0167.55.2.276.

Xie, D., Leong, F. L., & Feng, S. (2008). Culture-specific personality correlates of anxiety among Chinese and Caucasian college students. *Asian Journal of Social Psychology, 11,* 163–174. doi:10.1111/j.1467-839X.2008.00253.x.

Yorulmaz, O., Karanci, A., & Tekok-Kiliç, A. (2006). What are the roles of perfectionism and responsibility in checking and cleaning compulsions? *Journal of Anxiety Disorders, 20,* 312–327. doi:10.1016/j.janxdis.2005.02.009.

Zuroff, D. C., Blatt, S. J., Sotsky, S. M., Krupnick, J. L., Martin, D. J., Sanislow, C. A., & Simmens, S. (2000). Relation of therapeutic alliance and perfectionism to outcome in brief outpatient treatment of depression. *Journal of Consulting and Clinical Psychology, 68,* 114–124. doi:10.1037/0022-006X.68.1.114.

Chapter 9
Perfectionism and Eating Disorders

Tracey D. Wade, Anne O'Shea and Roz Shafran

Overview

The coupling of perfectionism and eating disorders has a very long history, with a case study emerging from the medieval years. St. Catherine of Siena (1347–1380) is thought to have suffered from anorexia nervosa. From the age of 16 years, she ate less and less until eventually she ate nothing but the daily Eucharist, maintaining this regime even in the face of disapproval from the clergy. She died in Rome at the age of 33, a death considered to be caused by the effects related to starvation. One of her writings gives us a clue to some of the issues that may have maintained this sustained and committed behaviour:

> Make a supreme effort to root out self-love from your heart and to plant in its place this holy self-hatred. This is the royal road by which we turn our backs on mediocrity, and which leads us without fail to the summit of perfection.

A more modern example of the co-occurrence of perfectionism and eating disorders comes from Jenni Schaefer, the author of "Goodbye Ed, Hello me; Recover from your eating disorder and fall in love with life":

> In the past, my brain could only compute perfection or failure—nothing in between. So words like competent, acceptable, satisfactory, and good enough fell into the failure category.

The purpose of this chapter is to examine the nature of the relationship between perfectionism and eating disorders, in terms of how this relationship is described in different theories, the evidence with respect to the direction of this relationship and the usefulness of interventions which seek to decrease perfectionism in terms

T. D. Wade (✉) · A. O'Shea
School of Psychology, Flinders University, GPO Box 2100, Adelaide, South Australia 5001, Australia
e-mail: tracey.wade@flinders.edu.au

R. Shafran
Institute of Child Health, University College London, London, UK

F. M. Sirois, D. S. Molnar (eds.), *Perfectionism, Health, and Well-Being,*
DOI 10.1007/978-3-319-18582-8_9

of their impact on disordered eating. Disordered eating and eating disorders cover a variety of different behaviours and attitudes, but the core features that are discussed in the current chapter include the following:

- The importance of control overeating, weight and shape in terms of determining self-worth;
- Objective binge eating, defined as eating a large amount of food in a circumscribed period of time (2 h) while experiencing a feeling of lack of control;
- Purging behaviours, which can include the use of self-induced vomiting, diuretics or laxatives for the purpose of controlling weight and shape;
- Extreme forms of non-purging behaviours such as driven exercise and fasting used primarily for the purpose of controlling weight and shape.

Theoretical Perspectives on Perfectionism and Eating Disorders

Hilde Bruch (1974), a pioneer in the field of eating disorders, noted that clients with eating disorders demonstrate "*superperfection*" and argued that the adolescent turns to body weight as a concrete source of self-definition and as a means of compensating for the lack of a clear identity as well as for associated feelings of powerlessness and incompetence. In 1978, Peter Slade developed a functional analytical model of anorexia nervosa in which he also hypothesised that, in the context of adolescent conflicts, interpersonal problems, and stress and failure experiences, the adolescent with low self-esteem and perfectionistic tendencies would feel a need to control completely, or attain success, in some aspect of life. One of the aspects of life most salient to young women is in the domain of body weight and size. He described this perfectionistic viewpoint in a very similar manner to that of Schaefer:

> [adolescents] *see events and their own achievements in black and white terms, such that anything else less than idealized, perfect success or attainment represents failure and lack of success* (p. 171).

Since this early theoretical emphasis on the role of perfectionism in increasing risk for eating disorders, a number of authors have attempted to develop testable theories that define how perfectionism may work together with other risk factors to cause and maintain eating disorders. We look at each of the most prominent theories in turn.

The Three-Factor Model First proposed by Vohs and colleagues in 1999, this model posited that self-esteem moderates the relationship between the interaction of perfectionism and perceived weight status (regardless of actual weight status), and changes in bulimic symptoms. In other words, perfectionists who perceived themselves as being overweight would exhibit higher levels of bulimic symptomology if their self-esteem was low, compared to perfectionists with weight concerns who have high self-esteem. Low self-esteem was seen to interfere with the attainment of desired goals, which in the context of frustration with respect to any weight-related goals (e.g. wanting to lose weight) can trigger negative mood in perfectionists and result in disordered eating. This model, after accounting for the effects of body mass index (BMI), was supported across a number of early studies (Vohs, Voelz et al., 2001; Vohs, Bardone, Joiner, Abramson, & Heatherton, 1999; Vohs, Heatherton, & Herrin, 2001).

Since being developed, the three-factor model has been revised in a number of ways. First, perceived weight status has been operationalised as body dissatisfaction (Vohs, Voelz et al., 2001) and more recently as weight and shape concern (Bardone-Cone et al., 2008) using the relevant subscales of the Eating Disorder Examination-Questionnaire (EDE-Q; Fairburn & Beglin, 1994). Second, recent studies have replaced the Bulimia subscale of the Eating Disorders Inventory (EDI; Clausen, Rosenvinge, Friborg, & Rokkedal, 2011) as the measure of bulimic behaviours with the number of episodes of binge eating and inappropriate compensatory behaviour as assessed by the EDE-Q (Bardone-Cone, Abramson, Vohs, Heatherton, & Joiner, 2006; Bardone-Cone et al., 2008). Third, given that independent attempts to replicate the model using self-esteem have persistently failed (Shaw, Stice, & Springer, 2004; Steele, Corsini, & Wade, 2007; Tissot & Crowther, 2008; Watson, Steele, Bergin, Fursland, & Wade, 2011), the three-factor model has replaced self-esteem with self-efficacy (Bardone-Cone et al., 2006; 2008). Self-efficacy was considered not as an alternative to self-esteem but rather as a more relevant component of the original construct of interest, namely doubt about one's ability to achieve and perceiving interference with goal attainment.

The inclusion of self-efficacy may show better replicability, with one study indicating it prospectively predicted bingeing but not purging behaviours (Bardone-Cone et al., 2006) where perfectionism was measured using the subscale from the EDI that includes a mix of items related to "socially prescribed" and "self-oriented" perfectionism (Hewitt & Flett, 1991). Bardone-Cone et al. (2008) found that a three-way interaction with both personal standards (PS) and concern over mistakes perfectionism from the Frost Multidimensional Perfectionism Scale (FMPS; Frost, Marten, Lahart, & Rosenblate, 1990) predicted increases in binge eating. That is, young women who reported self-critical reactions to a failure to attain goals and who were low in self-efficacy and had concerns about shape and weight experienced the most binge eating episodes, as shown in Fig. 9.1. The use of PS perfec-

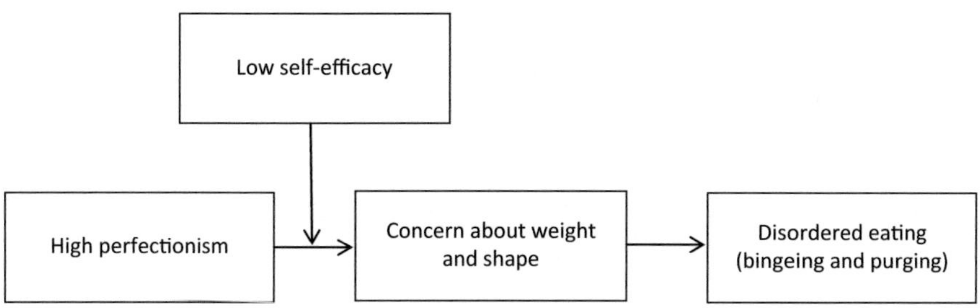

Fig. 9.1 The three-factor model

tionism in the interaction was also associated with more episodes of self-induced vomiting. In other words, young women who reported the importance of goal attainment and excellence and who were low in self-efficacy and had concerns about shape and weight experienced the most purging behaviour. To date, no treatments have been formulated based on this model.

The Transdiagnostic Theory of Eating Disorders The transdiagnostic theory of eating disorders is cognitive behavioural in nature and grew primarily from the cognitive behavioural theory of bulimia nervosa (Fairburn, 1997). A key aspect of the rationale for developing the theory was that cognitive behaviour therapy for bulimia nervosa was effective but that half of the patients were failing to make a full and lasting recovery (Fairburn, Shafran, & Cooper, 2003). One potential explanation was the narrow focus on specific psychopathology of eating, shape, weight and their control. The theory was therefore extended to incorporate four additional maintaining mechanisms derived from the literature—clinical perfectionism, core low self-esteem, mood intolerance and interpersonal difficulties (see Fig. 9.2).

Like the core psychopathology of eating disorders, "clinical perfectionism" was considered as a dysfunctional scheme for self-evaluation. It was defined as the overevaluation of striving for, and achievement of, personally demanding standards despite adverse consequences (Shafran, Cooper, & Fairburn, 2002). The application of these standards for eating, shape, weight and their control was suggested to in-

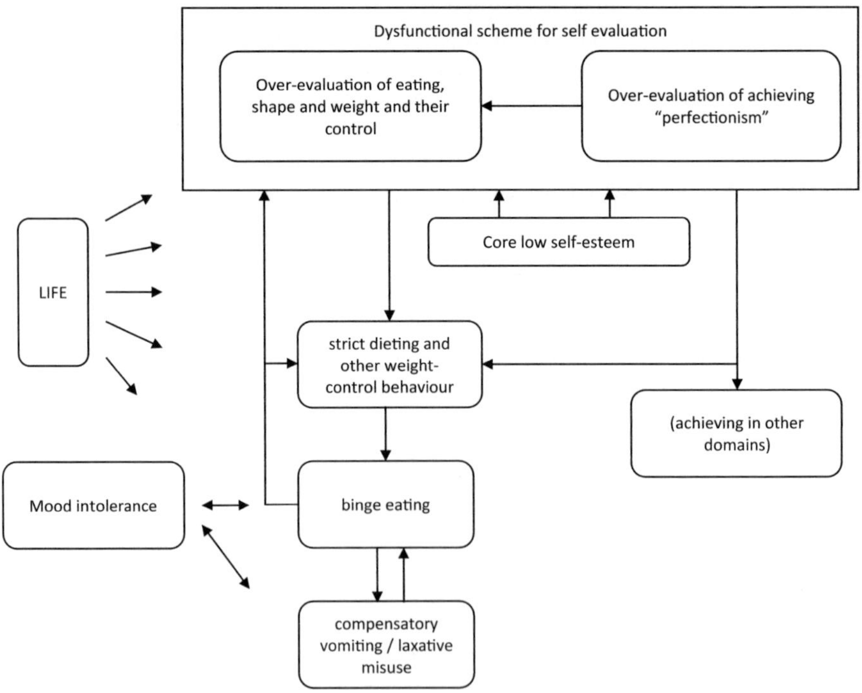

Fig. 9.2 Components of the transdiagnostic theory of eating disorders

teract with the eating disorder psychopathology and maintain it. In this account, the fears of "fatness", weight gain and overeating are considered as exemplars of the characteristic fear of failure of clinical perfectionism; shape and weight checking is viewed as counterproductive behavioural strategy and the characteristic self-criticism in patients with eating disorders viewed as arising from negatively biased appraisals of performance. The self-criticism was hypothesised to maintain negative self-evaluation which, in turn, was suggested to encourage even more determined striving to meet valued goals related to eating, shape and weight—thereby serving to maintain the eating disorder. It was therefore predicted that reducing clinical perfectionism would remove an additional maintaining mechanism for some patients who held this belief system and would improve the eating disorder.

It should be noted that in the original paper describing the transdiagnostic theory of eating disorders, the argument was made that eating disorders (anorexia nervosa, bulimia nervosa and eating disorder not otherwise specified) were maintained by shared, but distinctive, psychopathological processes with patients frequently migrating across diagnostic categories. It was therefore concluded that common mechanisms, including clinical perfectionism, are involved in the persistence of bulimia nervosa, anorexia nervosa and the atypical eating disorders.

The implication of the transdiagnostic theory of eating disorders for treatment is that clinicians should consider identifying and potentially addressing clinical perfectionism in the context of eating disorders when it appears to be a barrier to change. Data evaluating the transdiagnostic treatment indicate that patients with marked mood intolerance, clinical perfectionism, low self-esteem or interpersonal difficulties respond better to the treatment that incorporates techniques to address their specific difficulty (Fairburn et al., 2009). The treatment overall has promising results (Fairburn et al., 2009; Byrne, Fursland, Allen, & Watson, 2011; Dalle Grave et al., 2013; Dalle Grave, Calugi, Doll, Fairburn, 2013; Fairburn et al., 2015).

The Cognitive-Interpersonal Model of Anorexia Nervosa This model has been formulated specifically to help inform development of treatment for anorexia nervosa (Schmidt & Treasure, 2006), in line with principles encapsulated in the UK Medical Research Council's framework for the development of complex interventions (Craig et al., 2008). While no formal test of the model has been conducted, the development has involved an iterative translational process between basic research and model/treatment development, combining a top-down (i.e. theory-led, data-driven, quantitative) and bottom-up (i.e. patient and clinician experience-led, qualitative) approach (Schmidt, Wade, & Treasure, 2014), resulting in one revision of the model to date (Treasure & Schmidt, 2013).

The model proposes that anorexia nervosa typically arises in people who have anxious and perfectionist traits and is maintained by four broad factors (Schmidt et al., 2014) as shown in Fig. 9.3. The factors include: a rigid, detail-focused and perfectionist information processing style; impairments in the socio-emotional domain (such as avoidance of the experience and expression of emotions in the context of close relationships); the development of beliefs about the utility of anorexia nervosa; and inadvertent actions of close others that may serve to maintain the anorexia nervosa, e.g. high levels of expressed emotion, accommodation and enabling be-

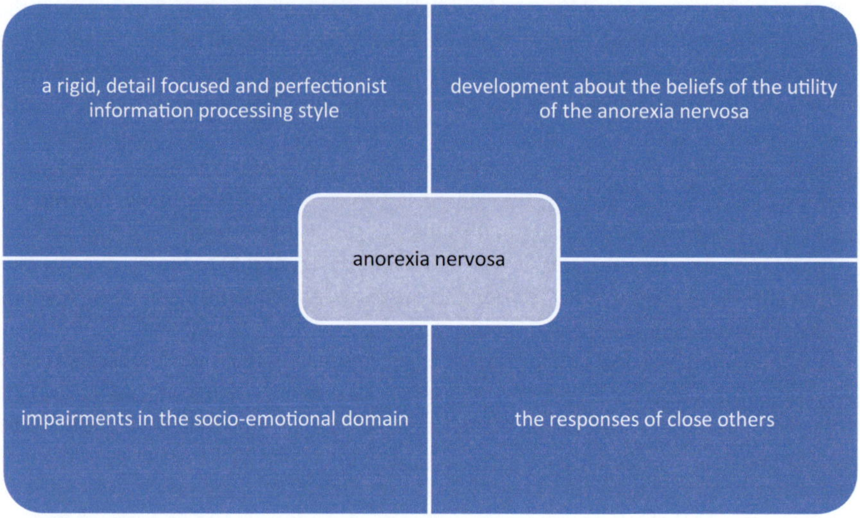

Fig. 9.3 Cognitive interpersonal model of anorexia nervosa

haviours. Starvation intensifies these problems, thereby forming a recursive loop between the consequences of starvation and these maintenance factors.

In terms of the specific relationship between perfectionism and eating, Schmidt and Treasure (2006) suggest the following:

> Individuals with these traits value perfection and fear making mistakes. They are excessively conscientious and cognitively rigid … The traits (being rigidly rule-bound, striving for perfection) can facilitate persistent dietary restriction and the control of appetite. A wish for simplicity and focus on details make this type of behaviour satisfying and may lead to the … belief 'anorexia nervosa makes me feel in control' (p. 349).

The type of perfectionism that they refer to is similar to the "global childhood rigidity" (Anderluh, Tchanturia, Rabe-Hesketh, Collier, & Treasure, 2009), which was found by Halmi and colleagues (2012) to be the predominate perfectionistic feature preceding development across all anorexia nervosa subtypes, including restricting, purging and binge eating subtypes. It has been proposed that childhood temperament including anxiety, obsessions and perfectionism may reflect neurobiological risk factors for developing anorexia nervosa, where restricted eating is used to moderate negative mood caused by skewed interactions between serotonin inhibitory and dopamine reward systems (Kaye, Wierenga, Bailer, Simmons, & Bischoff-Grethe, 2013).

The Maudsley Model of Treatment of Adults with anorexia nervosa (MANTRA) has been developed from this model, with a central focus on promoting more flexible thinking and less rigidity (Schmidt et al., 2014). MANTRA has been evaluated across two studies. The first of these was a small case series (Wade, Treasure, & Schmidt, 2011) where patients showed significant improvements at 12-month follow-up on eating disorder symptoms, weight and other variables with large to very large effect sizes in an intention-to-treat analysis. A larger pilot randomised controlled trial of 72 adult outpatients with anorexia nervosa compared MANTRA against Specialist Supportive Clinical Management (SSCM; McIntosh et al., 2005) and found overall significant improvements on weight, eating disorders symptoms, depression and anxiety, with no differences between these treatments (Schmidt et al., 2012). An exploratory analysis of 53 participants with more severe anorexia nervosa (BMI < 17.5) showed MANTRA patients to show further improvement in weight at 12-month follow-up, whereas those treated with SSCM did not (Schmidt et al., 2012). While further research on the efficacy of MANTRA is required, along with dismantling studies identifying the effective components, these findings may suggest the usefulness of tackling perfectionism in treating anorexia nervosa.

Evidence Supporting an Association Between Perfectionism and ED

Cross-Sectional Studies Systematic reviews suggest that perfectionism is a risk factor for eating disorders (Bardone-Cone et al., 2007; Jacobi, Hayward, de Zwaan, Kraemer, & Agras, 2004; Shafran & Mansell, 2001; Stice, 2002; Egan, Wade, & Shafran, 2011). It has been suggested that *both* healthy perfectionism (i.e. striving for achievement) and unhealthy perfectionism (i.e. self-criticism when goals are not achieved to what is considered to be an acceptable level) are associated with disordered eating (Bardone-Cone et al., 2007).

Currently, the majority of the evidence for the relationship between perfectionism and disordered eating rests on cross-sectional studies. Correlational studies have demonstrated that individuals with bulimia nervosa have significantly higher levels of perfectionism levels than healthy controls (Lilenfeld, Wonderlich, Riso, Crosby, & Mitchell, 2004). Retrospective case-control studies have also found significantly higher rates of childhood perfectionism in individuals with bulimia nervosa and anorexia nervosa than healthy controls (Fairburn, Cooper, Doll, & Welch, 1999; Fairburn, Welch, Doll, Davies, & O'Connor, 1997; Halmi et al., 2012). Childhood perfectionism is also recalled as being higher in individuals with anorexia nervosa compared to psychiatric controls (Pike et al., 2008; Machado, Gonçalves, Martins, Hoek, & Machado, 2014). Elevated concern over mistakes, a subscale of the FMPS that loads on the self-critical evaluative concerns (EC) construct, is associated with retrospectively reported eating disorders but not with other psychiatric disorders (Bulik et al., 2003). Females with a self-reported lifetime history of fasting or purging (i.e. self-induced vomiting or abuse of laxatives or diuretics) exhibit significantly higher levels of perfectionism than healthy controls (Forbush, Heatherton, & Keel, 2007).

Research also indicates that socially prescribed perfectionism (i.e. the need to attain standards perceived to be imposed by significant others), measured by the Hewitt and Flett Multidimensional Perfectionism Scale (HMPS; Hewitt & Flett, 1991), is significantly elevated in people with eating disorders (Bastiani, Rao, Weltzin, & Kaye, 1995; Cockell et al., 2002). Previous theorists (Bruch, 1974) have emphasised that both intrapersonal and interpersonal aspects of perfectionism are implicated in the emergence and continuance of eating disorder symptoms. Longitudinal research over 7 years of 13-year-old girls found that a "wish to be thinner" and mothers' ratings on perfectionism contributed most to the prediction of disturbed eating attitudes (Westerberg-Jacobson, Edlund, & Ghaderi, 2010). A study of 433 "trios" (a female with anorexia nervosa or "proband" and her mother and father) found that the most severe disordered eating in the proband was associated with mothers who also had elevations on eating disorder symptoms and anxious/perfectionistic traits (Jacobs et al., 2009). Elevated perfectionism in people in the social circle may not indicate perfectionistic pressures in the relationship but may rather indicate a genetic susceptibility, given that around 25–39 % of the variance of perfectionism can be accounted for by genetic effects (Wade & Bulik, 2007). While perfectionism in the father has not been implicated to date, the importance of paternal variables in terms of contribution to risk for eating disorders has been found across a variety of longitudinal studies, including paternal eating attitudes (Westerberg, Edlund, & Ghaderi, 2008) and importance of weight to father (Field et al., 2008), which may indicate some perfectionistic pressures specific to appearance and weight from the fathers or shared genetic vulnerability.

It should be noted that while it has been suggested that striving to achieve high standards does not play a role in the development of psychopathology generally (Stoeber & Otto, 2006), eating disorders have previously been singled out as being unique in terms of associations with both healthy and unhealthy perfectionism (Bardone-Cone et al., 2007). As mentioned earlier, binge eating in college-aged women has been shown to increase over time in the presence of two different types of perfectionism (Bardone-Cone et al., 2008), PS and EC. One study explicitly examined different clusters of these two types of perfectionism in young adolescents (Boone, Soenens, Braet, & Goossens, 2010) and their associations with eating disorder symptoms measured with the EDE-Q. Cluster analysis identified four groups of adolescents: (i) high PS and EC, (ii) high EC only, (iii) high PS and low EC and (iv) low PS and EC. The first cluster, around 15 % of the sample, experienced the highest levels of disordered eating across all four subscales of the EDE-Q. The way in which these two types of perfectionism may work together to increase risk for disordered eating requires further examination in longitudinal designs as we need to develop a better understanding of the contexts in which high standards can be damaging and when it can be protective.

Longitudinal Studies While some longitudinal studies have found that perfectionism is related to increases in eating disorder symptoms (e.g. Boone, Soenens, & Braet, 2010; Mackinnon et al., 2011), other studies have failed to confirm these findings (e.g. Gustafsson, Edlund, Kjellin, & Norring, 2009; Vohs, et al., 1999; Leon, Fulkerson, Perry, Keel, & Klump, 1999). Examination of simple relationships in this body of research is likely to contribute to these inconsistent findings as it has long been recognised that it is likely that more complex multivariate models will be required to properly understand the postulated effect of perfectionism on risk for disordered eating (Stice, 2002; Bardone-Cone et al., 2007). An example of these multivariate relationships is encapsulated in the three-factor model (Bardone-Cone et al., 2006; 2008) described above. In other words, perfectionism may only exert an effect on the development of disordered eating through its relationship with other important risk factors.

In addition to the three-factor model, several complex longitudinal models have been tested which show some promise. The first, in a sample of young adolescent girls (average age of 13 years) where three waves of data were collected over a 12-month period, showed body dissatisfaction moderated the effect of perfectionism on changes in importance of weight and shape (Boone, Soenens, & Luyten, 2014). Higher levels of both concern over mistakes and PS perfectionism with higher levels of body dissatisfaction at baseline significantly increased the importance of weight and shape at 12-month follow-up. Importance of weight and shape has been described as the "core psychopathology" of eating disorders (Cooper & Fairburn, 1993) and forms part of the diagnostic criteria for both anorexia nervosa and bulimia nervosa. It has been found to predict the growth of diagnostic threshold level of disordered eating behaviours in adolescents over a 12-month period (Wilksch & Wade, 2010). Mediational relationships were also investigated, but there was no support for a longitudinal mediational model where body dissatisfaction at 6-month follow-up was postulated to mediate the relationship between baseline perfectionism and overevaluation of weight and shape at 12-month follow-up.

A second study with 12- to 15-year-old boys and girls over a 12-month period, with three waves of data collected at 6-month intervals, did support mediational relationships (Boone, Vansteenkiste, Soenens, der Kaap-Deeder, & Verstuyf, 2014). Need frustration, measured with the balanced measure of psychological needs (Sheldon & Hilpert, 2012), was postulated to be a mediator of the relationship between self-critical perfectionism and the growth of binge eating symptoms. Need frustration refers to the frustration of needs of autonomy, competence and relatedness, and is thought to be of relevance to self-critical perfectionism where positive feelings after achievement are short-lived and replaced with a focus on the next demanding standard, and where attainment of goals can often be dismissed. In both boys and girls, higher levels of self-critical perfectionism at the first wave of assessment had a significant association with needs frustration at the second wave, which in turn had a significant association with the growth of tendencies to think about and engage in bouts of uncontrollable overeating as measured by the bulimia subscale of the EDI.

A third study has also examined longitudinal mediation pathways for risk for developing disordered eating in young adolescents (Wade, Wilksch, Paxton, Byrne, & Austin, submitted). Growth of the importance of weight and shape over a 12-month period in girls was predicted by the initial baseline level of concern over mistakes perfectionism and its relationship with higher levels of ineffectiveness subsequent to baseline and measured on three occasions. Ineffectiveness has previously been shown to predict the growth of the importance of weight and shape (Wilksch & Wade, 2010) and can be likened to the concept of self-efficacy, in that it was measured by the EDI with items related to feelings of inadequacy, insecurity, worthlessness and having no control over one's life. This is consistent with the most endorsed worries of women with anorexia nervosa which do not relate to the aspects of eating or weight but to issues that increase a sense of ineffectiveness such as rejection and abandonment, negative perceptions of self and experience of negative emotions (Sternheim et al., 2012). Interestingly, when baseline PS perfectionism was examined, there was no significant relationship with either levels of subsequent ineffectiveness or increases in the importance of weight and shape.

In summary, there is growing evidence of a longitudinal (i.e. causal) relationship between perfectionism and growth of either disordered eating or risk for disordered eating, in the presence of key variables, with the most promising being constructs that relate to self-efficacy and ineffectiveness. This echoes the focus formulated many years ago by Hilde Bruch (1974), where body weight becomes a means of self-definition and compensation for feelings of powerlessness and incompetence in the presence of perfectionism. The degree to which different types of perfectionism contribute to this risk requires further elucidation.

Studies of People Recovered from Eating Disorders Several studies have investigated people who have had an eating disorder and compared the levels of perfectionism with people who have never had an eating disorder and people who still have an eating disorder in order to understand if perfectionism influences development of disordered eating. The presence of elevated perfectionism in the recovered group compared to the healthy group would suggest one of the two things: first, dispositional perfectionism increased risk for development of an eating disorder, or second, the experience of an eating disorder has had a "scar effect" leaving the person more perfectionistic than before they developed the eating disorder.

Most research consistently shows perfectionism to be elevated in people with eating disorders and people recovering from eating disorders compared to healthy controls (Bastiani et al., 1995; Srinivasagam et al., 1995; Bardone-Cone, Sturm, Lawson, Robinson, & Smith, 2010; Halmi et al., 2000; Lilenfeld et al., 2000). However, other studies have suggested that recovery, when robustly defined, is associated with perfectionism levels that are no different from healthy controls (Bardone-Cone et al., 2010). The different definitions of recovery used in eating disorder research do pose considerable difficulties for making clear conclusions about a number of issues, including prediction of recovery and the study of mechanisms involved in recovery (Williams, Watts, & Wade, 2012). Although these latter findings may indicate that perfectionism is not a risk factor for eating disorders (i.e. does not cause eating disorders), it is still consistent with the suggestion that interventions that help decrease perfectionism may be key to making full recovery attainable (Bardone-Cone et al., 2010).

Experimental Studies A range of novel experimental designs have been employed to investigate the cognitive, affective and behavioural processes associated with perfectionism. For example, studies manipulating reactions to success and failure by providing contrived feedback on task performance have demonstrated the negatively biased appraisals of performance characteristic of perfectionists. While there is inconsistency regarding the type of perfectionism that is most problematic, studies by Besser and colleagues (Besser, Flett, & Hewitt, 2004; Besser, Flett, Hewitt, & Guez, 2008) suggest that perfectionists fail to internalise, or have difficulty processing, positive feedback and success. In fact, experimental studies investigating resetting of PS have demonstrated that perfectionists not only discount their success, but re-evaluate their PS as insufficiently demanding and raise their goals following success (Kobori, Hayakawa, & Tanna, 2009; Stoeber, Hutchfield, & Wood, 2008).

With respect to eating disorder psychopathology, specifically, the impact of perfectionism has been investigated in two nonclinical experimental studies. Shafran, Lee, Payne and Fairburn (2006) experimentally manipulated individual PS to investigate their influence on eating attitudes and behaviour. Participants were randomly allocated to either a high PS (perfectionist) or a low PS (non-perfectionist) condition. In the high PS condition, participants agreed to pursue the highest possible standards in everything, including thoughts, words and actions, for a 24 h period. In the low PS condition, participants agreed to perform at the minimum possible standard. Post manipulation, individuals in the high PS condition exhibited greater restriction of higher calorie foods and overall food consumption, as well as greater regret after eating, than individuals in the low PS group.

Boone, Soenens, Vansteenkiste and Braet (2012) extended this study in three ways. First, they examined the impact of trait perfectionism on the experimental manipulation of perfectionism by including a pre-manipulation measure of dispositional perfectionism. This consisted of the FMPS concern over mistakes and doubts about actions subscales to assess EC perfectionism and the FMPS personal standards subscale to assess PS perfectionism. Second, they also adopted a multidimensional approach to the manipulation of perfectionism. In addition to the two conditions manipulating high and low PS, a third condition was included to activate both PS and EC perfectionism. In this condition, participants agreed to pursue the highest possible standards to avoid failing or disappointing themselves or others. Third, this study examined the impact of the manipulation across broader range of eating disorder symptoms including items related to dietary restraint (e.g. attempted and actual restriction and restraint, reduced calories, reduced amount of food); body dissatisfaction (e.g. stomach too big, thighs not the right size, dissatisfied with shape of body); and binge eating (e.g. eating when upset, stuffed with food).

Both experimental manipulations induced increased levels of state PS and EC perfectionism compared to the non-perfectionist group, indicating that manipulating PS alone is sufficient to increase negative self-evaluation associated with EC perfectionism. In addition, both perfectionism groups experienced increases in restraint and binge eating symptomatology, but not body dissatisfaction compared to the non-perfectionist group. However, mediation analysis confirmed the causal role of state EC perfectionism only in eating disorder symptoms. While PS perfectionism was related to restraint, this correlation was not supported after controlling for the influence of EC perfectionism. EC perfectionism on the other hand was correlated with restraint, body dissatisfaction and binge eating. Further, state EC perfectionism was supported as a full mediator of the effect of the perfectionism manipulation on both restraint and binge eating. These findings were supported irrespective of trait perfectionism levels.

Based on this combined research, perfectionism is indicated as a causal risk factor for eating disorder psychopathology. Further, it suggests that perfectionism itself is malleable and may be sensitive not only to situational circumstances but also to interventions, and is therefore also a potential target for the treatment and prevention of eating disorders.

Prevention and Treatment Studies Research unambiguously indicates that perfectionism is not only treatable but that targeted cognitive behavioural interventions can significantly improve psychopathology. A recent meta-analysis (Lloyd, Schmidt, Khondoker, & Tchanturia, 2014) evaluated eight treatment studies employing cognitive behavioural techniques targeting perfectionism in individual therapy, guided self-help, web-based intervention or group therapy. Large pooled effect sizes were observed for improvements in perfectionism itself, and medium pooled effect sizes were observed for improvements in symptoms of anxiety and depression. To date, three studies have investigated the impact of treatment targeting perfectionism in clinical samples with eating disorders across a range of delivery formats.

Two of these studies have investigated the impact of group-based cognitive behaviour treatment for perfectionism within existing treatment programs. Lloyd, Fleming, Schmidt and Tchanturia (2014) evaluated a six-session treatment with women in an inpatient program for anorexia nervosa. Findings supported the efficacy of this form of treatment for improving perfectionism (with medium effect sizes). However, potential impacts on aspects of eating disorder psychopathology in comparison with treatment as usual were not reported. A study conducted by Goldstein and colleagues (2014) has evaluated the outcomes of group-based perfectionism therapy on both perfectionism and psychopathology. In this trial, seven sessions were delivered to a transdiagnostic eating disorder sample of patients with anorexia nervosa, bulimia nervosa or eating disorder not otherwise specified, within a day program treatment setting. Participants were randomly allocated to receive treatment as usual including a general cognitive-behavioural-based group, or treatment as usual with cognitive behavioural treatment for perfectionism. Both groups produced improvements in perfectionism and eating disorder psychopathology, with no differences between the groups. It is acknowledged by the authors that both cognitive behavioural groups in this study may have challenged aspects of perfectionism, and that ceiling effects associated with adding a small active component to an already successful treatment program (7 hours out of 136 overall treatment hours) may have masked a potential small effect.

Using a six-session guided self-help treatment program, Steele and Wade (2008) evaluated the impact of targeting perfectionism to reduce bulimic symptoms. Participants included women with either bulimia nervosa or eating disorder not otherwise specified with bingeing and purging. The study compared the effects of three guided self-help treatments: a cognitive behavioural perfectionism intervention with no eating disorder specific components; a traditional cognitive behavioural eating disorder intervention; and a placebo intervention including mindfulness techniques. Although there were no significant differences between the groups, effect sizes indicated a mixed picture. Effect sizes were larger for guided self-help targeting perfectionism than other conditions in improving excessive exercise, self-esteem and perfectionism, but smaller than the traditional eating disorder intervention for objective binge episodes, and equivalent for reducing purging and the global eating pathology. In particular, the perfectionism treatment demonstrated very large effect size for concerns about shape and weight, which represents one of the core aspects of eating disorder psychopathology.

While the majority of research examining perfectionism interventions resides in the treatment literature, one study has investigated this from a prevention perspective. Wilksch, Durbridge and Wade (2008) examined the benefits of a program targeting perfectionism in reducing eating disorder risk in high school females (mean age 15 years). Students participated in an eight-lesson program targeting perfectionism or media literacy, or classes as usual. Although neither program produced significant interaction effects of group and time for shape and weight concern, the perfectionism intervention had a greater impact on individuals at high risk for an eating disorder than either the media literacy or control groups at 3-month follow-up. Most promisingly, for those students with high levels of weight and shape concern who received the perfectionism intervention, positive rates of clinically significant improvement were observed for all variables beyond chance. In particular, more than half of these students experienced improvements in perfectionism (both PS and EC) and dieting, while only one participant experienced increased risk.

Altogether, the wider body of evidence indicates that perfectionism is not a stable trait but is malleable and sensitive to clinical interventions. Preliminary studies show promise that by reducing perfectionism, risk for nontargeted disorders including eating disorders may be reduced, and existing symptoms may also be improved while not being the primary focus of treatment.

Future Directions

While there has been a long history of linking perfectionism with eating disorders, and perfectionism appears in many theories explaining the aetiology and maintenance of eating disorders, compelling evidence relating to the direction of causality is only starting to appear in recent years. Two main issues require further clarification. First, we need to develop a better understanding of how perfectionism may increase risk for the development of an eating disorder, and second, we need to develop a better understanding of the comparative importance of modifying perfectionism in both prevention and treatment of eating disorders compared to other risk and maintenance factors.

With respect to this first issue, a number of specific questions need to be investigated. First, we need a better understanding of which perfectionism constructs relate to the development of different types of disordered eating in longitudinal studies. Various measures tapping into different perfectionism constructs exist, and the most useful measures in terms of predicting the development of disordered eating need to be identified. Second, further work is required to develop and test complex models that explain how perfectionism may increase risk for disordered eating. This will involve both exploration of potential moderators (for whom and under what conditions perfectionism becomes a risk factor) and mediators (mechanisms through which perfectionism exerts an effect on disordered eating). In particular, clearer identification of protective factors that can ameliorate the adverse effects of perfectionism is required, with a particular focus on self-efficacy and feelings of effectiveness. Third, longitudinal research is needed across different ages and populations, including young males, transition to adolescence, transition to adulthood and older women. It is likely that different models explaining the way in which perfectionism increases risk for disordered eating are required for these different groups.

The second issue, relating to the role of targeting perfectionism in interventions, is also associated with a number of specific questions that need to be addressed. First, more experimental studies are required to better understand the different ways in which manipulating perfectionism can change risk for disordered eating. Second, dismantling treatment studies are required to investigate the degree to which a focus on decreasing perfectionism can hasten and enhance recovery from an eating disorder. Third, matching of the format (online, guided, face to face) and content of perfectionism interventions is required. This will involve consideration of treatment moderators (Kraemer, Wilson, Fairburn, & Agras, 2002), that is, characteristics of the person who responds best to different formats and content. Fourth, more work is required in prevention with young adolescents and adults to understand the comparative importance of tackling perfectionism as opposed to other important risk factors for disordered eating.

References

Anderluh, M., Tchanturia, K., Rabe-Hesketh, S., Collier, D., & Treasure, T. (2009). Lifetime course of eating disorders: Design and validity testing of a new strategy to define the eating disorder phenotype. *Psychological Medicine, 39,* 105–114.

Bardone-Cone, A. M., Abramson, L. Y., Vohs, K. D., Heatherton, T. F., & Joiner T. E. (2006). Predicting bulimic symptoms: An interactive model of self-efficacy, perfectionism, and perceived weight status. *Behaviour Research and Therapy, 44,* 27–42.

Bardone-Cone, A. M., Wonderlich, S. A., Frost, R. O., Bulik, C. M., Mitchell, J. E., Uppala, S., & Simonich, H. (2007). Perfectionism and eating disorders: Current status and future directions. *Clinical Psychology Review, 27,* 384–405.

Bardone-Cone, A. M., Joiner, T. E., Crosby, R. D., Crow, S. J., Klein, M. H., le Grange, D., & Wonderlich, S. A. (2008). Examining a psychosocial interactive model of binge eating and vomiting in women with bulimia nervosa and subthreshold bulimia nervosa. *Behaviour Research and Therapy, 46,* 887–894.

Bardone-Cone, A. M., Sturm, K., Lawson, M. A., Robinson, D. P., & Smith, R. (2010). Perfectionism across stages of recovery from eating disorders. *International Journal of Eating Disorders, 43,* 139–148.

Bastiani, A. M., Rao, R., Weltzin, T., & Kaye, W. H. (1995). Perfectionism in anorexia nervosa. *International Journal of Eating Disorders, 17*(2), 147–152.

Besser, A., Flett, G. L., & Hewitt, P. L. (2004). Perfectionism, cognition, and affect in response to performance failure vs. success. *Journal of Rational-Emotive and Cognitive-Behavior Therapy, 22*(4), 297–324.

Besser, A., Flett, G. L., Hewitt, P. L., & Guez, J. (2008). Perfectionism, and cognitions, affect, self-esteem, and physiological reactions in a performance situation. *Journal of Rational-Emotive and Cognitive-Behavior Therapy, 26*(3), 206–228.

Boone, L., Soenens, B., Braet, C., & Goossens, L. (2010). An empirical typology of perfectionism in early-to-mid adolescents and its relation with eating disorder symptoms. *Behaviour Research and Therapy, 48*(7), 686–691.

Boone, L., Soenens, B., & Luyten, P. (2014). When or why does perfectionism translate into eating disorder pathology? A longitudinal examination of the moderating and mediating role of body dissatisfaction. *Journal of Abnormal Psychology, 123,* 412–418.

Boone, L., Soenens, B., Vansteenkiste, M., & Braet, C. (2012). Is there a perfectionist in each of us? An experimental study on perfectionism and eating disorder symptoms. *Appetite, 59,* 531–540.

Boone, L., Vansteenkiste, M., Soenens, B., der Kaap-Deeder, J., & Verstuyf, J. (2012). Self-critical perfectionism and binge-eating symptoms: A longitudinal test of the intervening role of psychological need frustration. *Journal of Counseling Psychology, 61,* 363–373.

Bruch, H. (1974). *Eating disorders: Obesity, anorexia nervosa and the person within.* London: Routledge & Kegan Paul.

Bulik, C. M., Tozzi, F., Anderson, C., Mazzeo, S. E., Aggen, S., & Sullivan, P. F. (2003). The relation between eating disorders and components of perfectionism. *The American Journal of Psychiatry, 160*(2), 366–368.

Byrne, S. M., Fursland, A., Allen, K. L., & Watson, H. (2011). The effectiveness of enhanced cognitive behavioural therapy for eating disorders: An open trial. *Behaviour Research and Therapy, 49*(4), 219–226.

Clausen, L., Rosenvinge, J. H., Friborg, O., & Rokkedal, K. (2011). Validating the EDI-3: A comparison of 561 female eating disorder patients and 878 females from the general population. *Journal of Psychopathology and Behavioral Assessment, 33,* 101–110.

Cockell, S. J., Hewitt, P. L., Seal, B., Sherry, S., Goldner, E. M., Flett, G. L., & Remick, R. A. (2002). Trait and self-presentational dimensions of perfectionism among women with anorexia nervosa. *Cognitive Therapy and Research, 26,* 745–758.

Cooper, P. J. & Fairburn, C. G. (1993). Confusion over the core psychopathology of bulimia nervosa. *International Journal of Eating Disorders, 13,* 385–389.

Craig, P., Dieppe, P., Macintyre, S., Mitchie, S., Nazareth, I., & Petticrew, M. (2008). Developing and evaluating complex interventions: The new medical research council guidance. *BMJ, 337,* a1655.

Dalle Grave, R., Calugi, S., Conti, M., Doll, H., & Fairburn, C. G. (2013). Inpatient cognitive behaviour therapy for anorexia nervosa: A randomized controlled trial. *Psychotherapy and psychosomatics, 82*(6), 390–398.

Dalle Grave, R., Calugi, S., Doll, H. A., & Fairburn, C. G. (2013). Enhanced cognitive behaviour therapy for adolescents with anorexia nervosa: an alternative to family therapy? *Behaviour research and therapy, 51*(1), R9–R12.

Egan, S. J., Wade, T. D., & Shafran, R. (2011). Perfectionism as a transdiagnostic process: A clinical review. *Clinical Psychology Review, 31*(2), 203–212.

Fairburn, C. G. (1997). Eating disorders. In D. M. Clark & C. G. Fairburn (Eds.), *Science and practice of cognitive behaviour therapy* (pp. 209–241). Oxford: Oxford University Press.

Fairburn, C. G., & Beglin, S. J. (1994). Assessment of eating disorders: Interview or self-report questionnaire? *International Journal of Eating Disorders, 16*(4), 363–370.

Fairburn, C. G., Welch, S. L., Doll, H. A., Davies, B. A., & O'Connor, M. E. (1997). Risk factors for bulimia nervosa: A community-based case control study. *Archives of General Psychiatry, 54,* 509–517.

Fairburn, C. G., Cooper, Z., Doll, H. A., & Welch, S. L. (1999). Risk factors for anorexia nervosa: Three integrated case-control comparisons. *Archives of General Psychiatry, 56*(5), 468–476.

Fairburn, C. G., Cooper, Z., & Shafran, R. (2003). Cognitive behaviour therapy for eating disorders: A "transdiagnostic" theory and treatment. *Behaviour research and therapy, 41*(5), 509–528.

Fairburn, C., Cooper, Z., Doll, H., O'Connor, M., Bohn, K., Hawker, D., Wales, J. A., & Palmer, R. (2009). Transdiagnostic cognitive-behavioral therapy for patients with eating disorders: A two-site trial with 60-week follow-up. *American Journal of Psychiatry, 166*(3), 311–319.

Fairburn, C. G., Bailey-Straebler, S., Basden, S., Doll, H. A., Jones, R., Murphy, R., & Cooper, Z. (2015). A transdiagnostic comparison of enhanced cognitive behaviour therapy (CBT-E) and interpersonal psychotherapy in the treatment of eating disorders. *Behaviour research and therapy, 70,* 64–71.

Field, A., Javaras, K. M., Aneja, P., Kitos, N., Camargo, C. A., Taylor, C. B., & Laird, N. M. (2008). Family, media, and peer predictors of becoming eating disordered. *Archives of Pediatric and Adolescent Medicine, 162,* 574–579.

Forbush, K., Heatherton, T. F., & Keel, P. K. (2007). Relationships between perfectionism and specific disordered eating behaviors. *International Journal of Eating Disorders, 40*(1), 37–41.

Frost, R. O., Marten, P., Lahart, C., & Rosenblate, R. (1990). The dimensions of perfectionism. *Cognitive Therapy and Research, 14,* 449–468.

Goldstein, M., Peters, L., Thorton, C. E., & Touyz, S. W. (2014) The treatment of perfectionism within the eating disorders: A pilot study. *European Eating Disorders Review, 22*(3), 217–221.

Gustafsson, S. A., Edlund, B., Kjellin, L., & Norring, C. (2009). Risk and protective factors for disturbed eating in adolescent girls—aspects of perfectionism and attitudes to eating and weight. *European Eating Disorders Review, 17,* 380–389.

Halmi, K. A., Sunday, S. P., Strober, M., Kaplan, A., Woodside, D. B., Fichter, M., et al. (2000). Perfectionism in anorexia nervosa: Variation by clinical subtype, obessionality, and pathological eating behaviour. *American Journal of Psychiatry, 157,* 1799–1805.

Halmi, K. A., Bellace, D., Berthod, S. A., Ghosh, S., Wade, B., Brandt, H. A., Bulik, C. M., Crawford, S., Fichter, M. M., Johnson, C. L., Kaplan, A., Kaye, W. H., Thornton, L., Treasure, J., Woodside, B. D., & Strober, M. (2012). An examination of early childhood perfectionism across anorexia nervosa subtypes. *International Journal of Eating Disorders, 45*(6), 800–807.

Hewitt, P. L., & Flett, G. L. (1991). Perfectionism in the self and social contexts: Conceptualization, assessment, and association with psychopathology. *Journal of Personality and Social Psychology, 60,* 456–470.

Jacobi, C., Hayward, C., de Zwaan, M., Kraemer, H. C., & Agras, S. (2004). Coming to terms with risk factors for eating disorders: Application of risk terminology and suggestions for a general taxonomy. *Psychological Bulletin, 130*(1), 19–65.

Jacobs, M. J., Roesch, S., Wonderlich, S. A., Crosby, R., Thornton, L., Wilfley, D. E., Berrettini, W. H., Brandt, H., Crawford, S., Fichter, M. M., Halmi, K. A., Johnson, C., Kaplan, A. S., Lavia, M., Mitchell, J. E., Rotondo, A., Strober, M., Woodside, D. B., Kaye, W. H., & Bulik, C. M. (2009). Anorexia nervosa trios: Behavioral profiles of individuals with anorexia nervosa and their parents. *Psychological Medicine, 39,* 451–461.

Kaye, W. H., Wierenga, C. E., Bailer, U. F., Simmons, A. N., & Bischoff-Grethe, A. (2013). Nothing tastes as good as skinny feels: The neurobiology of anorexia nervosa. *Trends in Neurosciences, 36,* 110–120.

Kobori, O., Hayakawa, M., & Tanno, Y. (2009). Do perfectionists raise their standards after success? An experimental examination of the revaluation of standard setting in perfectionism. *Journal of Behavior Therapy and Experimental Psychiatry, 40,* 515–521.

Kraemer, H. C., Wilson, G. T., Fairburn, C. G., & Agras, W. S. (2002). Mediators and moderators of treatment effects in randomised clinical trials. *Archives of General Psychiatry, 59,* 877–883.

Leon, G. R., Fulkerson, J. A., Perry, C. L., Keel, P. K., & Klump, K. L. (1999). Three to four year prospective evaluation of personality and behavioral risk factors for later disordered eating in adolescent girls and boys. *Journal of Youth and Adolescence, 28*(2), 181–196.

Lilenfeld, L. R., Stein, D., Bulik, C. M., Strober, M., Plotnicov, K., Pollice, C. et al. (2000). Personality traits among currently eating disordered, recovered and never ill first-degree relatives of bulimic and control women. *Psychological Medicine, 30,* 1399–1410.

Lilenfeld, L. R. R., Wonderlich, S. A., Riso, L. P., Crosby, R., & Mitchell, J. (2004). Eating disorders and personality: A methodological and empirical review. *Clinical Psychology Review, 26,* 299–320.

Lloyd, S., Fleming. C., Schmidt, U., & Tchanturia, K. (2014). Targeting perfectionism in anorexia nervosa using a group-based cognitive behavioural approach: A pilot study. *European Eating Disorders Review, 22*(5), 366–372.

Lloyd, S., Schmidt, U., Khondoker, M., & Tchanturia, K. (2014). Can psychological interventions reduce perfectionism? A systematic review and meta-analysis. *Behavioural and Cognitive Psychotherapy*, available on CJO2014. doi:10.1017/S1352465814000162.

Machado, B. C., Gonçalves, S. F., Martins, C., Hoek, H. W., & Machado, P. P. (2014). Risk factors and antecedent life events in the development of anorexia nervosa: A Portuguese case control study. *European Eating Disorders Review, 22,* 243–251.

Mackinnon, S. P., Sherry, S. B., Grahma, A. R., Stewart, S. H., Sherry, D. L., Allen, S. L., Fitzpatrick, S., & McGrath, D. S. (2011). Reformulating and testing the perfectionism model of binge eating among undergraduate women: A short-term, three-wave, longitudinal study. *Journal of Counselling Psychology, 58,* 630–646.

McIntosh, V. V., Jordan, J., Carter, F. A., Luty, S. E., McKenzie, J. M., Bulik, C. M., Frampton, C. M., & Joyce, P. R. (2005). Three psychotherapies for anorexia nervosa: A randomized, controlled trial. *American Journal of Psychiatry, 162,* 741–747.

Pike, K. M., Hilbert, A., Wilfley, D. E., Fairburn, C. G., Dohm, F.-A., Walsh, B. T., & Striegel-Moore, R. (2008). Toward an understanding of risk factors for anorexia nervosa: A case-control study. *Psychological Medicine, 38*(10), 1443–1453.

Schmidt, U., & Treasure, J. (2006). Anorexia nervosa: Valued and visible. A cognitive-interpersonal maintenance model and its implications for research and practice. *British Journal of Clinical Psychology, 45,* 343–366.

Schmidt, U., Oldershaw, A., Jichi, F., Sternheim, L., Startup, H., McIntosh, V., Jordan, J., Tchanturia, K., Wolff, G., Rooney, M., Landau, S., & Treasure, J. (2012). Out-patient psychological therapies for adults with anorexia nervosa: Randomised controlled trial. *British Journal of Psychiatry, 201,* 392–399.

Schmidt, U., Wade, T. D., & Treasure, J. (2014). The Maudsley Model of anorexia nervosa treatment for adults (MANTRA): Development, key features and preliminary evidence. *Journal of Cognitive Psychotherapy, 28,* 48–71.

Shafran, R., & Mansell, W. (2001). Perfectionism and psychopathology: A review of research and treatment. *Clinical Psychology Review, 21*(6), 879–906.

Shafran, R., Cooper, Z., & Fairburn, C. G. (2002). Clinical perfectionism: A cognitive-behavioural analysis. *Behaviour Research and Therapy, 40*(7), 773–791.

Shafran, R., Lee, M., Payne, E., & Fairburn, C. G. (2006). The impact of manipulating personal standards on eating attitudes and behaviour. *Behaviour Research and Therapy, 44*(6), 897–906.

Shaw, H. E., Stice, E., & Springer, D. W. (2004). Perfectionism, body dissatisfaction, and self-esteem in predicting bulimic symptomatology: Lack of replication. *International Journal of Eating Disorders, 36,* 41–47.

Sheldon, K., & Hilpert, J. (2012). The balanced measure of psychological needs (BMPN) scale: An alternative domain general measure of need satisfaction. *Motivation and Emotion, 36*(4), 439.

Slade, P. (1978). Towards a functional analysis of anorexia nervosa and bulimia nervosa. *British Journal of Clinical Psychology, 21,* 167–179.

Srinivasagam, N. M., Kaye, W. H., Plotnicov, K. H., Greeno, C., et al. (1995). Persistent perfectionism, symmetry, and exactness after long-term recovery from anorexia nervosa. *The American Journal of Psychiatry, 152*(11), 1630–1634.

Steele, A. L., & Wade, T. D. (2008). A randomised trial investigating guided self-help to reduce perfectionism and its impact on bulimia nervosa: A pilot study. *Behaviour Research and Therapy, 46*(12), 1316–1323.

Steele, A., Corsini, N., & Wade, T. D. (2007). The interaction of perfectionism, perceived weight status and self-esteem to predict bulimic symptoms: The role of 'benign' perfectionism. *Behaviour Research and Therapy, 45,* 1647–1655.

Sternheim, L., Startup, H., Saeidi, S., Morgan, J., Hugo, P., Russell, A., & Schmidt, U. (2012). Understanding catastrophic worry in eating disorders: Process and content characteristics. *Journal of Behavior Therapy and Experimental Psychiatry, 43,* 1095–1103.

Stice, E. (2002). Risk and maintenance factors for eating pathology: A meta-analytic review. *Psychological Bulletin, 128*(5), 825–848.

Stoeber, J., & Otto, K. (2006). Positive conceptions of perfectionism: Approaches, evidence, challenges. *Personality and Social Psychology Review, 10,* 295–319.

Stoeber, J., Hutchfield, J., & Wood, K. V. (2008). Perfectionism, self-efficacy, and aspiration level: Differential effects of perfectionistic striving and self-criticism after success and failure. *Personality and Individual Differences, 45*(4), 323–327.

Tissot, A. M., & Crowther, J. H. (2008). Self-orientated and socially prescribed perfectionism: Risk factors within an integrative model for bulimic symptomatology. *Journal of Social and Clinical Psychology, 27*(7), 734–755.

Treasure, J., & Schmidt, U. (2013). The cognitive-interpersonal maintenance model of anorexia nervosa revisited: A summary of the evidence for cognitive, socio-emotional and interpersonal predisposing and perpetuating factors. *Journal of Eating Disorders,* MS ID: 814225172874100.

Vohs, K. D., Bardone, A. M., Joiner, T. E., Abramson, L. Y., & Heatherton, T. F. (1999). Perfectionism, perceived weight status, and self-esteem interact to predict bulimic symptoms: A model of bulimic symptom development. *Journal of Abnormal Psychology, 108*(4), 695–700.

Vohs, K. D., Heatherton, T. F., & Herrin, M. (2001). Disordered eating and the transition to college: A prospective study. *International Journal of Eating Disorders, 29,* 280–288.

Vohs, K. D., Voelz, Z. R., Pettit, J. W., Bardone, A. M., Katz, J., Abramson, L. Y., Heatherton, T. F., & Joiner, T. E. (2001). Perfectionism, body dissatisfaction, and self-esteem: An interactive model of bulimic symptom development. *Journal of Social and Clinical Psychology, 20*(4), 476–497.

Wade, T. D., & Bulik, C. M. (2007). Shared genetic and environmental risk factors between undue influence of body shape and weight on self-evaluation and dimensions of perfectionism. *Psychological Medicine, 37,* 635–644.

Wade, T. D., Treasure, J., & Schmidt, U. (2011). A case series evaluation of the Maudsley Model for treatment of adults with anorexia nervosa. *European Eating Disorders Review, 19,* 382–389.

Wade, T. D., Wilksch, S. M., Paxton, S. J., Byrne, S. M., Austin, S. B. (submitted). How perfectionism and ineffectiveness influence growth of eating disorder risk in young adolescent girls. *Behaviour Research and Therapy, 66,* 56–63.

Watson, H. J., Steele, A. L., Bergin, J. L., Fursland, A., & Wade, T. D. (2011). Bulimic symptomatology: The role of adaptive perfectionism, shape and weight concern, and self-esteem. *Behaviour Research and Therapy, 49,* 565–572.

Westerberg, J., Edlund, B., & Ghaderi, A. (2008). A 2-year longitudinal study of eating attitudes, BMI, perfectionism, asceticism and family climate in adolescent girls and their parents. *Eating and Weight Disorders, 13,* 64–72.

Westerberg-Jacobson, J., Edlund, B., & Ghaderi, A. (2010). Risk and protective factors for disturbed eating: A 7-year longitudinal study of eating attitudes and psychological factors in adolescent girls and their parents. *Eating and Weight Disorders, 15,* e208–e218.

Wilksch, S. M., & Wade, T. D. (2010). Risk factors for clinically significant importance of shape and weight in adolescent females. *Journal of Abnormal Psychology, 119,* 206–215.

Wilksch, S. M., Durbridge, M. R., & Wade, T. D. (2008). A preliminary controlled comparison of programs designed to reduce risk of eating disorders targeting perfectionism and media literacy. *Journal of the American Academy of Child and Adolescent Psychiatry, 47*(8), 939–947.

Williams, S. E., Watts, T. K. O., & Wade, T. D. (2012). A review of the definitions of outcome used in the treatment of bulimia nervosa. *Clinical Psychology Review, 32,* 292–300.

Part III
Perfectionism, Health, and Well-Being in Context

Chapter 10
Perfectionists Do Not Play Nicely With Others: Expanding the Social Disconnection Model

Simon B. Sherry, Sean P. Mackinnon and Chantal M. Gautreau

"Not being perfect hurts," Sylvia Plath (Plath, 1993, p. 666)

"Every one should be really excellent," Steve Jobs (Jobs, 2008)

Humans are social animals. We spend roughly 80% of our time around others (Cacioppo, Fowler, & Christakis, 2009). For better or worse, relationships with others greatly impact us. In fact, positive relationships are vital to our well-being (Baumeister & Leary, 1995). However, some people have personality traits that impede their ability to participate in and benefit from stable, positive, and satisfying relationships. Life is difficult for such people. Being disconnected from others creates psychopathology by thwarting a basic need for close relationships.

Perfectionism is a personality trait robustly associated with both social problems and psychopathology. The social disconnection model (SDM; Hewitt, Flett, Sherry, & Caelian, 2006) is an integrative theoretical framework clarifying how perfectionism generates psychopathology through negative social behaviors (e.g., conflictual interactions), cognitions (e.g., seeing others as disappointed), and outcomes (e.g., romantic breakups). In the present chapter, our goal is to articulate an expanded SDM that addresses limitations of the original formulation of this model. We also present two case studies illustrating how the expanded SDM is applicable to two well-known perfectionists: Sylvia Plath and Steve Jobs. But first, we define perfectionism, outline the original SDM, and discuss research supporting it.

Simon B. Sherry was supported by a Social Sciences and Humanities Research Council of Canada Standard Research Grant. Sean Mackinnon was supported by a Social Sciences and Humanities Research Council of Canada postdoctoral fellowship.

S. B. Sherry (✉) · S. P. Mackinnon · C. M. Gautreau
Department of Psychology and Neuroscience, Dalhousie University, 1355 Oxford Street, PO BOX 15000, Halifax, Nova Scotia B3H 4R2, Canada
e-mail: simon.sherry@dal.ca

F. M. Sirois, D. S. Molnar (eds.), *Perfectionism, Health, and Well-Being*,
DOI 10.1007/978-3-319-18582-8_10

Defining Perfectionism

Perfectionism is a complex construct variably defined and redefined by researchers. Many perfectionism measures exist (Enns & Cox, 2002), with more continuing to be developed (e.g., dyadic perfectionism; Stoeber, 2012). Though researchers often debate the components of perfectionism, there is a growing consensus that many measures of perfectionism may be classified into one of the two latent constructs: perfectionistic concerns and perfectionistic strivings (Dunkley & Blankstein, 2000; Stoeber & Otto, 2006). Perfectionistic concerns are a latent construct comprising neurotic, self-critical components of perfectionism, such as doubts about personal abilities, strong negative reactions to perceived failure, beliefs that others demand perfection, and a perceived discrepancy between one's performance and excessively high standards. This higher-order latent construct represents a synthesis of constructs from diverse areas including personality/interpersonal (socially prescribed perfectionism; Hewitt & Flett, 1991), cognitive behavioral (concern over mistakes and doubts about actions; Frost, Marten, Lahart and Rosenblate, 1990), psychodynamic (self-criticism; Blatt, D'Afflitti, & Quinlan, 1976), and counseling psychology (discrepancy; Slaney, Rice, Mobley, Trippi, & Ashby, 2001). Ample evidence suggests that perfectionistic concerns are a risk factor for mental health problems, including depression, panic, generalized anxiety, social anxiety, bulimia nervosa, binge eating, suicide, and personality disorders (e.g., Cox, Clara, & Enns, 2009; Hewitt & Flett, 1991; Mackinnon et al., 2011; Roxborough et al., 2012). Perfectionistic concerns are also implicated in various physical health problems such as poor sleep, lower physical health (e.g., upset stomach), and sexual dysfunction (e.g., Molnar, Reker, Culp, Sadava, & DeCourville, 2006; Stoeber, Harvey, Almeida, & Lyons, 2013; Vincent & Walker, 2000). Given such evidence, most researchers view perfectionistic concerns as a maladaptive construct. In fact, perfectionistic concerns may be seen as a core vulnerability factor that cuts across many mental and physical health problems.

People high in perfectionistic concerns also tend to experience many interpersonal problems (Habke & Flynn, 2002). Indeed, it seems that perfectionistic concerns and a distressing sense of disconnection from and disharmony with other people go hand in hand (Sherry & Hall, 2009). Loneliness, problems with perceived social support, intense interpersonal conflicts, daily interpersonal hassles, feeling deficient in the eyes of other people, hostility, marital difficulties, relationship dissolution, and disagreeableness comprise only some of the interpersonal problems reported by people high in perfectionistic concerns (e.g., Hewitt et al., 2006; Mackinnon et al., 2012; Molnar, Sadava, Flett, & Colautti, 2012; Sherry et al., 2013). Overall then, people high in perfectionistic concerns appear to engage in interpersonally aversive behaviors and extreme social appraisals that hinder the development of stable and supportive relationships.

Perfectionistic strivings involve rigidly and unrealistically demanding perfection of oneself. Factor analyses suggest that perfectionistic strivings are strongly correlated with, but empirically distinct from, perfectionistic concerns (Dunkley

& Blankstein, 2000). There is a debate as to the adaptive or the maladaptive nature of perfectionistic strivings. Some authors argue perfectionistic strivings are positively related to psychopathology, especially as a risk factor for eating disorders (Bardone-Cone et al., 2007) or after a performance failure (Besser, Flett, & Hewitt, 2004). Other authors argue perfectionistic strivings are negatively correlated with psychopathology after partialling out shared covariation with perfectionistic concerns (Stoeber & Otto, 2006). Though this debate continues, it is generally agreed that perfectionistic strivings tend to be less strongly related to negative outcomes than perfectionistic concerns.

Other-oriented perfectionism is sometimes proposed as a third perfectionism dimension. Other-oriented perfectionism represents a tendency to harshly demand perfection from others (Hewitt & Flett, 1991). Though positively correlated with other perfectionism dimensions (Hewitt & Flett, 1991), other-oriented perfectionism is distinguished from perfectionistic concerns and strivings through its overlap with antisocial and narcissistic traits. For instance, Stoeber (in press) found that other-oriented perfectionism was uniquely related to facets of Machiavellianism, psychopathy, narcissism, and social dominance, and was associated with lower levels of agreeableness. Similarly, Sherry, Gralnick, Hewitt, Sherry, and Flett (2014) found other-oriented perfectionism was positively associated with narcissism beyond other facets of perfectionism. Other-oriented perfectionism has received comparatively less research attention overall, possibly because it has had mixed success predicting outcomes beyond perfectionistic concerns and strivings (Stoeber, in press). However, other-oriented perfectionism does have clear and important links with relationship conflict in romantic dyads when high perfectionistic standards are placed on one's romantic partner (Haring, Hewitt, & Flett, 2003; Stoeber, 2012), which suggests it is not a benign trait.

Outlining the Social Disconnection Model

Many perfectionists have major problems with social disconnection (i.e., conflict with and alienation from other people). In particular, people high in perfectionistic concerns generate social disconnection through neediness, overdependence on others, and hostile, rejecting interpersonal behaviors (Habke & Flynn, 2002), especially in response to perceived criticism or failure (Holm-Denoma, Otamendi, & Joiner, 2008). Indeed, people high in perfectionistic concerns may also attack others when their goals are thwarted because they believe love and acceptance is contingent on perfect performance (Blatt, 1995). People high in perfectionistic concerns also tend to seek acceptance and approval by excessively focusing on agentic accomplishments; however, through repeated disappointments, rejections, and conflicts, they find themselves socially disconnected and vulnerable to developing psychopathology.

The SDM (Hewitt et al., 2006) proposes three testable hypotheses regarding how people high in perfectionistic concerns become socially disconnected and psychologically distressed: (a) perfectionistic concerns confer vulnerability to psychopathology, such as depression, suicide, and eating problems; (b) perfectionistic concerns confer vulnerability to social disconnection; and (c) social disconnection mediates the link between perfectionistic concerns and psychopathology. Hewitt et al. (2006) also distinguished between subjective social disconnection (i.e., the psychological experience of isolation) and objective social disconnection (i.e., severed or impaired interpersonal relationships), though both are proposed as mediators. To date, most research on the SDM has focused on subjective social disconnection (e.g., perceived social support) as opposed to objective social disconnection (e.g., Sherry, Law, Hewitt, Flett, & Besser, 2008). In sum, the SDM proposes a mechanism for the perfectionism–psychopathology link: Perfectionistic concerns generate social disconnection, which, in turn, results in psychopathology.

The SDM is supported by research, with the strongest support for depression. Shahar, Blatt, Zuroff, Krupnick and Sotsky (2004) studied 144 patients with major depressive disorder and found pretreatment self-criticism led to reduced quality of the patient's social network and impairments in the therapeutic alliance, which, in turn, predicted less reduction in depressive symptoms posttreatment. Similarly, Dunkley, Sanislow, Grilo, and McGlashan (2006) found lower perceived social support and increased negative social interactions mediated the relationship between self-criticism and changes in depression in a 2-wave, 3-year longitudinal study of 96 clinic-recruited participants. Various other forms of social disconnection have been found to mediate the perfectionistic concerns–depressive symptoms relationship in longitudinal studies of student and community samples, including personality-dependent interpersonal stressors (Cox et al., 2009), dyadic conflict (Mackinnon et al., 2012), and interpersonal discrepancies (Sherry et al., 2013). Though much of the support for the SDM is found when predicting depressive symptoms, the SDM has also proven useful when predicting other outcomes. For instance, Molnar et al. (2012) found socially prescribed perfectionism was associated with lower levels of perceived social support which, in turn, was associated with poorer physical health in a cross-sectional sample of 538 undergraduates. When predicting binge eating, a 3-wave, 3-week longitudinal study of 200 undergraduate women, Mackinnon et al. (2011) found concern over mistakes had an indirect effect on binge eating through increased interpersonal discrepancies and decreased interpersonal esteem. Finally, Roxborough et al. (2012) found social hopelessness and being bullied mediated the relationship between socially prescribed perfectionism and suicide risk in a cross-sectional sample of 152 psychiatric outpatient children and adolescents. In sum, the SDM has enjoyed substantial support thus far.

Expanding the Social Disconnection Model

Despite promising empirical support for the SDM, there is a room for improvements to this emerging model. An expanded version of the SDM appears in Fig. 10.1, and our four proposed improvements to this model are now detailed.

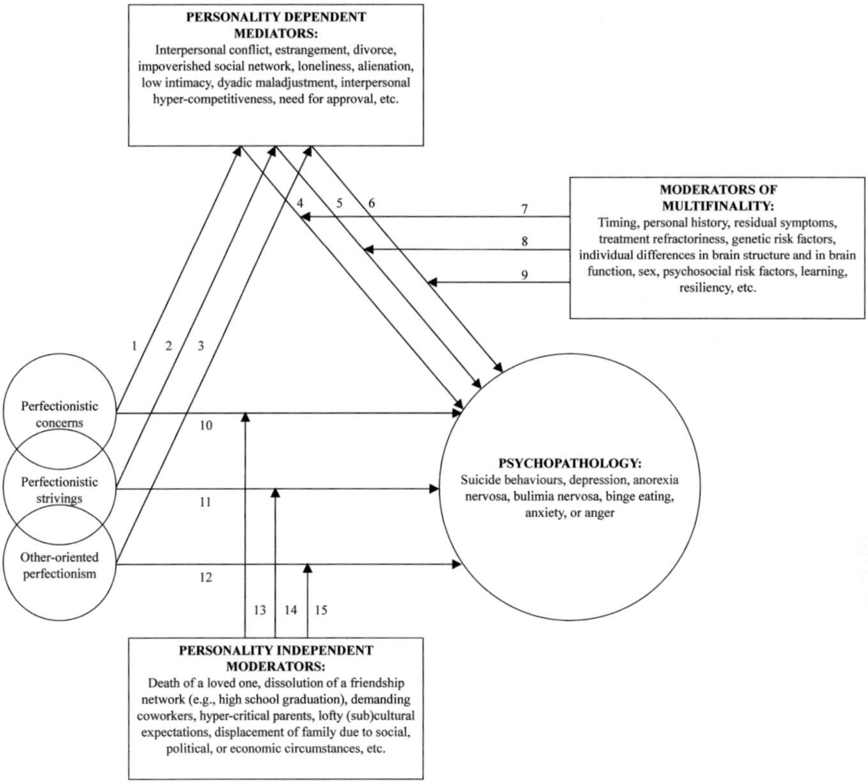

Fig. 10.1 The expanded social disconnection model

A Role for Perfectionistic Strivings and Other-Oriented Perfectionism

Building on theory and research reviewed above, Hewitt et al. (2006) conceptualized perfectionistic concerns as the main driver of perfectionists' interpersonal problems. While it is clearly appropriate to accord perfectionistic concerns a key role in perfectionists' interpersonal difficulties, we believe there is also an important role for perfectionistic strivings and other-oriented perfectionism in the SDM. People high in perfectionistic strivings have a compulsive, self-imposed need to be perfect and often lead an imbalanced life wherein self-definition (agency) is privileged over relatedness (communion). Expressed in terms of an undergraduate's existence, these people may spend too much time at the library and too little time with other people. Behaviors prototypical of people high in perfectionistic strivings (e.g., repetitive checking, avoiding mistakes, and compulsive overstriving) may result in a narrow, imbalanced set of life experiences where chances for social relations are missed or avoided (Frost et al., 1990; Graham et al., 2010). Given their often narrow behavioral repertoire, people high in perfectionistic strivings may simply not come into contact with opportunities to socialize: The relentless pursuit of perfection requires a lot of exclusion which may lead to a solitary existence. Considering the wider life course of people high in perfectionistic strivings, an extreme or a distorted concern with self-definition may occur and result in an asymmetrical course of development where agentic concerns trump communal concerns (Blatt, 1995).

People high in perfectionistic strivings are also hypercompetitive, manifesting a win-at-all-cost interpersonal style where others are viewed more as competitors than collaborators. Many theories of healthy, positive human development hold that people would ideally move toward a species preservation orientation wherein helping others, making a contribution, and a concern with humanity are paramount. For example, Adler (Ansbacher & Ansbacher, 1956) argued that well-adjusted people participate in what he termed the social interest (i.e., a feeling of community including contributions to society and cooperation with others). In contrast, many people high in perfectionistic strivings move toward a self-preservation orientation wherein individual competition, beating others, and being the absolute best are paramount (Flett, Hewitt, Blankstein, & Gray, 1998; Sherry, Hewitt, Flett, Lee-Baggley, & Hall, 2007). In addition to interpersonal problems, perfectionistic strivings are linked to psychopathology, including stress, anorexia nervosa and other eating disorders, body image disturbance, and suicide (Cockell et al., 2002). Thus, theory and research indicate perfectionistic strivings are linked with interpersonal problems and psychopathology, supporting the role of perfectionistic strivings in the SDM.

People high in other-oriented perfectionism ceaselessly demand perfection from others, a derogating and conflictual interpersonal style which contributes to psychopathology (Hewitt & Flett, 1991). Always demanding perfection from others strains relationships, with people high in other-oriented perfectionism acting hostile toward, dominant around, and disappointed with others (Sherry et al., 2007). Other-oriented perfectionists often suffer in romantic relationships. Such relationships are complicated by other-oriented perfectionists' rigid need for their partners to be perfect (Habke & Flynn, 2002). For example, Habke, Hewitt, and Flett (1999) found wives' other-oriented perfectionism was linked to lower sexual satisfaction in both husbands and wives.

Whereas people high in perfectionistic strivings appear to avoid interpersonal relationships, those high in other-oriented perfectionism seem to struggle in interpersonal relationships. People high in other-oriented perfectionism distress their partners. Indeed, the recipient of perfectionistic demands may suffer more than the source of perfectionistic demands. For instance, Hewitt, Flett, and Mikail, (1995) found that the spouses of people high in other-oriented perfectionism reported higher marital distress—even though the people high in other-oriented perfectionism were not martially distressed themselves. Beyond interpersonal problems, other-oriented perfectionism is tied to psychopathology, including anger and depression (Hewitt & Flett, 1990; Sherry et al., 2007). This chapter integrates other-oriented perfectionism into a broader model of social disconnection and psychopathology to encourage more research on this understudied construct.

In terms of a mediation model, the effect of perfectionistic strivings and other-oriented perfectionism on psychopathology may be highly indirect (e.g., no path between other-oriented perfectionism and depression). However, both perfectionistic strivings and other-oriented perfectionism may still generate social disconnection with important implications for psychopathology. Whereas the original SDM focuses only on perfectionistic concerns and social disconnection, the expanded SDM acknowledges the contribution of perfectionistic strivings and other-oriented perfectionism to social disconnection (see Fig. 10.1).

Personality-Dependent Mediators vs. Personality-Independent Moderators

Another proposed expansion to the SDM involves more clearly specifying the nature and the origins of the interpersonal problems experienced by perfectionists. Theory and research paint a picture of perfectionists as more than "passive recipients of situational influences" (Hammen & Shih, 2008, p. 410). In fact, perfectionists are often active agents who play a leading role in generating interpersonal problems that undermine their well-being (Hewitt et al., 2006; Sherry & Hall, 2009). Drawing on Hammen's (1991, 2006) notion of stress generation, in the expanded SDM, we distinguish between personality-dependent and personality-independent interpersonal problems. Personality-dependent interpersonal problems are something perfectionists do to themselves (e.g., rigid demandingness resulting in interpersonal conflict), whereas personality-independent interpersonal problems are something that happens to perfectionists (e.g., a mother gets cancer). That is, personality-dependent interpersonal problems are mediator variables that explain processes or mechanisms. Such variables help us understand how or why perfectionists experience problems. In contrast, personality-independent interpersonal problems are moderator variables that help us understand when and under what conditions perfectionists are likely to experience problems (see Fig. 10.1). Both personality-dependent and personality-independent interpersonal problems are important to understanding perfectionists and their problems. Acknowledging this distinction in the expanded SDM will allow for a clearer, more rigorous, and differentiated test of the SDM.

Combining the SDM and the Diathesis-Stress Model Using Moderated Mediation

As highlighted above and presented in Fig. 10.1, the expanded SDM distinguishes between personality-dependent interpersonal problems (mediators) and personality-independent interpersonal problems (moderators). Historically, researchers were required to make a choice between testing moderation models and testing mediation models. It was also never really clear why a researcher might consider a variable (e.g., interpersonal problems) as a moderator in one study (e.g., Chang, Sanna, Chang, & Bodem, 2008) and a mediator in another study (e.g., Sherry et al., 2008). By focusing on interpersonal problems as a mediating variable (e.g., Mackinnon et al., 2012), and largely ignoring interpersonal problems as a moderating variable, the original SDM shares this limitation. On a conceptual level, this implies perfectionists are primarily the authors of their own misery, a viewpoint that pays insufficient attention to (the seemingly arbitrary) life events that may conceivably happen to any person at any time independent of his/her personality (e.g., a spouse getting cancer or economic downturn leading to job loss). However, case studies and clinical observations (Blatt, 1995) suggest perfectionists deal not only with interpersonal problems directly linked with their personality (personality-dependent stressors that mediate the relation between perfectionism and psychopathology; see Fig. 10.1 for examples) but also with interpersonal problems largely beyond their direct control (personality-independent stressors that moderate the relation between perfectionism and psychopathology; see Fig. 10.1 for examples). In the terms familiar to perfectionism researchers, in this chapter we propose the integration of an established explanation for perfectionists' difficulties (i.e., the diathesis stress model, which focuses on moderation) with an emerging explanation for perfectionists' difficulties (i.e., the SDM, which focuses on mediation).

The diathesis stress model (also sometimes called the matching hypothesis, the specific vulnerability hypothesis, or the congruence hypothesis) holds that, for those high in perfectionism to get depressed, the stressor has to "hit close to home" (Hewitt & Flett, 1993, 2002). To illustrate, for people high on perfectionistic concerns, interpersonal stressors may be especially ego-involving. When those high in perfectionistic concerns encounter an interpersonal stressor, they are likely to get distressed in one way or another (e.g., depression). However, the SDM focuses only on the mediating effects of stressors on the relation between perfectionism and psychopathology. Statistical advances (i.e., moderated mediation) no longer require researchers to choose between testing moderation models and mediation models (see Fig. 10.1; Edwards & Lambert, 2007). Instead, moderated mediation models allow for integration of two explanations for when and why perfectionists experience psychopathology. That is, moderated mediation models allow for a conceptual integration of the social disconnection model with the diathesis stress model. Using a moderated mediation framework, the expanded SDM includes both personality-dependent mediators (as did the original SDM) and personality-independent moderators (consistent with diathesis stress models; see Fig. 10.1).

The Issue of Multifinality

The original SDM is silent on the issue of multifinality, even though the diverse interpersonal problems encountered by perfectionists are unlikely to lead to just one outcome. When applied to the SDM, the concept of multifinality suggests perfectionists experiencing similar interpersonal problems may diverge toward various outcomes (Cicchetti & Rogosch, 1996; Nolen-Hoeksema & Watkins, 2011). We have preliminary evidence for the SDM being relevant to diverse outcomes. The SDM is supported in relation to suicide behavior, depressive symptoms, social anxiety, alcohol-related problems, binge eating, and poorer physical health (e.g., Hewitt et al., 2006; Molnar et al., 2012; Nepon, Flett, Hewitt, & Molnar, 2011; Sherry & Hall, 2009; Sherry et al., 2012; Sherry et al., 2008). However, it is presently unclear when and why interpersonally distressed perfectionists travel divergent trajectories. If perfectionists begin from more or less the same interpersonally distressed starting point, we need to understand when and why some perfectionists progress to divergent endpoints such as subclinical variants of a disorder (e.g., symptoms of depression), full-blown, frank expressions of a disorder (e.g., major depressive disorder), one disorder and not another (e.g., generalized anxiety disorder vs. major depressive disorder), or comorbid, multiproblem outcomes (e.g., generalized anxiety disorder, major depressive disorder, and suicide behaviors all in one individual at one time).

In seeking to understand pathways of multifinality, it is also important to understand when and why some perfectionists may on some occasions escape unscathed from interpersonal problems (as clearly not all perfectionists will experience symptoms in response to interpersonal problems all the time). Whereas the SDM is focused primarily on risk factors (e.g., factors that increase the likelihood of perfectionism resulting in negative outcomes), future studies should also attend to protective factors (i.e., factors that may slow or even prevent perfectionism from resulting in negative outcomes). We need to study pathways from perfectionism to psychopathology *and* pathways from perfectionism to resilience.

There are certain psychosocial environments and biological predispositions reliably linked to psychopathology (Nolen-Hoeksema & Watkins, 2011). In terms of the expanded SDM (see Fig. 10.1), moderators of multifinality are factors that change the strength or the direction of the relation between personality-dependent mediators and psychopathology. Possibilities abound when it comes to specifying possible moderators of multifinality. To guide the identification of such moderators, we propose investigators might consider three broad classes of moderators of multifinality: personal variables, biological variables, and environmental variables. Regarding personal variables, timing (e.g., conflict with a romantic partner at age 14 vs. conflict with a romantic partner at age 64), personal history (e.g., past suicide attempts), residual symptoms (e.g., depressive symptoms remaining after treatment), and treatment refractoriness (e.g., not responding to appropriate treatment) are all candidate moderators of multifinality. To provide an illustrative example involving personal history as a moderator of multifinality, a conflict with a boss at work (i.e., a personality-dependent mediator) is especially likely to result in a suicide attempt (i.e., psychopathology), given a personal history of suicide attempts (Joiner et al., 2005). With respect to biological variables, genetic risk factors (e.g., family history of depression), individual differences in brain structure and in brain function (e.g., error-related negativity), and sex (male vs. female) are other possible moderators of multifinality. Using genetic risk factors as an example of a moderator of multifinality, the relationship between relationship dissolution and depression may be especially strong for women who inherited a dysfunctional *5-HTTLPR* gene from the maternal side of her family (Anguelova, Benkelfat & Turecki, 2003). In terms of environmental variables, psychosocial risk factors (e.g., poverty), learning (e.g., history of rewards and punishments), and resiliency (e.g., resourcefulness) are other possible moderators of multifinality. For instance, using learning as a moderator of multifinality, a dispute between spouses may be especially likely to result in depressive symptoms for one partner when the other partner typically gives care and attention to depressive behavior (i.e., positively reinforcing avoidance behavior; Hopko, Magidson and Lejuez, 2011). While we do not believe that there are innumerable moderators of multifinality for perfectionists (Nolen-Hoesksema & Watkins, 2011), we do believe that there are probably several multivariate pathways that split into several outcomes (e.g., emotional distress, suicide behaviors, or eating disorders).

In summary, the expanded SDM is more inclusive in that it includes perfectionistic concerns, as well as perfectionistic strivings and other-oriented perfectionism. This expanded model also distinguishes between personality-dependent and personality-independent moderators, bringing greater precision to this conceptual model. The expanded SDM is also integrative in nature, drawing on moderated mediation models to subsume the diathesis stress model within its conceptual framework. This expanded model also sheds light on how interpersonally distressed perfectionists may travel divergent trajectories of symptom development. The expanded SDM also has clinical utility, something we hope to demonstrate by applying this model to the lives of two (in)famous interpersonally distressed perfectionists.

Applying the Expanded SDM to Sylvia Plath's Life

Sylvia Plath is a Pulitzer Prize-winning novelist and poet. Many accounts of Plath describe perfectionism as a core feature of her personality integral to her depression and suicide (e.g., Shulman, 1998). Plath had high levels of perfectionistic strivings and perfectionistic concerns, a combination theorized to have decreased well-being and poor psychological adjustment (Gaudreau & Thompson, 2010; Fig. 10.2a, paths 10 and 11). Plath's striving for perfection began early in life, with one high school teacher describing her as the type of student to argue that an A- should be an A (Gill, 2008). Indeed, Plath was a self-proclaimed perfectionist, and described her perfectionism as "a demon who wants me to run away screaming if I am going to be flawed, fallible" (Kukil, 2000; October 1, 1957). An ex-boyfriend of Plath noted: "[She was] driven by her demons to succeed [and] neglected aspects of her life other than the academic." (Lameyer, 1977, pg. 41 cited in Shulman, 1998). Plath's perfectionism led to numerous personality-dependent mediators that contributed to her psychological problems (Fig. 10.2a, paths 1 and 2). Plath's journal reveals crippling feelings of loneliness and perceived disconnection from others: "Alone, going alone among strangers. Month by month, colder shoulders. No eyes met mine. […] Alone. Loneliness burned" (Kukil, 2000; January 22, 1958). Other authors note more objective forms of social disconnection: Plath had a sharp tongue

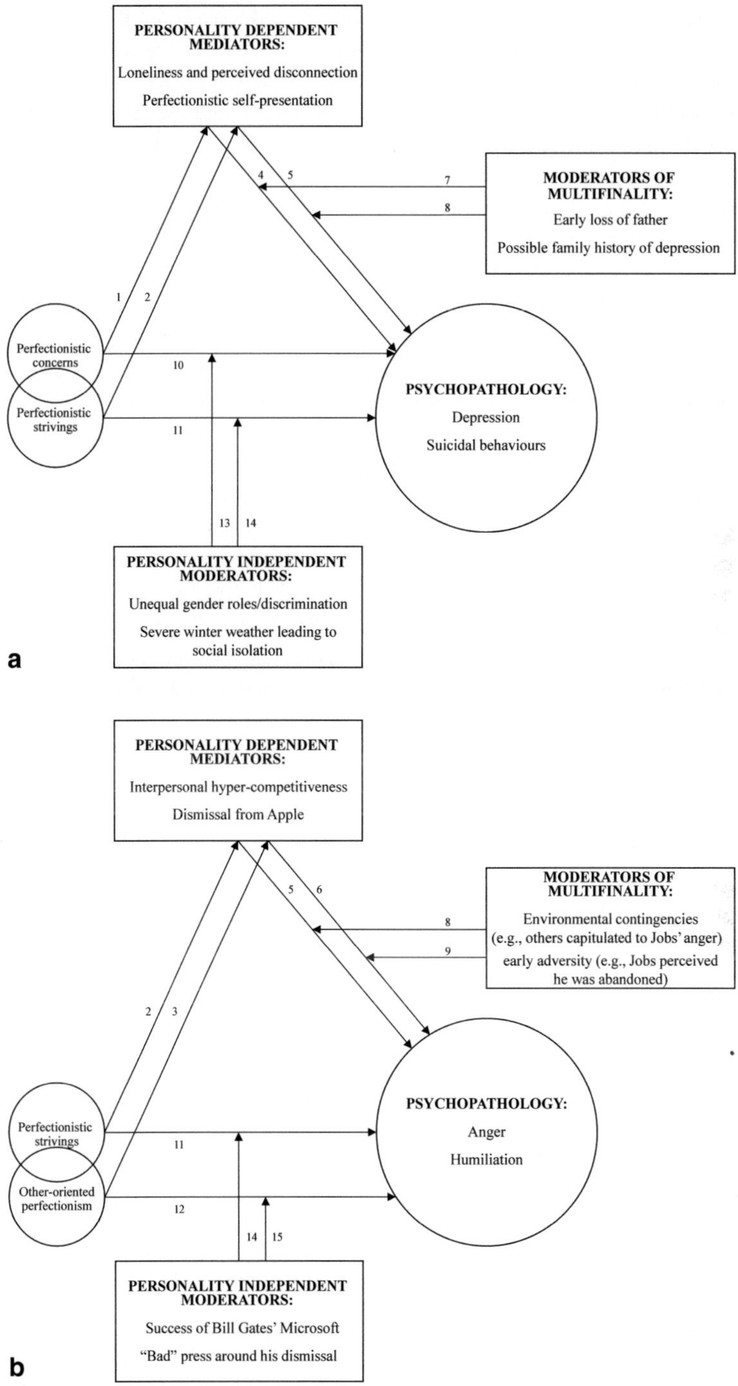

Fig. 10.2 The expanded SDM applied to the lives of Sylvia Plath (**a**) and Steve Jobs (**b**)

and was known to be demanding, inconsiderate, and temperamental when stressed (Shulman, 1998). Indeed, Plath kept distance between herself and others through perfectionistic self-presentation strategies; by creating a perfect façade, which she believed others would like, she was difficult to know personally, and rarely let her guard down even among close others (Lester, 1998). These perfectionistic self-presentation strategies made her loathe to ask for support from others, even from her husband: "Keep quiet with Ted about worries. […] Even with Ted I must learn to be very calm and happy" (Kukil, 2000; November 5, 1957). These interpersonal problems led to depression and suicidal ideation (Fig. 10.2a, paths 4 and 5).

For Plath, psychological problems manifested primarily as symptoms of depression and, tragically, her suicide in 1963. Within the expanded SDM, several moderators of multifinality contribute to these outcomes (Fig. 10.2a, paths 7 and 8). Plath's father died after complications from surgery when she was 8 years old, a traumatizing event that made Plath feel betrayed and abandoned (Lester, 1998; Shulman, 1998). Plath also had a history of prior suicide attempts (a known risk factor for suicide; Jenkins, Hale, Papanastassiou, Crawford and Tyrer, 2002), including one attempt in 1953 where she overdosed on sleeping pills after her application for a high-level creative writing course was unsuccessful (Gill, 2008). Plath's family history is also suggestive of a genetic link. Notably, her father was noted to have a "morbid personality" in recently released FBI reports that many believe provide evidence of Otto Plath's difficulties with depression (Alberge, 2012). Moreover, her son Nicholas Hughes also suffered from depression, and ultimately committed suicide on May 19, 2009 (Wilkinson, 2009).

There were also identifiable personality-independent moderators (Fig. 10.2a, paths 13 and 14). During Plath's life, cultural pressures surrounding the prescribed gender roles for women were immense. Hammer (2001) notes that Plath struggled to meet the competing demands of career success and motherhood. Indeed, the glass ceiling was a source of considerable frustration for a high-achieving, perfectionistic woman like Plath, who insisted on "having it all" (Hammer, 2001, p. 66). Moreover, around a year before her death, Ted Hughes had an affair with a mutual acquaintance, which was devastating for Plath (Lester, 1998). There were also numerous other life stressors in the month preceding her suicide in 1963, including a severe bout of influenza, social isolation (she was in a 2-month queue to receive a telephone in her new flat), childcare shortages, and an exceptionally severe winter (Gill, 2008). Along with the other components of the expanded SDM, these personality-independent moderators provide a compelling, theory-driven explanation for Plath's symptoms of depression and ultimate suicide.

Applying the Expanded SDM to Steve Jobs' Life

Perfectionism is a defining feature of Apple founder and visionary designer, Steve Jobs', personality (Isaacson, 2011). Jobs' biography suggests he was particularly high on perfectionistic strivings and other-oriented perfectionism (Isaacson, 2011). His perfectionistic strivings are evident in his work with Apple. He believed his products were life-changing and revolutionary (Burrows, 2004), and relentlessly obsessed over even the smallest detail of his products, refining them until they were "perfect" (Gladwell, 2011). Jobs said, "That's my job—to make sure everything is great" (Moisescot, 2012). His pursuit of perfection was often inefficient; he once spent 6 months tweaking scroll bars for a computer operating system (Surowiecki, 2011).

While Jobs is often described as an angry, mercurial man, it is unclear whether his perfectionistic strivings directly manifested into anger (see Fig. 10.2b, path 11). What is clear is that Jobs' hypercompetitiveness greatly contributed to his anger, and Jobs was explosively angry when he felt subordinate to others in competition. Jobs' perfectionistic strivings led to many interpersonal problems. In striving for perfection, Jobs was hypercompetitive (personality-dependent mediator; see Fig. 10.2b, path 2), viewing others as competitors, not collaborators. His hypercompetitiveness also fuelled to his anger (see Fig. 10.2b, path 5). Good enough was never good enough for Jobs; he was notorious for throwing temper tantrums and showing intense anger toward those who disagreed with him, or tried to get him to lower his standards (Barondes, 2011; Moisescot, 2012). In 2010, Jobs received an e-mail from writer Ryan Tate critiquing Jobs for describing the iPad as a revolutionary product. At the end of a vitriolic e-mail response, Jobs replied, "By the way, what have you done that's so great?" (Rainy, 2011).

The relationship between Jobs' hypercompetitiveness and anger was made worse by environmental contingencies rewarding Jobs' anger (moderator of multifinality; see Fig. 10.2b, path 8). Dating back to Jobs' childhood, when Jobs got angry, others would act to quickly appease his anger by agreeing with or accommodating to his impossible standards (Moisescot, 2012). His anger was reinforced by the favourable consequences it produced. Because others capitulated to Jobs' anger, the relationship between his hypercompetitiveness and anger was especially strong. Such environmental contingencies help to explain why Jobs' hypercompetitiveness manifested in anger rather than something else (e.g., depression).

Jobs was also involved in a lifelong competition with Microsoft's Bill Gates. During the 1980s and the 1990s, Apple sales lagged behind Microsoft and IBM. In fact, some Apple computers were widely considered as failures by insiders in the computer industry (personality-independent moderator; see Fig. 10.2b, path 14; Streitfield, 2011). During this time, Apple was subordinate to Microsoft in terms of both market share and public popularity. Being high in perfectionistic strivings, with its "if-you're-not-first-you're-worst" mentality, made Jobs' anger at the success of Bill Gates' Microsoft even worse.

Jobs also demanded perfectionism from others (Isaacson, 2011). He expected his coworkers to live up to his high expectations and to manufacture products that were well ahead of their time (Gates, 2011). "He was a tough customer, very demanding. There's a passion for perfection, and he divides everybody into heroes and dunces" (Isaacson, 2011). His other-oriented perfectionism led him to derogate others, to experience feelings of disappointment and dissatisfaction with others, and to engage in frequent conflicts with others. For example, he would often send his food back multiple times at restaurants and interviewed 67 nurses when he was ill before he found 3 nurses he could tolerate (Gladwell, 2011). In media accounts, Jobs is variously described as tyrannical, derogatory, insensitive, manipulative, a bully, mean, merciless, judgmental, frighteningly cold, and unreasonable (e.g., Gladwell, 2011; Isaacson, 2011). Jobs' frequent conflict with coworkers eventually resulted in being dismissed in 1985 from Apple, the corporation he created (see Fig. 10.2b, path 3; Gladwell, 2011). His dismissal resulted in strong feelings of humiliation for Jobs (see Fig. 10.2b, path 6; Isaacson, 2011). This humiliation was made worse by the sense of abandonment he already felt after his biological parents gave him up for adoption as an infant (moderator of multifinality; see Fig. 10.2b, path 9). Jobs' dismissal from Apple was also very public, resulting in a lot of "bad press" (personality-independent moderator; Jobs, 2005) and exacerbating his humiliation (see Fig. 10.2b, path 15). While it is unclear whether Jobs' other-oriented perfectionism led directly to his humiliation (see Fig. 10.2b, path 12), his prickly traits clearly contributed to his dismissal and his humiliation. His case also illustrates the expanded SDM and shows how social disconnection leads to psychopathology (e.g., anger and humiliation) for someone high in both perfectionistic strivings and other-oriented perfectionism.

Limitations and Future Directions

Despite the advances offered in the expanded SDM, there are still limitations to the model. For example, perfectionism both arises from and contributes to a dysfunctional interpersonal environment (Blatt, 1995). Our model focuses mostly on experiences in the proximal interpersonal environment (i.e., events close to the present moment). Future studies should also take into account developmental experiences in the distal interpersonal environment (i.e., events in the distant past). These include risk factors such as parental psychological control, exposure to parental psychopathology, physical, sexual, and emotional abuse, neglect, and harsh parenting (e.g., Flett, Hewitt, Oliver, & Macdonald, 2002). We would not be surprised to find a resemblance between developmental experiences in the distal interpersonal environment (e.g., growing up with a critical, demanding father) and activating experiences in the proximal interpersonal environment (e.g., having a critical, demanding boss at work). This correspondence between distal and proximal environments may be guided by a personality-based pattern of selection (Buss, 1987), wherein perfectionists select environments (e.g., the people they interact with) that are generally congruent with their early upbringing and disposition.

The social disconnection model is an explicitly interpersonal model tested to date with largely intrapersonal methods. In future research on the expanded SDM, perfectionism should be studied in actual interpersonal contexts, such as within families, romantic relationships, and workplaces. How does a daughter's perfectionistic strivings contribute to her depression? And, at the same time, how does her father's other-oriented perfectionism contribute to her depression? In other words, perfectionism and perfectionists are embedded in a much wider interpersonal context, a context which is not often studied by perfectionism research, despite many theoretical writings suggesting the importance of this context.

Clinical Implications

Perfectionism represents an interpersonal trait that predisposes people to interpersonal problems, which may then result in depression, disordered eating, generalized anxiety, or other problems (e.g., social anxiety). The SDM and its growing research base help to clarify the characterological and the interpersonal context in which mental and physical health problems occur for perfectionists. Since interpersonal problems play a leading role in the onset and the maintenance of perfectionists' difficulties, clinicians are advised to closely examine their client's long-term social history and current social functioning during assessment. Such an examination will point toward treatment targets (e.g., a need to modify demandingness).

The SDM also provides a theoretical support for interpersonal therapy as one treatment choice when working with distressed perfectionists. This therapy involves modifying important interpersonal problems such as interpersonal disputes, deficits, transitions, and losses (Klerman, Weissman, Rounsaville, & Chevron, 1984). By improving key elements of their interpersonal functioning and by developing a more supportive social network, people high in perfectionism may reduce their vulnerability to various mental and physical health problems (Klerman et al. 1984). Interpersonal therapy may also provide a way to assist distressed perfectionists in forging a more positive social identity, forming positive, stable relationships, and integrating into wider social communities (e.g., a university campus).

Concluding Remarks

Building on Hewitt et al. (2006), the expanded SDM brings a greater clarity and coherence to our understanding of interpersonally distressed perfectionists and their problems. This model provides a framework for understanding, researching, assessing, and treating interpersonally distressed perfectionists so that Sylvia Paths, Steve Jobs, and other perfectionists of our world can build more satisfying relationships and lead longer, more satisfying lives.

References

Alberge, D. (2012, Aug 17). FBI files on Sylvia Plath's father shed new light on poet. *The Guardian*. http://www.theguardian.com/books/2012/aug/17/sylvia-plath-otto-father-files.

Anguelova, M. M., Benkelfat, C. C., & Turecki, G. (2003). A systematic review of association studies investigating genes coding for serotonin receptors and the serotonin transporter: I. Affective disorders. *Molecular Psychiatry, 8,* 574–591. doi:10.1038/sj.mp.4001328.

Ansbacher, H., & Ansbacher, R. (1956). *The individual psychology of Alfred Adler*. Oxford: Basic Books.

Bardone-Cone, A. M., Wonderlich, S. A., Frost, R. O., Bulik, C. M., Mitchell, J. E., Uppala, S., & Simonich, H. (2007). Perfectionism and eating disorders: Current status and future directions. *Clinical Psychology Review, 27,* 384–405. doi:10.1016/j.cpr.2006.12.005.

Barondes, S. (2011, Nov 5). Why was Steve Jobs sometimes so mean? [Web log post]. http://www.psychologytoday.com/blog/making-sense-people/201111/why-was-steve-jobs-sometimes-so-mean. Accessed 10 June 2014.

Baumeister, R. F., & Leary, M. R. (1995). The need to belong. *Psychological Bulletin, 117,* 497–529. doi:10.1037/0033-2909.117.3.497.

Besser, A., Flett, G. L., & Hewitt, P. L. (2004). Perfectionism, cognition, and affect in response to performance failure vs success. *Journal of Rational-Emotive and Cognitive-Behavior Therapy, 22,* 301–328. doi:10.1023/B:JORE.0000047313.35872.5c.

Blatt, S. J. (1995). The destructiveness of perfectionism: Implications for the treatment of depression. *American Psychologist, 50,* 1003–1020. doi:10.1037/0003-066X.50.12.1003.

Blatt, S. J., D'Afflitti, J. P., & Quinlan, D. M. (1976). Experiences of depression in normal young adults. *Journal of Abnormal Psychology, 85,* 383–389. doi:10.1037/0021-843X.85.4.383.

Burrows, P. (2004, Oct). Steve Jobs: He thinks different. *Bloomberg Business Week Magazine.* http://www.businessweek.com/stories/2004-10-31/steve-jobs-he-thinks-different.

Buss, D. M. (1987). Selection, evocation, and manipulation. *Journal of Personality and Social Psychology, 53,* 1214–1221.

Cacioppo, J. T., Fowler, J. H., & Christakis, N. A. (2009). Alone in the crowd: The structure and spread of loneliness in a large social network. *Journal of Personality and Social Psychology, 97,* 977–991. doi:10.1037/a0016076.

Chang, E. C., Sanna, L. J., Chang, R., & Bodem, M. R. (2008). A preliminary look at loneliness as a moderator of the link between perfectionism and depressive and anxious symptoms in college students: Does being lonely make perfectionistic strivings more distressing? *Behaviour Research and Therapy, 46,* 877–886. doi:10.1016/j.brat.2008.03.012.

Cicchetti, D., & Rogosch, F. A. (1996). Equifinality and multifinality in developmental psychopathology. *Development and Psychopathology, 8,* 597–600. doi:10.1017/S0954579400007318.

Cockell, S. J., Hewitt, P. L., Seal, B., Sherry, S. B., Goldner, E. M., Flett, G. L., et al. (2002). Trait and self-presentational dimensions of perfectionism among women with anorexia nervosa. *Cognitive Therapy and Research, 26,* 745–758.

Cox, B. J., Clara, I. P., & Enns, M. W. (2009). Self-criticism, maladaptive perfectionism, and depression symptoms in a community sample: A longitudinal test of the mediating effects of person-dependent stressful life events. *Journal of Cognitive Psychotherapy, 23,* 336–349. doi:10.1891/0889 8391.23.4.330.

Dunkley, D. M., & Blankstein, K. R. (2000). Self-critical perfectionism, coping, hassles, and current distress: A structural equation modeling approach. *Cognitive Therapy and Research, 24,* 713–730. doi:10.1023/A:1005543529245.

Dunkley, D. M., Sanislow, C. A., Grilo, C. M., & McGlashan, T. H. (2006). Perfectionism and depressive symptoms 3 years later: Negative social interactions, avoidant coping, and perceived social support as mediators. *Comprehensive Psychiatry, 47,* 106–115. doi:10.1016/j.comppsych.2005.06.003.

Edwards, J. R., & Lambert, L. (2007). Methods for integrating moderation and mediation: A general analytical framework using moderated path analysis. *Psychological Methods, 12,* 1–22. doi:10.1037/1082-989X.12.1.1.

Enns, M. W., & Cox, B. J. (2002). The nature and assessment of perfectionism: A critical analysis. In G. L. Flett & P. L. Hewitt (Eds.), *Perfectionism: Theory, research, and treatment* (pp. 33–62). Washington, DC: American Psychological Association. doi:10.1037/10458-002.

Flett, G. L., Hewitt, P. L., Blankstein, K. R., & Gray, L. (1998). Psychological distress and the frequency of perfectionistic thinking. *Journal of Personality and Social Psychology, 75,* 1363–1381. doi:10.1037/0022-3514.75.5.1363.

Flett, G. L., Hewitt, P. L., Oliver, J. M., & Macdonald, S. (2002). Perfectionism in children and their parents: A developmental analysis. In G. L. Flett & P. L. Hewitt (Eds.), *Perfectionism: Theory, research, and treatment* (pp. 89–132). Washington, DC: American Psychological Association. doi:10.1037/10458-004.

Frost, R. O., Marten, P., Lahart, C., & Rosenblate, R. (1990). The dimensions of perfectionism. *Cognitive Therapy and Research, 14,* 449–468. doi: 10.1007/BF01172967.

Gates, C. (2011, Oct). Perfectionist Steve Jobs 'difficult' to work with. *Business Day*. http://www.stuff.co.nz/business/world/5746098/Perfectionist-Steve-Jobs-difficult-to-work-with.

Gaudreau, P., & Thompson, A. (2010). Testing a 2 × 2 model of dispositional perfectionism. *Personality and Individual Differences, 48,* 532–537. doi:10.1016/j.paid.2009.11.031.

Gill, J. (2008). *The Cambridge introduction to Sylvia Plath*. Cambridge: Cambridge University Press.

Gladwell, M. (2011, Nov). The tweaker. *The New Yorker*. http://www.newyorker.com/reporting/2011/11/14/111114fa_fact_gladwell?currentPage=all.

Graham, A. R., Sherry, S. B., Stewart, S. H., Sherry, D. L., McGrath, D., Fossum, K., & Allen, S. L. (2010). The existential model of perfectionism and depressive symptoms: A short-term, four-wave longitudinal study. *Journal of Counseling Psychology, 57,* 423–438. doi:10.1037/a0020667.

Habke, A. M., & Flynn, C. A. (2002). Interpersonal aspects of trait perfectionism. In G. L. Flett & P. L. Hewitt (Eds.), *Perfectionism: Theory, research, and treatment* (pp. 151–180). Washington, DC: American Psychological Association. doi:10.1037/10458-006.

Habke, A. M., Hewitt, P. L., & Flett, G. L. (1999). Perfectionism and sexual satisfaction in intimate relationships. *Journal of Psychopathology and Behavioral Assessment, 21,* 307–322. doi:10.1023/A:1022168715349.

Hammen, C. (1991). Generation of stress in the course of unipolar depression. *Journal of Abnormal Psychology, 100,* 555–561. doi:10.1037/0021-843X.100.4.555.

Hammen, C. (2006). Stress generation in depression: Reflections on origins, research, and future directions. *Journal of Clinical Psychology, 62,* 1065–1082. doi:10.1002/jclp.20293.

Hammen, C., & Shih, J. H. (2008). Stress generation and depression. In K. S. Dobson & D. A. Dozois (Eds.), *Risk factors in depression* (pp. 409–428). San Diego: Elsevier Academic Press. doi:10.1016/B978-0-08-045078-000018-6.

Hammer, L. (2001). Plath's lives. *Representations, 75,* 61–88. http://www.jstor.org/stable/10.1525/rep.2001.75.1.61.

Haring, M., Hewitt, P. L., & Flett, G. L. (2003). Perfectionism, coping, and quality of intimate relationships. *Journal of Marriage and Family, 65,* 143–158. doi:10.1111/j.1741-3737.2003.00143.x.

Hewitt, P. L., & Flett, G. L. (1990). Perfectionism and depression: A multidimensional analysis. *Journal of Social Behavior and Personality, 5,* 423–438.

Hewitt, P. L., & Flett, G. L. (1991). Perfectionism in the self and social contexts: Conceptual assessment, and association with psychopathology. *Journal of Personality and Social Psychology, 60,* 456–470. doi:10.1037/0022-3514.60.3.456.

Hewitt, P. L., & Flett, G. L. (1993). Dimensions of perfectionism, daily stress, and depression: A test of the specific vulnerability hypothesis. *Journal of Abnormal Psychology, 102,* 58–65. doi:10.1037/0021-843X.102.1.58.

Hewitt, P. L., & Flett, G. L. (2002). Perfectionism and stress processes in psychopathology. In G. L. Flett & P. L. Hewitt (Eds.), *Perfectionism: Theory, research, and treatment* (pp. 255–284). Washington, DC: American Psychological Association. doi:10.1037/10458-011.

Hewitt, P. L., Flett, G. L., & Mikail, S. F. (1995). Perfectionism and relationship adjustment in pain patients and their spouses. *Journal of Family Psychology, 9,* 335–347. doi:10.1037/0893-3200.9.3.335.

Hewitt, P. L., Flett, G. L., Sherry, S. B., & Caelian, C. (2006). Trait perfectionism dimensions and suicidal behavior. In T. E. Ellis (Ed.), *Cognition and suicide: Theory, research, and therapy* (pp. 215–235). Washington, DC: American Psychological Association.

Holm-Denoma, J. M., Otamendi, A., & Joiner, T. E. (2008). On self-criticism as interpersonally maladaptive. In E. C. Chang (Ed.), *Self-criticism and self-enhancement: Theory, research, and clinical implications* (pp. 73–86). Washington, DC: American Psychological Association. doi:10.1037/11624-005.

Hopko, D. R., Magidson, J. F., & Lejuez, C. W. (2011). Treatment failure in behavior therapy: Focus on behavioral activation for depression. *Journal of Clinical Psychology, 67,* 1106–1116. doi:10.1002/jclp.20840.

Isaacson, W. (2011). *Steve Jobs*. New York: Simon & Schuster.

Jenkins, G. R., Hale, R., Papanastassiou, M., Crawford, M. J., & Tyrer, P. (2002). Suicide rate 22 years after parasuicide: Cohort study. *British Medical Journal, 325,* 1155. doi:10.1136/bmj.325.7373.1155.

Jobs, S. (Speaker). (2005). Steve Jobs'2005 Stanford Commencement Address. http://news.stanford.edu/news/2005/june15/videos/987.html. Accessed 12 June 2014.

Jobs, S. (2008). Steve Jobs speaks out/Interviewer: Betsy Morris. *Fortune*. http://money.cnn.com/galleries/2008/fortune/0803/gallery.jobsqna.fortune/index.html.

Joiner, T. R., Conwell, Y., Fitzpatrick, K., Witte, T. K., Schmidt, N. B., Berlim, M. T., Rudd, M., et al. (2005). Four studies on how past and current suicidality relate even when 'everything but the kitchen sink' is covaried. *Journal of Abnormal Psychology, 114,* 291–303. doi:10.1037/0021-843X.114.2.291.

Klerman, G. L., Weissman, M. M., Rounsaville, B., & Chevron, E. (1984). *Interpersonal psychotherapy of depression*. New York: Basic Books.

Kukil, K. V. (Ed.). (2000). *The journals of Sylvia Plath 1950–1962*. London: Faber and Faber.

Lameyer, G. (1977). *Sylvia plath: The woman and her work*. New York: Dodd, Mead, and Company.

Lester, D. (1998). Theories of suicidal behavior applied to Sylvia Plath. *Death Studies, 22,* 655–666. doi:10.1080/074811898201344.

Mackinnon, S. P., Sherry, S. B., Graham, A. R., Stewart, S. H., Sherry, D. L., Allen, S. L., Fitzpatrick, S., McGrath, D. S. (2011). Reformulating and testing the perfectionism model of binge eating among undergraduate women: A short-term, three-wave longitudinal study. *Journal of Counseling Psychology, 58,* 630–646. doi:10.1037/a0025068.

Mackinnon, S. P., Sherry, S. B., Antony, M. M., Stewart, S. H., Sherry, D. L., & Hartling, N. (2012). Caught in a bad romance: Perfectionism, conflict, and depression in romantic relationships. *Journal of Family Psychology, 26,* 215–225. doi:10.1037/a0027402.

Moisescot, R. (2012, March). Steve at work. All About Steve Jobs. http://allaboutstevejobs.com/persona/steveatwork.php. Accessed 12 June 2014.

Molnar, D. S., Reker, D. L., Culp, N. A., Sadava, S. W., & DeCourville, N. H. (2006). A mediated model of perfectionism, affect, and physical health. *Journal of Research in Personality, 40,* 482–500. doi:10.1016/j.jrp.2005.04.002.

Molnar, D. S., Sadava, S. W., Flett, G. L., & Colautti, J. (2012). Perfectionism and health: A mediational analysis of the roles of stress, social support and health-related behaviours. *Psychology and Health, 27,* 846–864. doi:10.1080/08870446.2011.630466.

Nepon, T., Flett, G. L., Hewitt, P. L., & Molnar, D. S. (2011). Perfectionism, negative social feedback, and interpersonal rumination in depression and social anxiety. *Canadian Journal of Behavioural Science, 43,* 297–308. doi:10.1037/a0025032.

Nolen-Hoeksema, S., & Watkins, E. R. (2011). A heuristic for developing transdiagnostic models of psychopathology: Explaining multifinality and divergent trajectories. *Perspectives on Psychological Science, 6,* 589–609. doi:10.1177/1745691611419672.

Plath, S. (1993). From diary. In P. Rose (Ed.), *The Norton book of women's lives* (pp. 664–670). New York: W. W. Norton and Company.

Rainy, S. (2011, Nov). The critics who have taken on Steve Jobs. *The Telegraph*. http://www.telegraph.co.uk/technology/steve-jobs/8899695/The-critics-who-have-taken-on-Steve-Jobs.html.

Roxborough, H. M., Hewitt, P. L., Kaldas, J., Flett, G. L., Caelian, C. M., Sherry, S., & Sherry, D. L. (2012). Perfectionistic self-presentation, socially prescribed perfectionism, and suicide in youth: A test of the perfectionism social disconnection model. *Suicide and Life-Threatening Behavior, 42,* 217–233. doi:10.1111/j.1943-278X.2012.00084.x.

Shahar, G., Blatt, S. J., Zuroff, D. C., Krupnick, J. L., & Sotsky, S. M. (2004). Perfectionism impedes social relations and response to brief treatment for depression. *Journal of Social and Clinical Psychology, 23,* 140–154. doi:10.1521/jscp.23.2.140.31017.

Sherry, S. B., & Hall, P. A. (2009). The perfectionism model of binge eating: Tests of an integrative model. *Journal of Personality and Social Psychology, 96,* 690–709.

Sherry, S. B., Hewitt, P. L., Flett, G. L., Lee-Baggley, D. L., & Hall, P. A. (2007). Trait perfectionism and perfectionistic self-presentation in personality pathology. *Personality and Individual Differences, 42,* 477–490. doi:10.1016/j.paid.2006.07.026.

Sherry, S. B., Law, A., Hewitt, P. L., Flett, G. L., & Besser, A. (2008). Social support as a mediator of the relationship between perfectionism and depression: A preliminary test of the social disconnection model. *Personality and Individual Differences, 45,* 339–344.

Sherry, S. B., Hewitt, P. L., Stewart, S. H., MacKinnon, A. L., Mushquash, A. R., Flett, G. L., et al. (2012). Social disconnection and hazardous drinking mediate the link between perfectionistic attitudes and depressive symptoms. *Psychopathology and Behavioral Assessment, 34,* 370–381.

Sherry, S. B., MacKinnon, A. L., Fossum, K., Antony, M. M., Stewart, S. H., Sherry, D. L., Nealis, L. J., Mushquash, A. R., et al. (2013). Perfectionism, discrepancies, and depression: Testing the perfectionism social disconnection model in a short-term, four-wave longitudinal study. *Personality and Individual Differences, 54,* 692–697. doi:10.1016/j.paid.2012.11.017.

Sherry, S. B., Gralnick, T. M., Hewitt, P. L., Sherry, D. L., & Flett, G. L. (2014). Perfectionism and narcissism: Testing unique relationships and gender differences. *Personality and Individual Differences, 61–62,* 52–56. doi:10.1016/j.paid.2014.01.007.

Shulman, E. (1998). Vulnerability factors in Sylvia Plath's suicide. *Death Studies, 22,* 597–613. doi:10.1080/074811898201317.

Slaney, R. B., Rice, K. G., Mobley, M., Trippi, J., & Ashby, J. S. (2001). The revised almost perfect scale. *Measurement and Evaluation in Counseling and Development, 34,* 130–145.

Stoeber, J. (2012). Dyadic perfectionism in romantic relationships: Predicting relationship satisfaction and longterm commitment. *Personality and Individual Differences, 53,* 300–305. doi:10.1016/j.paid.2012.04.002.

Stoeber, J. (in press). How other-oriented perfectionism differs from self-oriented and socially prescribed perfectionism. *Journal of Psychopathology and Behavioral Assessment.* doi:10.1007/s10862-013-9397-7.

Stoeber, J., & Otto, K. (2006). Positive conceptions of perfectionism: Approaches, evidence, challenges. *Personality and Social Psychology Review, 10,* 295–319. doi:10.1207/s15327957pspr1004_2.

Stoeber, J., Harvey, L. N., Almeida, I., & Lyons, E. (2013). Multidimensional sexual perfectionism. *Archives of Sexual Behavior, 42*(8), 1593–1604. doi:10.1007/s10508-013-0135-8.

Streitfield, D. (2011, Oct). Defending life's work with words of a tyrant. *The New York Times.* http://www.nytimes.com/2011/10/07/technology/steve-jobs-defended-his-work-with-a-barbed-tongue.html?_r=0.

Surowiecki, J. (2011, Oct). How Steve Jobs changed. *The New Yorker.* http://www.newyorker.com/talk/financial/2011/10/17/111017ta_talk_surowiecki#ixzz2IolpDpC7.

Vincent, N. K., & Walker, J. R. (2000). Perfectionism and chronic insomnia. *Journal of Psychosomatic Research, 49,* 349–354. doi:10.1016/S0022-3999(00)00175-6.

Wilkinson, P. (2009, March 23). Tragic poet Sylvia Plath's son kills himself. *CNN.* http://www.cnn.com/2009/SHOWBIZ/books/03/23/plath.son.suicide/index.html.

Chapter 11
Perfectionism in Academic Settings

Kenneth G. Rice, Clarissa M. E. Richardson and Merideth E. Ray

Perfectionism in Academic Settings

> Once Upon a Time…I was Perfect.
> Some people can't wait for high school to end. The constant comparison between students, the need to be the best, the idea that average is not even good enough to make it on a scale of excellence. It's no secret that [School Name] High School is one of the most challenging and rewarding educational facilities in [the state]. Students file out of a classroom after a test and complain of how bad they did, when really they might have gotten a B-. Outside in the real world, adults wish that trivial events like these were the least of their worries, but to a high schooler, what goes on between these brick walls [is] everything.
> When trying to get into college, students try to rack up the number of clubs and hours of community service to place on their college admissions applications. But the perfection doesn't lie in numbers, it is reflected in the effort put forth by every student in the school.

These comments in a high school yearbook capture in a succinct and personal way the central elements of perfectionism as they have been described for decades by clinicians, researchers, and journalists. The student points to the relevance of striving to be "the best" and the downstream implications of effort and credentials established during high school. She alludes to the distortions that might befall perfectionists, the pernicious ways in which they might interpret their performance and how the intensity and distress engendered by those interpretations may not

The authors are grateful to Jana Mohammad Al-Nahhas, Angela Montfort, and Marieke van Nuenen for their assistance with this chapter.

K. G. Rice (✉) · M. E. Ray
Department of Counseling and Psychological Services, Georgia State University, P. O. Box 3980, Atlanta, GA 30302-3980, USA
e-mail: kgr1@gsu.edu

C. M. E. Richardson
Department of Psychology, University of Florida, Gainesville, USA

F. M. Sirois, D. S. Molnar (eds.), *Perfectionism, Health, and Well-Being,*
DOI 10.1007/978-3-319-18582-8_11

match up well with the perspectives of others; where some see adequacy in a B-, the perfectionistic student sees that level of performance as painful inadequacy. Indeed, excellence as a performance criterion, as she suggests, leaves no room for average performance. Interestingly, another part of the picture she paints shows that the personal experience of perfectionism is embedded in contextual considerations, features in the educational setting that might foster and maintain perfectionistic qualities among students, such as quality of school, emphasis on social comparison, developmental era, and salience of self-other evaluations.

As the title indicates, this chapter is concerned with the intersection of perfectionism and academics and is meant to be selective rather than exhaustive. We draw partly on other recent contributions summarizing key findings in areas of perfectionism and performance (e.g., Stoeber, 2012a) and attempt to broaden the coverage into some other academically relevant material. However, Bong, Hwang, Noh, and Kim (2014) recently pointed out that the literature blending perfectionism and academics is not as developed as one might expect, especially in achievement-oriented contexts such as schools and universities. There may be good reasons for the limited development of this literature. Perfectionism and academic settings represent two deceptively simple concepts or topics that quickly give way to complex variations, there is not uniform agreement regarding how perfectionism should be understood or measured, and there are wide-ranging indicators and contexts that can be framed within a broader topic of academic settings.

Academic Settings

It is important to understand the scope of academic settings. Academic settings could mean primary, secondary, postsecondary (college, university), and professional training, and/or other educational contexts. Academic settings could also include the parties involved in such settings, such as students, teachers/professors, other staff, and administrators. These settings may be nested in higher-level contexts, such as districts, states, and countries. There are potentially interesting combinations of person and context, such as students studying in a foreign country or performance and other academic-related issues for gender or racial minority students pursuing educational degrees in majors that historically have had extreme rates of gender or racial imbalance. "Academic settings" as an emphasis carries with it an implicit attention to more obvious academic variables such as performance indicators (grades), academic behaviors, motivation, performance under pressure/stress, and extensions of academic topics such as academic self-efficacy, commitment to academic pursuits, and career decision-making. Our focus in this chapter will be on grades and a handful of other relevant academic outcomes. Limited attention will be given to variables pertaining to development, social and personal factors, relationships, social connection and support, athletics, leadership, and mental health.

Definitional and Measurement Considerations for Perfectionism

As it appears in the literature, perfectionism can be considered either a unidimensional or multidimensional personality characteristic. Perfectionism can refer to something global about a person and the ways in which she or he acts across multiple situations or it can refer to something specific about a person within a specific performance situation. Perfectionism might be viewed by some as clearly problematic, unhealthy, and maladaptive, but perhaps more controversial is the view that perfectionism may be adaptive or maladaptive depending on the combination of characteristics deemed central to the construct and the outcomes that can be traced to those characteristics within a particular context.

There is little doubt that what can be described as the clinical or maladaptive view is the dominant perspective. Witness the content of chapters comprising Flett and Hewitt's (2002) edited volume and the definitional and content emphases comprising the chapters in this current volume. Shafran, Cooper, and Fairburn (2002) defined "clinical perfectionism" as the "overdependence of self-evaluation on the determined pursuit of personally demanding, self-imposed, standards in at least one highly salient domain, despite adverse consequences" (p. 778). Pacht (1984, p. 387) wrote, "The insidious nature of perfectionism leads me to use the label only when describing a kind of psychopathology."

Our main concerns with the clinical view are simply stated as: (a) Cause (perfectionism) and effect (psychological distress) have not been well differentiated within several threads of the measurement and more substantive research literature and (b) a critical reading of the existing research has simply not supported a unilateral "destructiveness" (Blatt, 1995) of perfectionism. Our sense of what is and is not known about perfectionism leads us to a more balanced view regarding its possible realties, and our conclusion is that perfectionism, like other personality characteristics, might yield space for adaptation and positive outcomes if one knows how and where to look for such outcomes. As clinicians and clients will bear witness, perfectionism can portend adversity-related outcomes, but there is reasonable doubt that perfectionism reflects either a unitary entity or is tantamount to a kind of psychopathology. Factor analyses of measures based on unidimensional conceptualizations (e.g., Clinical Perfectionism Questionnaire; Fairburn, Cooper, & Shafran, 2003) reveal two correlated, but empirically distinct perfectionism factors of personal standards and self-evaluation. Multiple studies have found support for the correlation between these two factors ($r=.39$ & $r=.37$; Dickie, Surgenor, Wilson, & McDowall, 2012; Stoeber & Damian, 2014). Labels vary, but two dimensions (strivings or standards and maladaptive evaluation or perfectionistic concerns) also often emerge in factor analyses based on multidimensional measures of perfectionism and appear to be differentially related to a variety of outcomes (e.g., Aldea & Rice, 2006; Dunkley, Blankstein, Halsall, Williams, & Winkworth, 2000; Stoeber & Otto, 2006). Consequently, studies support a multifaceted view of perfectionism and indicate that perfectionism is not synonymous with psychopathology.

In contrast to measures that can be traced to conceptual models emphasizing "perfectionism is pathology," the Almost Perfect Scale-Revised (APS-R; Slaney, Mobley, Trippi, Ashby, & Jonson, 1996; Slaney, Rice, Mobley, Trippi, & Ashby, 2001) represents a parsimonious conceptualization and measurement of perfectionism that permits potentially healthy *or* unhealthy expressions of perfectionism. The APS-R subscales measure self-performance expectations (Standards) and gap or degree of self-critical evaluation in one's perceived ability to live up to expected standards (Discrepancy); a third subscale, Order, measures preferences for order and organization, but is less central in understanding core dimensions of perfectionism (Stoeber & Otto, 2006). Unlike subscales from other measures or results from second-order factor analyses, the two APS-R scores are generally orthogonal or, at most, minimally correlated with one another. This suggests that standards and self-evaluation regarding the ability to meet standards can, at least in many Western samples tested thus far, represent two distinct perfectionism dimensions.

One key consideration seems to be whether performance standards, even extremely high ones, are reasonable and motivating *or* unreasonable and debilitating. This is an important point often missed in arguments against an adaptive expression of perfectionism. The contemporary thinking among some in what might be called the "adaptive camp" is that elevated standards are not viewed as isomorphic with adaptive perfectionism. Instead, the idea is that *standards, combined with high levels of self-criticism or combined with low levels of self-criticism, and the association between those alignments and other adjustment criteria, support differentiating adaptive from maladaptive perfectionism.* This more nuanced view can be discerned from several research threads.

In their recent review, Lo and Abbott (2013; see also Stoeber & Otto, 2006) noted that several models of perfectionism emphasize standards or standard setting as not only a key element of perfectionism, but a key focus or target of intervention. Ostensibly, the argument is that standards are unrealistically high among (maladaptive) perfectionists, so a reasonable course of action would be lowering them. One limitation of that premise is that determining whether standards are realistic can be challenging and at least implicitly assumes that methods for assessing perfectionism are up to that task, or that a referee exists who can make that conclusion.

Another and probably related problem is that people often like their personal standards, find them motivating, and want to retain them. Indeed, Stoeber and Hotham (2013) found that the perfectionistic characteristics that many researchers and clinicians might regard as maladaptive are experienced as socially desirable in a general, nonclinical sample, such as most samples located within academic settings. Even clinically distressed individuals, with perfectionism as a cause or correlate of their psychological distress, might question the need to change an aspect of personality that has potentially positive motivational and outcome consequences for them (Egan, Piek, Dyck, Rees, & Hagger, 2013). Some experiments indicate that clinically perfectionistic participants most commonly choose to retain their standards, regardless of positive (success) or negative (failure) consequences of the standards (Egan, Dick, & Allen, 2012). If they do choose to change their standards for themselves, clients might be more likely to set standards *higher* following failure, though interestingly athletes have been more likely to set subsequent standards *lower* in response to failure (Egan et al., 2013).

Similar to others (e.g., Stoeber, 2012a), we believe the current status of research evidence supports the proposition that perfectionism can be (a) understood as multidimensional, (b) organized under minimally two higher-order dimensions of standards or striving for expected levels of performance and self-critical evaluation concerns linked to reaching those standards, and (c) further understood as adaptive or maladaptive in light of the valence of variables associated with or stemming from perfectionism, as well as the context within which the relative value or cost of perfectionism is being evaluated.

Perfectionism Measurement

Measuring these two major forms or expressions of perfectionism may not be as easy as one might imagine. Although the desired endpoint from a measure of perfectionism might be reliable and valid scores representing two major perfectionism dimensions, the starting point in measurement decisions can lead the researcher to a long, daunting list of options. Excluding short versions of previously published scales, we counted 19 measures presented or published in peer-reviewed journals. Some of the scales assess general perfectionism traits, whereas others measure perfectionism associated with specific activities, behaviors, and attitudes. Despite the large number of perfectionism scales available, chances are good that results based on any two or more of them can be reduced to two higher-order dimensions: perfectionistic striving or high standards for performance and perfectionistic concerns, such as worry about making mistakes and negative self-evaluation about reaching one's standards (Rice, Richardson, & Tueller, 2014).

Whether those two dimensions will substantially overlap depends on selection of the measures and subscales/facets that will comprise the factors. Not only do both dimensions have perhaps obvious implications for academic performance, but the bulk of the measures themselves were developed using mostly student samples, with validity criteria relevant to academics, emotional well-being, and interpersonal functioning of students. In that respect alone, many of the measures would have a strong warrant for use in academic contexts. One limitation, however, is the complete reliance on individual self-report responses to questionnaire items as the method by which perfectionism is assessed. Samples may produce striving or standards scores restricted in range and skewed in distribution. Many respondents rate their performance expectations using mostly the high end of scale ranges, and such response styles may be immune to attempts to expand response ranges and balance self-views (Rice & Richardson, 2014). Self-reports of personality characteristics may also be affected by emotional states (Bagby, Buis, & Nicholson, 1995), although the limited research on that point suggests that self-critical perfectionism as assessed by the APS-R was not substantially affected by state changes in depression (e.g., Sherry, Mackinnon, Macneil, & Fitzpatrick, 2013). Thus, accurately detecting different kinds of perfectionists and associations with various criterion variables may be attenuated by method limitations. One implication is that future research should be less reliant on self-report and instead incorporate alternatives such as informant reports (Connelly & Ones, 2010) or implicit measures to gauge perfectionism (De Cuyper, Pieters, Claes, Vandromme, & Hermans, 2013).

Analysis Approaches and Select Findings

Subscales and Correlational Approaches

Along with measurement limitations associated with item or scale responses, another complexity in the measurement and analysis of perfectionism concerns at least several ways the separate, combined, and interactive effects between the two major perfectionism dimensions have been examined. Often, subscale scores or perfectionism factors have been used as predictors of pertinent academic mediators or outcomes. Some generally consistent findings indicate that perfectionistic striving or standards is positively associated with academic performance, often operationalized by self-reported cumulative grade point average (GPA; Accordino, Accordino, & Slaney, 2000). Effects involving associations between perfectionistic concerns or indicators of self-critical perfectionism (i.e., Discrepancy) and GPA seem more variable than those observed with measures of perfectionistic standards and, when significant, typically are inversely associated and relatively small in effect size (Rice & Ashby, 2007; Slaney et al., 2001). Some studies have found trends toward gender and racial/ethnic differences in perfectionism–performance associations. For example, Blankstein and Winkworth (2004) found that, for women, none of the perfectionism dimensions they examined significantly predicted final semester grade in a psychology course. However, the degree to which men perceived others as having perfectionistic expectations for them (socially prescribed perfectionism) predicted lower final grades, whereas self-oriented perfectionism predicted higher final grades. Castro and Rice (2003) found that none of the perfectionism dimensions they tested were associated with GPA for White students. However, endorsing higher personal standards was significantly associated with self-reported GPA for Asian American students, but not for African Americans, and self-doubt was inversely associated with GPA for both Asian and African American students. Although there might be moderators of the associations between perfectionism and GPA, there is consistent evidence that regardless of that association, those with higher scores on self-critical perfectionism report less satisfaction with their grades (Grzegorek, Slaney, Franze, & Rice, 2004; Mobley, Slaney, & Rice, 2005; Wang, 2012).

Other studies of academic indicators other than self-reported GPA find similar effects. For example, Brown et al. (1999) intensively studied effects of personal standards (perfectionistic strivings) and concerns about making mistakes (perfectionistic concerns) on academic behaviors and outcomes for a small group of female students completing a psychology course. Both perfectionism dimensions were positively associated with the weekly number of hours studying and the likelihood of discussing grades with instructors. Perfectionistic concerns, but not strivings, were associated with perceptions of greater course difficulty and, as might be expected, more negative moods before exams. Higher scores on personal standards, but not perfectionistic concerns, were associated with better course grades.

Other studies have examined indicators such as keeping up with academic demands, evaluation of academic performance, achievement motivation, work ethic, and academic self-confidence. In general, those studies find that perfectionistic concerns are negative predictors and high performance standards are positive predictors, with similar findings in terms of direction and medium effect sizes found in middle school (Nounopoulos, Ashby, & Gilman, 2006), high school (Accordino et al., 2000), and college students (Rice, Vergara, & Aldea, 2006).

Partial Correlation Approaches

In the "partialled" approach to perfectionism analyses, the effects of one perfectionism indicator are evaluated after statistically controlling, or partialling, the effects associated with the other indicators. The idea is relatively straightforward. After effects of dimensions can be partialled from each other, what should remain is a "purer" form of each dimension, such as perfectionistic strivings not confounded by concerns or vice versa (see Hill, 2014, for a thoughtful critique of this approach).

Eum and Rice (2011) examined the association between residualized APS-R Standards and Discrepancy scores and several academic indicators for college students. Adaptive perfectionism (Standards controlling for Discrepancy) was positively associated with mastery and performance approach goal orientations, whereas maladaptive perfectionism (Discrepancy controlling for Standards) was positively associated with mastery and performance avoidance goal orientations, and also positively associated with performance approach orientations. Only maladaptive perfectionism was associated (strongly) with cognitive test anxiety. Both perfectionism dimensions were not significantly associated with GPA or a word recall performance measure.

Another interesting research example of the partialling approach suggests that at least some academic outcomes might be immune to suppression issues suggested by Hill (2014), or not as affected by suppression as are indicators of emotional well-being. Stoeber and Rambow (2007) studied ninth graders and found that none of the generally moderate and positive associations between perfectionism and academic indicators, such as hope of success, motivation, and achievement, changed when striving and negative reactions to imperfection were partialled. However, the initial negligible association between striving and depression ($r = .04$) was substantially affected when negative reactions to imperfection were controlled in the analyses ($r = -.29$). Stoeber and Rennert (2008) observed similar findings in a study of teacher stress and burnout, and in another more recent study of student emotional adjustment (Stoeber, Kobori, & Brown, 2014). In sum, a few studies suggest that partialling one form of perfectionism from another may reveal associations between standards and some constructs associated with academic outcomes, but perhaps not with more direct indicators of performance.

Dimensional Interaction Approaches

Gaudreau and Thompson (2010) described a 2 × 2 model of perfectionism in which the relative merits or costs for personal standards (strivings) and evaluative concerns would be better represented by the multiplicative interaction term than by categorical or classification approaches. Although testing the interaction between different perfectionism-related dimensions is not necessarily a new idea (e.g., Blatt, Quinlan, Pilkonis, & Shea, 1995), a few studies have followed the 2 × 2 approach to examine perfectionism effects on academic variables.

In the initial study, Gaudreau and Thompson (2010) found that the standards by concerns interaction accounted for significant variability in five of the criterion variables they measured, three of which were more directly linked to academic issues, such as concurrent academic self-determination and goal progress 4 weeks after the initial assessment. Follow-up analyses indicated that "pure" personal standards (high standards and low evaluative concerns) were associated with the highest levels of self-determination, academic satisfaction, and goal progress compared with predicted values for the other three combinations of standards and concerns. Pure evaluative concerns (low standards and high concerns) were associated with the lowest levels of academic outcomes. The "mixed" perfectionism combination of high standards and high evaluative concerns was associated with self-determination and satisfaction that were at least somewhat higher than detected with pure evaluative concerns, and lower than the other combinations, but academic goal progress effects were similar to non-perfectionism (low standards and low concerns). In contrast, Altstötter-Gleich, Gerstenberg, and Brand (2012) found that performance (concentration accuracy) was *highest* for those with elevated levels of perfectionistic concerns and low levels of striving, or what Gaudreau and Thompson referred to as pure evaluation concerns.

Classification Approaches

Cluster Analysis Rather than comparing the effects of perfectionism dimensions, other analytic approaches compare groups of perfectionists and non-perfectionists using cluster analysis (e.g., Parker, 1997; Rice & Mirzadeh, 2000) and latent class (latent profile) models (e.g., Gilman, Rice, & Carboni, 2014; Rice, Lopez, & Richardson, 2013). Some cluster analysis studies of perfectionism (e.g., Parker & Mills, 1996; Parker, 1997) have examined whether types of perfectionists and non-perfectionists could be identified with cluster analysis. Parker's contribution also was important because he studied a large group of over 800 academically-talented sixth graders; a question regarding whether striving could be unrealistically high would be particularly relevant for such a sample (Parker, 2002). He found support for three clusters of students, labeled "healthy" or "unhealthy" perfectionists, or "non-perfectionists" based on group comparisons with other measures of personality and self-esteem. He found significant but small differences between the clusters on verbal and math achievement scores, and more practically important differences on other criterion measures. For example, "healthy" perfectionists had a "moderately high level of personal standards, which is probably indicative of focused and realistic standards … scored the least neurotic, the most extroverted, the most agreeable, and the most conscientious … descriptors suggest individuals who are organized, dependable, and socially skilled… conscientious, goal and achievement oriented, predictable, well adjusted, and socially at ease" (p. 555). Compared with the other clusters, "unhealthy" perfectionists scored the highest on all perfectionism indicators and were highest on neuroticism and lowest on agreeableness. Interestingly, this group also produced the most classification errors, suggesting a less clear separation of this cluster from others, or greater within-cluster variation than might be present with other clusters.

Subsequent, similar research generally supported three- or four-cluster solutions among a wide range of samples gathered in academic settings. Rice and Mirzadeh (2000) found support for a three-cluster solution in college students. They reported that adaptive perfectionists (high levels of personal standards and lower concerns about making mistakes or self-doubt) were more likely than maladaptive perfectionists (high standards and high concerns about mistakes and self-doubt) to report substantially higher ($d = .89$) satisfaction with academic experiences and performance, even after controlling for effects attributable to depression. Gilman and Ashby (2003) reported a three-cluster solution in their study of middle school students and found that their adaptive perfectionist cluster had significantly higher average GPAs (3.52) compared with the GPAs of the maladaptive (3.12) and non-perfectionist (2.85) clusters. Dixon, Lapsley, and Hanchon (2004) studied academically gifted high school students and found support for a four-cluster typology they labeled mixed-adaptive, mixed-maladaptive, pervasive, and self-assured. Their "mixed-adaptive" cluster (e.g., with high standards and moderate concerns about making mistakes) had the highest levels of academic competence compared with the other clusters that were less differentiated on that indicator. Rice and Ashby (2007) studied over 1500 undergraduates and also found support for a three-cluster model. Adaptive perfectionists had significantly, though modestly, higher average cumulative GPAs (3.41) compared with maladaptive (3.22) and non-perfectionists (3.22) (see Rice & Slaney, 2002 for similar results).

Interestingly, in other studies using self-reported GPA, differences between all three clusters on that performance criterion have *not* been observed (Mobley et al., 2005), or adaptive and maladaptive clusters have not been significantly different on GPA but both have reported significantly higher GPAs than non-perfectionists (Grzegorek et al., 2004). Different studies using grades or test scores as the indicators of academic achievement also do not necessarily find differences between clusters. For example, Wang, Yuen, and Slaney (2009) studied over 500 Hong Kong high school students and did not find significant between-cluster differences on three self-reported grades obtained on the Hong Kong Certificate of Education Examination.

Four clusters have been found in several studies (e.g., Rice, Ashby, & Gilman, 2011; Wang, Slaney, & Rice, 2007). In general, the fourth cluster appears to represent a highly self-critical but low standards group. Although an "evaluative concerns" cluster might have value, Rice et al. (2011) argued that the cluster is probably a more differentiated group of distressed non-perfectionists than maladaptive perfectionists. For example, Sironic and Reeve (2012) found that the fourth cluster they identified was comparable to non-perfectionists and scored lower than adaptive and maladaptive perfectionists on self-regulation strategies (planning, monitoring, and regulating knowledge acquisition).

Latent Class and Mixture Modeling Approaches Latent class and mixture modeling in studies of perfectionism might be considered an *upgrade* over cluster analysis (see Hallquist & Wright, 2014). Recent work in this area blends dimensional with categorical models of perfectionism and provides methods for testing whether score patterns or distributions exist that can be reliably explained by latent classes. Moreover, although stated as "or," the choice has represented a false and limiting dichotomy between one model over the other; mixture models allow for both, and thus far at least, the available evidence supports a combination of dimensions and groups (Rice et al., 2014; Rice & Richardson, 2014; but see Broman-Fulks, Hill, & Green, 2008). Building from that descriptive complexity, more questions can also be addressed by mixture modeling approaches, such as whether those classes or groups of people with varying patterns of perfectionism scores have different outcomes on criterion indicators, whether classes are stable over time, and in the case of growth mixture modeling, whether classes can further be formed on the basis of different change trajectories. Thus, latent profile and mixture models can provide a level of sophisticated statistical sensitivity to the area of perfectionism which may produce a more nuanced perspective on the construct and its implications.

Herman and colleagues conducted latent profile analyses (Herman, Trotter, Reinke, & Ialongo, 2011) and subsequently growth mixture modeling analyses (Herman, Wang, Trotter, Reiunke, & Ialongo, 2013) on a large sample of African American sixth graders. Herman et al. (2011) found support for four latent classes. The Critical (Maladaptive) group had significantly *higher* average GPA (3.02) compared with the Non-Critical (Adaptive) (2.58) and the Non-Striving (2.53) groups, but was not significantly different from the Non-Perfectionists (2.83). There were no between-class differences on concurrent reading scores, or on reading and math tests administered when the children were in first grade. Follow-up results revealed four patterns or trajectories from 6th- through 12th-grade-associated maladaptive perfectionism scores (the striving subscale was dropped). Sixth grade reading skills were generally higher for children subsequently identified in the "Increasing" and "Low" perfectionism classes compared with the "Decreasing" and "High" classes.

Of particular value was the detection of variation in trajectories, suggesting developmental patterns of stability and change in perfectionism.

Rice et al. (2014) used factor mixture modeling based on two perfectionism factors (Standards, Discrepancy) and multiple latent class models with the factors. Using a large sample of college students, they determined that the addition of latent classes improved fit over the pure dimensional model and that the three-class model represented the most interpretable configuration. There were no differences between the perfectionist classes on self-reported GPA (adaptive $M=3.44$, maladaptive $M=3.37$), and the adaptive group had significantly higher GPA compared with the non-perfectionists ($M=3.31$).

Summary

Different avenues for conceptualization and data analysis have been applied to understanding the structure and implications of perfectionism. Although there are exceptions, in general, results suggest that adaptive dimensions and components of perfectionism (e.g., strivings or high performance standards without corresponding self-criticism) are associated with positive academic indicators such as self-reported GPA, satisfaction with academic performance, keeping up with academic demands, effective study habits, mastery goal orientations, and self-determination. Conversely, maladaptive dimensions and components of perfectionism (e.g., perfectionistic concerns or self-criticism combined with high performance expectations) often are positively associated with perceived course difficulty, negative moods before exams, and test anxiety, and inversely associated with more positive academic indicators. Some effects are present as early as middle school. High performance standards appear to provide motivation for performance, but when paired with more maladaptive components of perfectionism, it is possible that self-criticism will hinder motivation and pursuit of goals leading to eventual poor academic performance. Research on perfectionism in high demand science, technology, engineering, and math disciplines recently has examined potential mechanisms through which perfectionism positively or negatively affects academic outcomes.

Science, Technology, Engineering, and Math (STEM)

Here we summarize some of our recent research that is relevant to the "academic settings" focus of this chapter. Our interests concern the role that perfectionism may play in several aspects of adjustment, persistence, and performance, and other outcomes for students pursuing a college major in one of the STEM fields. We attend to studies that involve students and familiar academic criterion indicators such as grades and course-level performance, and also examine indicators such as science self-efficacy and academic adjustment.

In a large sample of engineering students ($N=450$; 52% women) (Rice et al., 2013), adaptive perfectionists (identified with latent profile analyses) had significantly higher levels of science self-efficacy and higher STEM GPAs compared with maladaptive and non-perfectionists. Compared with men, presumably adaptively perfectionistic women had *lower* Science Self-Efficacy scores, although adaptively perfectionistic women were comparably strong academic performers in STEM courses. In courses where women have been historically underrepresented, maladaptively perfectionistic women had an average GPA that was .51 points *less* than the GPAs of maladaptively perfectionistic men in those courses, but in courses where women and men have been comparably represented, no gender differences in grades were observed.

Building on this and other related work (e.g., Rice, Lopez, Richardson, & Stinson, 2013), we recently completed a yearlong study of academic stress among freshmen STEM majors. Our particular focus adapted the stress-generation and stress-enhancement models of perfectionism (Flett & Hewitt, 2002) to change processes relevant to STEM majors. The stress-generation model positions perfectionism as a precursor to experiences of subsequent stress (i.e., perfectionists are likely to create their own stress, possibly by reacting more strongly than others might to challenging experiences). The stress-enhancement model positions perfectionism as a moderator of stress effects on some relevant outcome (i.e., perfectionism intensifies stress effects). To evaluate these models, we gathered self-reported academic stress at three time points during each of the first two semesters (fall and spring) for the freshmen. We also analyzed specific course grade data and other academic information from institutional records.

The combination of Time 1 perfectionism and end-of-year (Time 6) reports of academic and personal problems produced a reliable latent class structure of three student groups (see Fig. 11.1): adaptive perfectionists with high standards and the lowest levels of problems, maladaptive perfectionists with elevations across all perfectionism and problem subscales, and non-perfectionists with the lowest standards levels and perfectionist concerns and adjustment problems generally midway between adaptive and maladaptive perfectionists. Rather than stress-generation, a stress-maintenance model might more aptly describe the stress patterns for the three classes (see Fig. 11.2). The adaptive perfectionists had significantly low and relatively stable academic stress over the year, whereas maladaptive and non-perfectionists had higher, but also stable, levels of stress. In general, female STEM students reported more stress than men, and more academic problems. Women were also more likely to be in the maladaptive perfectionist class than in the other groups.

Our focus for testing the stress-enhancement model was on academic performance operationalized as grades in STEM courses. We calculated a represented GPA (RGPA) based on courses in areas where women and men have been more evenly represented (life sciences, social sciences) and an underrepresented GPA (UGPA) based on courses where women have traditionally been underrepresented (e.g., engineering, computing sciences). We also covaried high school GPA and SAT-Math scores in the analyses. Adaptive perfectionists had significantly higher

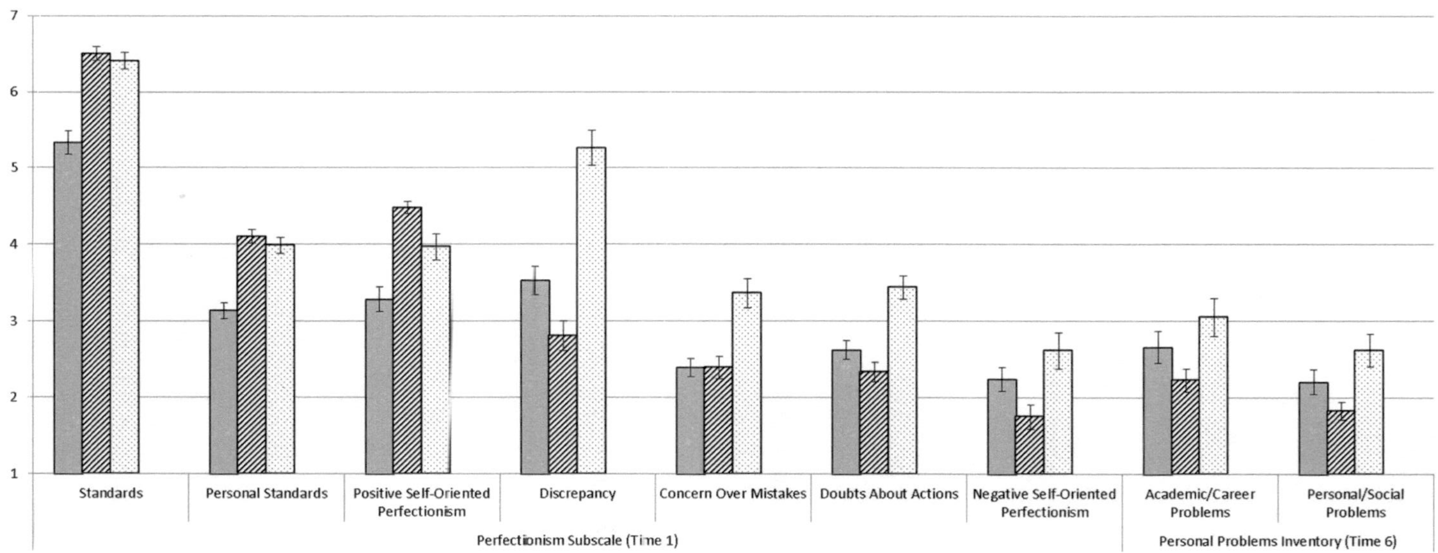

Fig. 11.1 Average (unstandardized) scores on the perfectionism and freely estimated distal outcomes (problem subscales) for the three latent classes. The scale ranges were different for measures: Standards and Discrepancy (1–7); Personal Standards, Concern over Mistakes, Doubts About Actions, Positive and Negative Self-Oriented Perfectionism (1–5); and Academic/Career and Personal/Social Problems (1–6). *Shaded bars* represent non-perfectionists, *bars with diagonal pattern* represent adaptive perfectionists, and *bars with dotted pattern* represent maladaptive perfectionists. *Error bars* represent 95 % confidence intervals

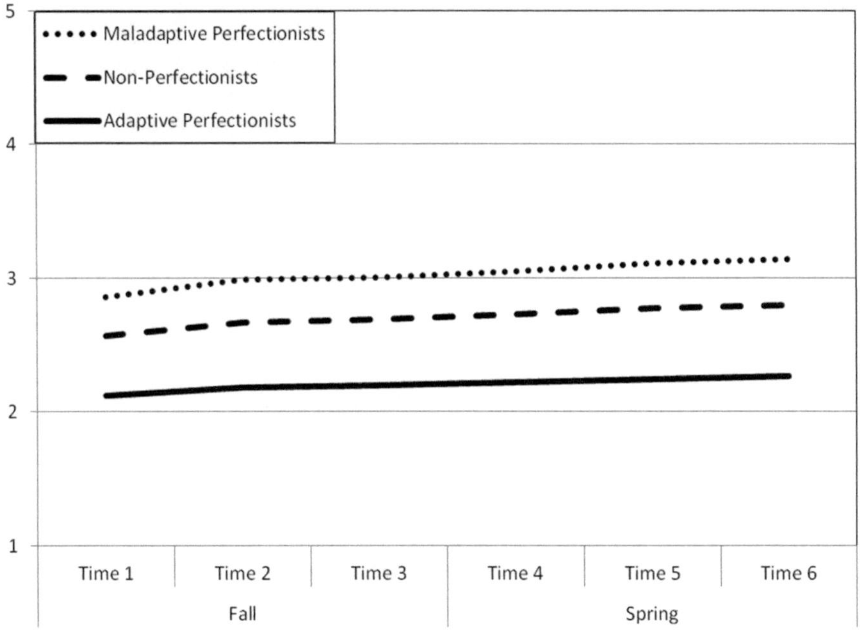

Fig. 11.2 Plot of the change in academic stress for the three latent classes

GPAs on both indicators compared with maladaptive and non-perfectionists; differences approximated small to medium effect sizes. Female adaptive perfectionists had UGPAs that were about .20 grade points lower than their male counterparts, but no other gender x perfectionism differences emerged for UGPA or RGPA. Overall, the higher academic performance of adaptive perfectionists and comparable but lower performance of the maladaptive and non-perfectionists were more consistent with stress-dampening effects of adaptive perfectionism rather than stress-enhancing effects of maladaptive perfectionism.

Perhaps the lower levels of perceived academic stress over the year reported by the adaptive perfectionists reflected better stress-reactivity abilities, possibly through better problem-solving, deployment of academic skills to manage the demands, and motivating rather than impairing personal standards and expectations. Our focus was on academic performance as the primary outcome, but it was clear from the maladaptive profile (standards combined with extremely high perfectionistic concerns, more academic problems, and higher stress) that this group may not seem much different from non-perfectionists in terms of grades but likely is having considerable difficulty managing other aspects of emotional and social adjustment during this important first year of STEM study. Consequently, we are pursuing two threads of additional research on STEM students, one that involves testing interventions aimed at enhancing their stress-regulation skills and another evaluating longer term, beyond first-year consequences of earlier assessed perfectionism and stress.

Intervention Implications

Given our assumptions about what is maladaptive about perfectionism, we can identify potential targets for interventions in an academic setting. Those involving a reduction in self-criticism and enhancement of capacities to regulate emotions and cognitions in response to stress, failure, and disappointment may be more beneficial than those aimed at lowering standards (Rice et al., 2011), perhaps especially for women pursuing academic paths in which they are numerically and historically underrepresented. So-called adaptive perfectionists already seem to possess good emotion regulatory capacities when confronted with stress (Richardson, Rice, & Devine, 2014), and maladaptive perfectionists do not (Aldea & Rice, 2006). Also, given that maladaptive perfectionists are more likely to engage in avoidance coping rather than active or problem-solving coping (Dunkley et al., 2000), it may be important to consider providing educational sessions on active and problem-solving coping, which may decrease academic and personal/social problems. We further believe that high standards can serve personal and social good. Interventions might well serve individuals and society if they work to maintain or increase standards rather than reduce them, provided those interventions are accompanied by components that keep self-criticism low or in check, and emotion regulation appropriately up- or downregulated given situational demands. Perhaps it is also important to consider providing adequate support, encouragement, and opportunities for social engagement within the academic context, which may serve as a buffer for stress that can decrease distress and academic problems among maladaptive perfectionists (Dunkley et al., 2000). This may be of particular importance in fields in which women are typically underrepresented. Further, interventions aimed at reducing stereotype threat effects, such as a self-affirming writing assignments (Bowen, Wegmann, & Webber, 2013), may also serve to buffer the negative effects of perfectionism and gender.

Recommendations for Future Research

Anachronistic views of perfectionism have given way to multidimensional, categorical, and multivalenced understandings of the construct. Numerous studies generally converge on some forms or types of perfectionism as being healthy or adaptive, and distinct from other forms or types of perfectionism that seem unhealthy or maladaptive. As clearly shown in our recent work on STEM students and in other research (e.g., Chang, 1998), contexts and outcomes must be considered in any understanding of perfectionism. Our central arguments in this chapter have been that (1) these dimensions and types should be differentiated using the best available contemporary modeling techniques, (2) methods for doing so are likely to yield different groupings and ultimately conclusions based on measurement and conceptualization allegiances, and (3) perfectionism has important implications for predicting academic-relevant outcomes.

"That's Nice Dear but You're Starting Too Late!"

During a measurement development project (Rice & Preusser, 2002), we held meetings with school officials and teachers to describe the goal of creating a scale useful in detecting perfectionism in 9- to 10-year-old children. A teacher in attendance shared that, although she supported the effort, she thought a scale for 9- to 10-year-olds might be late if what we wanted to do was detect perfectionism and possibly intervene in some way. She remarked that teachers (and parents) see signs of perfectionism at earlier ages among children who, for example, have exaggerated reactions when they make a mistake or seem overly sensitive to any kind of correction or feedback. Those comments were prescient and as relevant today as they were then.

Among other implications, the teacher's comments speak to measurement diversity, contextual and developmental considerations, and globalization of perfectionism. A central measurement concern involves a good indicator of high performance expectations or standards (striving) and a second measure tapping self-criticism of performance. There is a strong tendency in the USA to endorse high levels of standards (Rice & Richardson, 2014). We are not yet advocating the abandonment of self-reports, but would encourage measurement advances that provide more range and variability in self-expectations tethered to performance scenarios.

Other approaches could include ratings of a target subject made by someone familiar with the subject, particularly if that familiarity has occurred within a sustained performance context. Although there have been some attempts to integrate romantic partners in dyadic, multilevel approaches to understanding perfectionism and its implications (e.g., Stoeber, 2012b), reports from parents, teachers, coaches, and managers, or from siblings, fellow students, teammates, roommates, and others seem conspicuously absent from the research. Less self-report and more behavioral observation or behavioral anchoring or other-reports may be especially helpful in perfectionism research involving children or others less familiar with self-report questionnaires. As Lievens (2014) recently pointed out, personality measurement could be improved with assessment strategies used in occupational settings (e.g., framing items as linked to specific contexts). These are not new ideas in the more general areas of personality assessment but have only minimally been examined in studies of perfectionism. The use of other-reports and other less straightforward measures certainly complicates study design, analysis, and interpretation, therefore, future work should carefully evaluate improvements in measurement precision, sensitivity, and specificity, along with incremental validity to determine whether the costs of more complicated approaches are worth the effort, in light of their scientific benefits.

Finally, it should be noted that our examination of perfectionism in academic settings was limited for the most part to Western samples and variables such as grades and academic adjustment. We also avoided extensive coverage of emotion regulation tendencies, physiological stress reactivity, and interpersonal issues that also would be relevant to understanding perfectionism in academic settings. However, such a decision separates potentially inseparable aspects of students, teachers, and others in academic settings. For instance, many students experience mild to substantial psychological impediments to their learning. A comprehensive understanding of academic outcomes may emerge through the dual effects of perfectionistic concerns on more traditional psychological indicators (e.g., depression, anxiety) and perfectionistic striving on more traditional performance outcomes (e.g., grades, study habits). Our most recent thinking is that emotion up- and downregulation approaches may be a primary mechanism linking expressions (and types) of perfectionism to both sets of outcomes. Complex interdisciplinary and multimethod blending of these ideas has already begun and is likely to be an important part of the future of perfectionism research.

References

Accordino, D. B., Accordino, M. P., & Slaney, R. B. (2000). An investigation of perfectionism, mental health, achievement, and achievement motivation in adolescents. *Psychology in The Schools, 37*(6), 535–545. doi:10.1002/1520-6807(200011)37:6<535::AID-xcPITS6>3.0.CO;2-O

Aldea, M. A., & Rice, K. G. (2006). The role of emotional dysregulation in perfectionism and psychological distress. *Journal of Counseling Psychology, 53*(4), 498–510. doi:10.1037/0022-0167.53.4.498.

Altstötter-Gleich, C., Gerstenberg, F. R., & Brand, M. (2012). Performing well-Feeling bad? Effects of perfectionism under experimentally induced stress on tension and performance. *Journal of Research in Personality, 46*(5), 619–622. doi:10.1016/j.jrp.2012.05.010.

Bagby, R., Buis, T., & Nicholson, R. A. (1995). Relative effectiveness of the standard validity scales in detecting fake-bad and fake-good responding: Replication and extension. *Psychological Assessment, 7*(1), 84–92. doi:10.1037/1040-3590.7.1.84.

Blankstein, K. R., & Winkworth, G. R. (2004). Dimensions of perfectionism and levels of attributions for grades: Relations with dysphoria and academic performance. *Journal of Rational-Emotive and Cognitive-Behavior Therapy, 22*(4), 271–299. doi:10.1023/B:JORE.0000047312.20212.30.

Blatt, S. J. (1995). The destructiveness of perfectionism: Implications for the treatment of depression. *American Psychologist,* 50(12), 1003–1020. doi:10.1037/0003-066X.50.12.1003.

Blatt, S. J., Quinlan, D. M., Pilkonis, P. A., & Shea, M. (1995). Impact of perfectionism and need for approval on the brief treatment of depression: The National Institute of Mental Health Treatment of Depression Collaborative Research Program revisited. *Journal of Consulting and Clinical Psychology, 63*(1), 125–132. doi:10.1037/0022-006X.63.1.125.

Bong, M., Hwang, A., Noh, A., & Kim, S. (2014). Perfectionism and motivation of adolescents in academic contexts. *Journal of Educational Psychology*. doi:10.1037/a0035836.

Bowen, N. K., Wegmann, K. M., & Webber, K. C. (2013). Enhancing a brief writing intervention to combat stereotype threat among middle-school students. *Journal of Educational Psychology, 105,* 427–435. doi: 10.1037/a0031177.

Broman-Fulks, J. J., Hill, R. W., & Green, B. A. (2008). Is perfectionism categorical or dimensional? A taxometric analysis. *Journal of Personality Assessment, 90*(5), 481–490.

Brown, E. J., Heimberg, R. G., Frost, R. O., Makris, G. S., Juster, H. R., & Leung, A. W. (1999). Relationship of perfectionism to affect, expectations, attributions and performance in the classroom. *Journal of Social and Clinical Psychology, 18*(1), 98–120. doi:10.1521/jscp.1999.18.1.98.

Castro, J. R., & Rice, K. G. (2003). Perfectionism and ethnicity: Implications for depressive symptoms and academic achievement. *Cultural Diversity and Ethnic Minority Psychology, 9,* 64–78. doi:10.1037/1099-9809.9.1.64.

Chang, E. C. (1998). Cultural differences, perfectionism, and suicidal risk in a college population: Does social problem solving still matter? *Cognitive Therapy and Research, 22,* 237–254.

Connelly, B. S., & Ones, D. S. (2010). Another perspective on personality: Meta-analytic integration of observers' accuracy and predictive validity. *Psychological Bulletin, 136*(6), 1092–1122. doi:10.1037/a0021212.

De Cuyper, K., Pieters, G., Claes, L., Vandromme, H., & Hermans, D. (2013). Indirect measurement of perfectionism: Construct and predictive validity. *Journal of Social and Clinical Psychology, 32,* 844–858. doi:10.1521/jscp.2013.32.8.844.

Dickie, L., Surgenor, L. J., Wilson, M., & McDowall, J. (2012). The structure and reliability of the Clinical Perfectionism Questionnaire. *Personality and Individual Differences, 52*(8), 865–869. doi:10.1016/j.paid.2012.02.003.

Dixon, F. A., Lapsley, D. K., & Hanchon, T. A. (2004). An empirical typology of perfectionism in gifted adolescents. *Gifted Child Quarterly, 48,* 95–106.

Dunkley, D. M., Blankstein, K. R., Halsall, J., Williams, M., & Winkworth, G. (2000). The relation between perfectionism and distress: Hassles, coping, and perceived social support as mediators and moderators. *Journal of Counseling Psychology, 47,* 437–453. doi:10.1037/AW22-0167.47.4.437.

Egan, S. J., Dick, M., & Allen, P. J. (2012). An experimental investigation of standard setting in clinical perfectionism. *Behaviour Change, 29,* 183–195. doi:10.1017/bec.2012.16.

Egan, S. J., Piek, J. P., Dyck, M. J., Rees, C. S., & Hagger, M. S. (2013). A clinical investigation of motivation to change standards and cognitions about failure in perfectionism. *Behavioural and Cognitive Psychotherapy, 41,* 565–578.

Eum, K., & Rice, K. G. (2011). Test anxiety, perfectionism, goal orientation, and academic performance. *Anxiety, Stress and Coping: An International Journal, 24*(2), 167–178. doi:10.1080/10615806.2010.488723.

Fairburn, C. G., Cooper, Z., & Shafran, R. (2003). Cognitive behaviour therapy for eating disorders: A 'transdiagnostic' theory and treatment. *Behaviour Research and Therapy, 41*(5), 509–528. doi:10.1016/S0005-7967(02)00088-8.

Flett, G. L., & Hewitt, P. L. (2002). Perfectionism and maladjustment: An overview of theoretical, definitional, and treatment issues. In G. L. Flett & P. L. Hewitt (Eds.), *Perfectionism: Theory, research, and treatment* (pp. 5–31). Washington, DC: American Psychological Association. doi:10.1037/10458-001.

Gaudreau, P., & Thompson, A. (2010). Testing a 2 × 2 model of dispositional perfectionism. *Personality and Individual Differences, 48*(5), 532–537. doi:10.1016/j.paid.2009.11.031.

Gilman, R., & Ashby, J. S. (2003). A first study of perfectionism and multidimensional life satisfaction among adolescents. *Journal of Early Adolescence, 23*(2), 218–235. doi:10.1177/0272431603023002005.

Gilman, R., Rice, K. G., & Carboni, I. (2014). Perfectionism, perspective taking, and social connection in adolescents. *Psychology in the Schools, 51*(9), 947–959. doi:10.1002/pits.21793.

Grzegorek, J. L., Slaney, R. B., Franze, S., & Rice, K. G. (2004). Self-criticism, dependency, self-esteem, and grade point average satisfaction among clusters of perfectionists and non-perfectionists. *Journal of Counseling Psychology, 51,* 192–200. doi:10.1037/0022-0167.51.2.192.

Hallquist, M. N., & Wright, A. C. (2014). Mixture modeling methods for the assessment of normal and abnormal personality, part I: Cross-sectional models. *Journal of Personality Assessment, 96*(3), 256–268. doi:10.1080/00223891.2013.845201.

Herman, K. C., Trotter, R., Reinke, W. M., & Ialongo, N. (2011). Developmental origins of perfectionism among African American youth. *Journal of Counseling Psychology, 58,* 321–334. doi:10.1037/a0023108.

Herman, K. C., Wang, K., Trotter, R., Reinke, W. M., & Ialongo, N. (2013). Developmental trajectories of maladaptive perfectionism among African American adolescents. *Child Development, 84,* 1633–1650. doi:10.1111/cdev.12078.

Hill, A. P. (2014). Perfectionistic strivings and the perils of partialling. *International Journal of Sport and Exercise Psychology, 12,* 302–315.

Lievens, F. (2014, July). *Contextualizing personality assessment: Why (not)*? Paper presented at the 17th European Conference on Personality, Lausanne, Switzerland.

Lo, A., & Abbott, M. (2013). The impact of manipulating expected standards of performance for adaptive, maladaptive, and non-perfectionists. *Cognitive Therapy and Research, 37,* 762–778. doi:10.1007/s10608-013-9528-1.

Mobley, M., Slaney, R. S., & Rice, K. G. (2005). Cultural validity of the Almost Perfect Scale-Revised for African-American college students. *Journal of Counseling Psychology, 52,* 629–639. doi:10.1037/0022-0167.52.4.629.

Nounopoulos, A., Ashby, J. S., & Gilman, R. (2006). Coping resources, perfectionism, and academic performance among adolescents. *Psychology in the Schools, 43*(5), 613–622. doi:10.1002/pits.20167.

Pacht, A. R. (1984). Reflections on perfection. *American Psychologist, 39*(4), 386–390. doi:10.1037/0003-066X.39.4.386.

Parker, W. D. (1997). An empirical typology of perfectionism in academically talented children. *American Educational Research Journal, 34*, 545–562. doi:10.2307/1163249.

Parker, W. D. (2002). Perfectionism and adjustment in gifted children. In G. L. Flett & P. L. Hewitt (Eds.), *Perfectionism: Theory, research, and treatment* (pp. 133–148). Washington, DC: American Psychological Association. doi:10.1037/10458-005.

Parker, W. D., & Mills, C. J. (1996). The incidence of perfectionism in gifted students. *Gifted Child Quarterly, 40*(4), 194–199. doi:10.1177/001698629604000404.

Rice, K. G., & Ashby, J. S. (2007). An efficient method for classifying perfectionists. *Journal of Counseling Psychology, 54,* 72–85. doi:10.1037/0022-0167.54.1.72.

Rice, K. G., & Mirzadeh, S. A. (2000). Perfectionism, attachment, and adjustment. *Journal of Counseling Psychology, 47,* 238–250. doi: 10.1037/0022-0167.47.2.238.

Rice, K. G., & Preusser, K. J. (2002). The Adaptive/Maladaptive Perfectionism Scale. *Measurement and Evaluation in Counseling and Development, 34,* 210–222.

Rice, K. G., & Slaney, R. B. (2002). Clusters of perfectionists: Two studies of emotional adjustment and academic achievement. *Measurement and Evaluation in Counseling and Development, 35*(1), 35–48.

Rice, K. G., & Richardson, C. M. E. (2014). Classification challenges in perfectionism. *Journal of Counseling Psychology, 61,* 641–648.

Rice, K. G., Vergara, D. T., & Aldea, M. A. (2006). Cognitive-affective mediators of perfectionism and college student adjustment. *Personality and Individual Differences, 40*(3), 463–473. doi:10.1016/j.paid.2005.05.011.

Rice, K. G., Ashby, J. S., & Gilman, R. (2011). Classifying adolescent perfectionists. *Psychological Assessment, 23,* 563–577. doi:10.1037/a0022482.

Rice, K. G., Lopez, F. G., & Richardson, C. E. (2013). Perfectionism and performance among STEM students. *Journal of Vocational Behavior, 82,* 124–134. doi:10.1016/j.jvb.2012.12.002.

Rice, K. G., Lopez, F. G., Richardson, C. E., & Stinson, J. M. (2013). Perfectionism moderates stereotype threat effects on STEM majors' academic performance. *Journal of Counseling Psychology, 60*(2), 287–293. doi:10.1037/a0032052.

Rice, K. G., Richardson, C. M. E., & Tueller, S. (2014). The short form of the revised almost perfect scale. *Journal of Personality Assessment, 96,* 368–379. doi: 10.1080/00223891.2013.838172.

Richardson, C. E., Rice, K. G., & Devine, D. P. (2014). Perfectionism, emotion regulation, and the cortisol stress response. *Journal of Counseling Psychology, 61,* 110–118. doi:10.1037/a0034446.

Shafran, R. R., Cooper, Z. Z., & Fairburn, C. G. (2002). Clinical perfectionism: A cognitive-behavioural analysis. *Behaviour Research and Therapy, 40*(7), 773–791. doi:10.1016/S0005-7967(01)00059-6.

Sherry, S. B., Mackinnon, S. P., Macneil, M. A., & Fitzpatrick, S. (2013). Discrepancies confer vulnerability to depressive symptoms: A three-wave longitudinal study. *Journal of Counseling Psychology, 60,* 112–126. doi:10.1037/a0030439.

Sironic, A., & Reeve, R. A. (2012). More evidence for four perfectionism subgroups. *Personality and Individual Differences, 53*(4), 437–442. doi:10.1016/j.paid.2012.04.003.

Slaney, R. B., Mobley, M., Trippi, J., Ashby, J., & Johnson, D. G. (1996). *The Almost Perfect Scale-Revised.* Unpublished manuscript, The Pennsylvania State University, University Park, PA.

Slaney, R. B., Rice, K. G., Mobley, M., Trippi, J., & Ashby, J. S. (2001). The revised Almost Perfect Scale. *Measurement and Evaluation in Counseling and Development, 34,* 130–145.

Stoeber, J. (2012a). Perfectionism and performance. In S. M. Murphy (Ed.), *The Oxford handbook of sport and performance psychology* (pp. 294–306). New York: Oxford University Press. doi:10.1093/oxfordhb/9780199731763.013.0015.

Stoeber, J. (2012b). Dyadic perfectionism in romantic relationships: Predicting relationship satisfaction and longterm commitment. *Personality and Individual Differences, 53*(3), 300–305. doi:10.1016/j.paid.2012.04.002.

Stoeber, J., & Damian, L. E. (2014). The clinical perfectionism questionnaire: Further evidence for two factors capturing perfectionistic strivings and concerns. *Personality and Individual Differences, 61-62,* 38–42. doi:10.1016/j.paid.2014.01.003.

Stoeber, J., & Hotham, S. (2013). Perfectionism and social desirability: Students report increased perfectionism to create a positive impression. *Personality and Individual Differences, 55,* 626–629. doi:10.1016/j.paid.2013.04.023.

Stoeber, J., & Otto, K. (2006). Positive conceptions of perfectionism: Approaches, evidence, and challenges. *Personality and Social Psychology Review, 10,* 295–319. doi:10.1207/s15327957pspr1004_2.

Stoeber, J., & Rambow, A. (2007). Perfectionism in adolescent school students: Relations with motivation, achievement, and well-being. *Personality and Individual Differences, 42*(7), 1379–1389. doi:10.1016/j.paid.2006.10.015.

Stoeber, J., & Rennert, D. (2008). Perfectionism in school teachers: Relations with stress appraisals, coping styles, and burnout. *Anxiety, Stress and Coping: An International Journal, 21*(1), 37–53. doi:10.1080/10615800701742461.

Stoeber, J., Kobori, O., & Brown, A. (2014). Examining mutual suppression effects in the assessment of perfectionism cognitions: Evidence supporting multidimensional assessment. *Assessment, 21,* 647–660.

Wang, K. T. (2012). Personal and family perfectionism of Taiwanese college students: Relationships with depression, self-esteem, achievement motivation, and academic grades. *International Journal of Psychology, 47*(4), 305–314. doi:10.1080/00207594.2011.626050.

Wang, K. T., Slaney, R. B., & Rice, K. G. (2007). Perfectionism in Chinese university students from Taiwan: A study of psychological well-being and achievement motivation. *Personality and Individual Differences, 42,* 1279–1290.

Wang, K. T., Yuen, M., & Slaney, R. B. (2009). Perfectionism, depression, loneliness, and life satisfaction: A study of high school students in Hong Kong. *The Counseling Psychologist, 37*(2), 249–274. doi:10.1177/0011000008315975.

Chapter 12
Perfectionism in Employees: Work Engagement, Workaholism, and Burnout

Joachim Stoeber and Lavinia E. Damian

Perfectionism in Employees

Perfectionism is a personality disposition characterized by striving for flawlessness and setting exceedingly high standards for performance accompanied by tendencies for overly critical evaluations (Frost, Marten, Lahart, & Rosenblate, 1990; Hewitt & Flett, 1991). Perfectionism is a prevalent disposition. Most people have at least one domain in life in which they are perfectionistic (Stoeber & Stoeber, 2009). Furthermore, the domain of life most affected by perfectionism is work, be it academic work (school, university) or professional work (Slaney & Ashby, 1996; Stoeber & Stoeber, 2009). There are many ways in which perfectionism can affect work. For example, perfectionists' exceedingly high standards of performance—seldom, if ever, is anything good enough—have been associated with reduced productivity and lower efficiency (Sherry, Hewitt, Sherry, Flett, & Graham, 2010; Stoeber & Eysenck, 2008). In addition, perfectionists tend to have a lower tolerance of ambiguity which may lead to reduced work satisfaction (Fairlie & Flett, 2003; Wittenberg & Norcross, 2001). Furthermore, perfectionists worry and ruminate more about work than non-perfectionists making it difficult for perfectionists to switch off and relax after work, and this may negatively affect their work–life balance, health, and well-being (Flaxman, Ménard, Bond, & Kinman, 2012; Mitchelson, 2009). Consequently, individual differences in perfectionism play an important role when regarding health and well-being in employees.

Despite perfectionism being most prevalent in the work domain, perfectionism research so far has mainly focused on students, athletes, and clinical samples paying relatively little attention to employees. The present chapter aims to redress this

J. Stoeber (✉)
School of Psychology, University of Kent, Canterbury, Kent CT2 7NP, UK
e-mail: J.Stoeber@kent.ac.uk

L. E. Damian
Department of Psychology, Babeş-Bolyai University, Cluj-Napoca, Romania

F. M. Sirois, D. S. Molnar (eds.), *Perfectionism, Health, and Well-Being*,
DOI 10.1007/978-3-319-18582-8_12

imbalance by focusing on perfectionism in employees (including students working part-time) and how perfectionism relates to three key variables in peoples' working life—work engagement, workaholism, and burnout—that have shown close associations with employee health and well-being.

Perfectionistic Strivings and Perfectionistic Concerns

Before looking at perfectionism's relationships with work engagement, workaholism, and burnout, however, we need to have a closer look at perfectionism itself to better understand the findings of the literature. The reason is that perfectionism is not a unitary characteristic. Instead, perfectionism has different facets and is therefore best conceptualized as a multidimensional personality disposition (see Enns & Cox, 2002, for a review).

To capture the multidimensional nature of perfectionism, researchers have developed a number of scales measuring the different facets of perfectionism. This diversity is welcome from a research perspective and has produced many important insights into the differential relationships of multidimensional perfectionism. However, the multiplicity of perfectionism scales poses a challenge for readers unfamiliar with the literature who may find it difficult to achieve a good understanding of the findings from different studies using different scales. Fortunately, there is converging evidence that the various aspects of multidimensional perfectionism form two superordinate factors (Frost, Heimberg, Holt, Mattia, & Neubauer, 1993; see also Bieling, Israeli, & Antony, 2004). The first factor has been termed *perfectionistic strivings* (or personal standards perfectionism) and captures those aspects of perfectionism associated with striving for perfection and setting exceedingly high standards of performance. The second factor has been termed *perfectionistic concerns* (or evaluative concerns perfectionism) and captures those aspects of perfectionism associated with concerns over making mistakes, fear of negative evaluation by others, feelings of discrepancy between one's expectations and performance, and negative reactions to imperfection (see Stoeber & Otto, 2006, for a comprehensive review). Table 12.1 gives an overview of multidimensional perfectionism scales and which of their subscales' scores represent indicators of the two factors.

The differentiation between the two factors is of central importance to the understanding of perfectionism. Whereas the two factors typically show large-sized positive correlations[1]—most people who show elevated levels of perfectionistic strivings also show elevated levels of perfectionistic concerns—they show different, sometimes opposite, patterns of associations. Perfectionistic concerns are typically associated with negative characteristics, processes, and outcomes (e.g., neuroticism, avoidant coping, negative affect), indicating that perfectionistic concerns capture maladaptive aspects of perfectionism. In contrast, perfectionistic strivings are often associated with positive characteristics, processes, and outcomes (e.g.,

[1] Following Cohen (1992), correlations with absolute values of 0.10, 0.30, and 0.50 are considered small-, medium-, and large-sized.

Table 12.1 Indicators of perfectionistic strivings and perfectionistic concerns: examples

Scale	Perfectionistic strivings	Perfectionistic concerns
FMPS	Personal standards	Concern over mistakes
	Pure personal standards[a]	Concern over mistakes + doubts about actions[b]
HF-MPS	Self-oriented perfectionism[c]	Socially prescribed perfectionism
APS-R	High standards	Discrepancy
PI	Striving for excellence	Concern over mistakes
MIPS	Striving for perfection	Negative reactions to imperfection

Scales are listed in chronological order of their first publication.

FMPS Frost Multidimensional Perfectionism Scale (Frost et al., 1990); *HF-MPS* Hewitt–Flett Multidimensional Perfectionism Scale (Hewitt & Flett, 1991); *APS-R* revised Almost Perfect Scale (Slaney, Rice, Mobley, Trippi, & Ashby, 2001); *PI* Perfectionism Inventory (R. W. Hill et al., 2004); *MIPS* Multidimensional Inventory of Perfectionism in Sport (Stoeber, Otto, Pescheck, Becker, & Stoll, 2007; for adaptations outside sport, see, e.g., Stoeber & Rennert, 2008)

[a] See DiBartolo, Frost, Chang, LaSoto, and Grills (2004)

[b] See Stöber (1998)

[c] Particularly the subscale capturing perfectionistic striving (see Stoeber & Childs, 2010)

conscientiousness, problem-focused coping, positive affect), indicating that perfectionistic strivings capture aspects of perfectionism that may have an adaptive component (Stoeber & Otto, 2006).

However, there are two important things to note. First, because the two factors show considerable overlap, the positive associations of perfectionistic strivings are often suppressed by the negative associations of perfectionistic concerns.[2] Consequently, perfectionistic strivings' positive associations may only become apparent when the overlapping variance between strivings and concerns is taken into account and partial correlations or multiple regressions are calculated (R. W. Hill, Huelsman, & Araujo, 2010; Stoeber & Otto, 2006; see also Gaudreau, 2012). Second, the negative associations of perfectionistic concerns are usually stronger than the positive associations of perfectionistic strivings. Consequently, in studies computing an "overall perfectionism" score (i.e., lumping strivings and concerns together), perfectionism usually shows negative associations indicative of perfectionistic concerns. Furthermore, whereas perfectionistic concerns often suppress the positive associations of perfectionistic strivings, perfectionistic strivings rarely suppress the negative associations of perfectionistic concerns (or only to a much smaller degree; R. W. Hill et al., 2010). Hence, it is relatively safe to examine perfectionistic concerns without statistically controlling for perfectionistic strivings. In contrast, examining perfectionistic strivings without statistically controlling for perfectionistic concerns may lead to erroneous conclusions about perfectionistic strivings' maladaptiveness—which will become clear further below where we review the findings on perfectionism in employees and burnout.

[2] For an in-depth discussion of these suppression effects and how to interpret them, the interested reader is referred to Stoeber, Kobori, and Brown (in press).

Work Engagement, Workaholism, and Burnout

Work engagement, workaholism, and burnout are key variables in occupational and organizational psychology research on employee health and well-being. The reason is that all three have shown to predict indicators of employee well-being such as positive affect, life satisfaction, work satisfaction, and—as an inverse indicator—negative affect (cf. Diener, Suh, Lucas, & Smith, 1999). Moreover, they have been shown to be closely related to people's work–life balance which is a construct that is receiving growing interest in the literature because it predicts individual health and well-being (Matuska, 2010). In this, work engagement has been associated with better employee well-being (positive relationships with positive affect and satisfaction, negative relationships with negative affect), whereas workaholism and burnout have been associated with poorer employee well-being (negative relationships with positive affect and satisfaction, positive relationships with negative affect) (e.g., Schaufeli, Taris, & van Rhenen, 2008). In addition, workaholism and burnout have been associated with poorer physical health (e.g., Clark, Michel, Zhdanova, Pui, & Baltes, in press; Shirom & Melamed, 2005; Wojdylo, Baumann, Buczny, Owens, & Kuhl, 2013).

Perfectionism is a personality disposition predicting individual differences in work engagement, workaholism, and burnout. Hence, it is important to gain a better understanding of how perfectionism is related to work engagement, workaholism, and burnout and examine whether the two superordinate factors of perfectionism—perfectionistic strivings and perfectionistic concerns—show differential relationships with each of these important work-related outcomes.

Perfectionism and Work Engagement

Work engagement is a state of mind in which employees consider their work to be personally meaningful, feel positive toward their work, and are involved in, committed to, and enthusiastic and passionate about their work (see Attridge, 2009, for a review). Over the past 10 years, work engagement has become a key concept in organizational and occupational psychology and human resource management (where it is often referred to as "employee engagement"). The reason is that work engagement has shown positive relationships not only with employee well-being, but also with a whole range of other desirable outcomes at work such as work motivation and job performance (e.g., Bakker & Bal, 2010; Christian, Garza, & Slaughter, 2011; van Beek, Taris, & Schaufeli, 2011). Consequently, employees who are engaged are an important human resource for employers (van Beek et al., 2011). Therefore, it comes as no surprise that research on work engagement is flourishing and that work engagement is receiving increased attention also from practitioners, employers, and policy makers.

To measure work engagement, the great majority of studies has used a conceptualization of work engagement differentiating three aspects: vigor, dedication, and absorption (e.g., Schaufeli, Salanova, González-Romá, & Bakker, 2002). Vigor captures the effort that employees invest in their work and the energy they experience when working. Dedication captures the meaning and involvement in work and the purpose that employees experience when working. Absorption captures the extent to which employees are fully concentrated and engrossed in their work, sometimes to the extent that they have difficulties detaching themselves from their work. Vigor and dedication constitute the core aspects of work engagement representing positive energy and involvement in work, whereas absorption is a more ambivalent aspect (cf. Schaufeli & Salanova, 2011).

Are perfectionists more engaged in their job than non-perfectionists? Despite the surge of interest in work engagement over the past decade, there is a dearth of studies on perfectionism and work engagement. To our knowledge, only four studies so far have examined the relationships of perfectionism in employees with work engagement. All studies found perfectionistic strivings to be associated with higher levels of work engagement, whereas perfectionistic concerns were not consistently associated with lower work engagement. The first study (Childs & Stoeber, 2010) examined a sample of employees from various sectors (e.g., public sector, law firms, retail). Taking a differentiated look at the perfectionism–engagement relationship, the study investigated perfectionistic strivings and perfectionistic concerns and looked at the three aspects of work engagement individually. When bivariate correlations were examined, perfectionistic strivings showed positive correlations with all aspects of work engagement: vigor, dedication, and absorption. In contrast, perfectionistic concerns showed a negative correlation with vigor but nonsignificant correlations with dedication and absorption. However, when the overlap with perfectionistic strivings was controlled for in multiple regressions, perfectionistic concerns also showed a negative relationship with dedication.

The remaining three studies did not investigate the different aspects of work engagement, but only examined overall work engagement (combining vigor, dedication, and absorption). The second study (Tziner & Tanami, 2013) examined a sample of employees working in the public sector. As in the first study, only perfectionistic strivings showed a positive correlation with work engagement. In contrast, perfectionistic concerns showed no significant negative correlation. The third study (Wojdylo et al., 2013) examined a sample of employees from different occupations (e.g., office workers, teachers). Unfortunately, the study regarded only perfectionistic concerns, not perfectionistic strivings. When correlations were examined, perfectionistic concerns showed no significant negative correlation with work engagement. The fourth and final study (Ozbilir, Day, & Catano, in press) examined a sample of Canadian and Turkish employees from different sectors (e.g., education, health care, administration). When the data were collapsed across nationalities, perfectionistic strivings showed a positive correlation with work engagement. Moreover, perfectionistic concerns showed a negative correlation with work engagement, suggesting that employees high in perfectionistic concerns may show lower work engagement than employees low in perfectionistic concerns.

In sum, the findings suggest that only perfectionistic strivings consistently show positive relationships with work engagement, whereas perfectionistic concerns are either unrelated to work engagement or show negative relationships. Because the same pattern—that is, perfectionistic strivings being associated with higher levels of work engagement and perfectionistic concerns being associated with lower levels or unrelated to work engagement—has been found in studies with students that examined perfectionism and academic engagement (e.g., Shih, 2012; Zhang, Gan, & Cham, 2007), we are confident about the validity of this suggestion despite the small number of studies on perfectionism and work engagement.

Perfectionism and Workaholism

In contrast to work engagement, workaholism has been described as an uncontrollable need to work incessantly and is characterized by working excessively and compulsively (Schaufeli et al., 2008). In the words of Oates (1971), who is credited for coining the term, a workaholic is a person "whose need for work has become so excessive that it creates noticeable disturbance or interference with his bodily health, personal happiness, and interpersonal relations, and with his smooth social functioning" (p. 4). A recent meta-analysis conducted by Clark et al. (in press) found workaholism to be associated with high levels of burnout at work and low levels of satisfaction with life outside work. Furthermore, workaholism was associated with low levels of emotional well-being and high levels of psychological distress. In addition, workaholism was associated with high levels of psychosomatic symptoms and physical health complaints which have been linked to workaholics' not getting enough leisure time, physical exercise, and sleep (see also Burke, 2000; Ng, Sorensen, & Feldman, 2007; Robinson, 2000; Snir & Harpaz, 2006). Consequently, workaholism is not a positive characteristic indicating a healthy passion and enthusiasm for one's work, but an unhealthy characteristic that can have ruinous consequences for an individual's emotional, social, and physical well-being.

Perfectionism has long been closely linked to workaholism, so close that Spence and Robbins's (1992) multidimensional conceptualizations of workaholism considered perfectionism a key characteristic of workaholism differentiating workaholics from people who are enthusiastic about their work, but do not feel compulsively driven to work. Perhaps this is the reason why there is a significant number of studies that have investigated perfectionism and workaholism in employees, so Clark and colleagues (in press) could use data from 10 studies for their meta-analysis.[3] Using only findings from studies examining overall perfectionism and workaholism (not differentiating perfectionistic strivings and perfectionistic concerns), the meta-analysis aggregated data involving more than 2,700 employees and found perfectionism to show an estimated population correlation of $\rho = 0.55$ with workaholism, which represents a large-sized effect confirming the close relationship between perfectionism and workaholism.

But how does the relationship look if perfectionistic strivings and perfectionistic concerns are differentiated? To our knowledge, five studies have investigated the

[3] The cutoff date of Clark et al.'s literature search was July 2013, so their meta-analysis did not include Stoeber, Davis, and Townley (2013), Tziner and Tanami (2013), and Mazzetti, Schaufeli, and Guglielmi (2014). Moreover, it missed Taris, van Beek, and Schaufeli (2010).

perfectionism–workaholism relationship differentiating between the two superordinate factors of perfectionism. The first study (Clark, Lelchook, & Taylor, 2010) examined perfectionism and workaholism in students working part-time, additionally controlling for relevant demographic variables (e.g., gender, age, years in occupation) and the Big Five personality factors (see John & Srivastava, 1999). At the level of bivariate correlations, both perfectionistic strivings and perfectionistic concerns showed positive correlations with workaholism. Moreover, when regression analyses were computed controlling for the overlap between the two perfectionism factors (as well as the demographic variables and the Big Five), perfectionistic strivings and perfectionistic concerns showed significant positive regression weights,[4] indicating that both perfectionism factors contributed to the prediction of workaholism (and explained variance in workaholism beyond the Big Five). The second study (Taris, van Beek, & Schaufeli, 2010) examined perfectionism and workaholism in employees working in the head office of a retail organization, additionally controlling for relevant demographic variables (e.g., gender, age, salary level), job demands, and job control (Karasek, 1979). At the level of bivariate correlations, both perfectionistic strivings and perfectionistic concerns again showed positive correlations with workaholism. However, when regression analyses were computed statistically controlling for the overlap between the two perfectionism factors (as well as the demographic variables, job demands, and job control), only perfectionistic concerns were associated with higher levels of workaholism, indicating that perfectionistic concerns contributed to the prediction of workaholism beyond job demands and job control. Furthermore, when a mediation analysis[5] was conducted, workaholism was found to be a mediator of the positive relationship between perfectionistic concerns and the exhaustion component of burnout (perfectionistic concerns → workaholism → exhaustion), suggesting that workaholism may be responsible for the link between perfectionistic concerns and exhaustion (detailed further below).

The third study focusing on the perfectionism–workaholism relationship is Tziner and Tanami's (2013) study mentioned previously which examined a sample of employees working in the public sector. Like the previous two studies, the study found perfectionistic strivings and perfectionistic concerns to show positive correlations with workaholism. This was different in the fourth study (Stoeber, Davis, & Townley, 2013) which examined a sample of employees working in a professional services company and students working part-time. In addition, the study investigated employees' self-regulated work motivation (Tremblay, Blanchard, Taylor, Pelletier, & Villeneuve, 2009) within the framework of self-determination theory (Deci & Ryan, 1985; Ryan & Deci, 2000). Differently from the previous studies, only perfectionistic strivings showed positive relationships with workaholism in both the bivariate correlations and the multiple regressions, but not perfectionistic

[4] Regression weights are similar to partial correlations, with positive regression weights indicating a positive relationship and negative regression weights a negative relationship (Cohen, Cohen, West, & Aiken, 2003).

[5] A mediation analysis is a statistical procedure probing whether the relationship between two variables X and Y can be explained by a third variable called mediator (X → mediator → Y; see Baron & Kenny, 1986).

concerns. Moreover, the study found that the relationship between perfectionistic strivings and workaholism was mediated by identified and introjected regulation of work motivation (perfectionistic strivings → identified/introjected regulation → workaholism). According to self-determination theory, identified regulation is characterized by personal importance and conscious valuing of reasons for work, and introjected regulation is characterized by ego involvement motivated by internal rewards and punishments. Because identified regulation is a form of autonomous motivation, whereas introjected regulation is a form of controlled motivation, the findings suggest that high levels of combined autonomous–controlled motivation may be responsible for the perfectionism–workaholism relationship regarding perfectionistic strivings.

The final study (Mazzetti, Schaufeli, & Guglielmi, 2014) examined perfectionism and workaholism in employees subscribing to a newsletter of a training and consultancy agency, additionally controlling for overwork climate. Overwork climate was defined as employees' perception of "their work environments to be characterized by a climate that expects them to perform overwork (i.e., working beyond set work hours, doing unpaid overtime work, taking work home, and working during weekends or holidays)" (p. 11). When bivariate correlations were regarded, perfectionistic strivings showed a positive correlation with workaholism. Moreover, when moderated regression analyses were conducted investigating interaction effects, the positive relationship between perfectionistic strivings and workaholism was moderated by a significant interaction with overwork climate: Perfectionistic strivings showed a significant positive correlation with workaholism only in employees who perceived their organization to expect overworking. In employees who did not have this perception, perfectionistic strivings were unrelated to workaholism.

Whereas Mazzetti et al.'s (2014) study makes an important contribution to the search for moderators of the perfectionism–workaholism relationship,[6] the study only measured perfectionistic strivings, but not perfectionistic concerns. Hence, it is unclear whether perfectionistic strivings would have shown the same effects had the overlap with perfectionistic concerns been controlled for (cf. Taris et al., 2010). Still, taking the findings of the other studies into account—particularly Stoeber and colleagues' (2013) study which controlled for perfectionistic concerns—we believe that it is justified to conclude that both perfectionistic strivings and perfectionistic concerns show positive relationships with workaholism.

Perfectionism and Burnout

Job burnout is a complex syndrome that is commonly conceptualized as being comprised of three components: exhaustion, cynicism, and inefficacy (see Maslach, Schaufeli, & Leiter, 2001, for a comprehensive review). Exhaustion

[6] For an explanation of moderators and how they differ from mediators, see again Baron and Kenny (1986).

(also called emotional exhaustion) is usually regarded the core component of burnout and is characterized by a feeling of being overextended and a depletion of one's emotional resources (feeling emotionally "drained"). Cynicism—in earlier research referred to as depersonalization—represents the interpersonal component of burnout and is characterized by a negative, detached, and depersonalized attitude toward one's work, coworkers, and the people who one's work is directed at (e.g., customers, clients/patients, students). Inefficacy—also referred to as ineffectiveness, reduced efficacy, or reduced personal accomplishment—is the self-evaluation component of burnout and is characterized by feelings of declining competence and productivity at work and of increased inability to solve problems that arise in one's work (Maslach et al., 2001). Besides being associated with health problems and reduced well-being, burnout has been associated with a range of problems on the job such as absenteeism, high turnover, low work morale, and reduced job performance (e.g., reduced quality of patient care) as well as marital and family problems (see Maslach et al., 2001; Shirom, 2002; and Taris, 2006, for reviews). Hence, it is understandable that researchers have sought to identify contextual (e.g., job characteristics) and personal factors (e.g., personality dispositions) that predict burnout in employees. One of the personality dispositions they identified to predict burnout in employees was perfectionism.

Even though research on perfectionism in employees is limited, there is a substantial number of studies that have investigated the relationships between perfectionism and job burnout. Moreover, the majority of studies has differentiated perfectionistic strivings and perfectionistic concerns when examining the relationships (e.g., Caliskan, Arikan, & Saatci, 2014; Chang, 2012; Childs & Stoeber, 2010, 2012; Craiovan, 2014; Fairlie & Flett, 2003; Hrabluik, Latham, & McCarthy, 2012; Kazemi & Ziaaddini, 2014; Li, Hou, Chi, Liu, & Hager, 2014; Mitchelson & Burns, 1998; Ozbilir et al., in press; Philp, Egan, & Kane, 2012; Schwenke, Ashby, & Gnilka, 2014; Stoeber & Rennert, 2008; Taris et al., 2010; Tashman, Tenenbaum, & Eklund, 2010; Van Yperen, Verbraak, & Spoor, 2011).

What did the studies find? A number of them found perfectionistic concerns to show positive relationships with burnout and its components, whereas perfectionistic strivings showed no significant relationships. Mitchelson and Burns (1998), for example, examined a sample of women working in sales and other occupations. Perfectionistic concerns showed positive correlations with exhaustion and cynicism (but not inefficacy), whereas perfectionistic strivings showed nonsignificant correlations with all three components. Fairlie and Flett (2003) examined perfectionism and emotional exhaustion in a sample of employees (including students) working over 20 hours per week. Differently from the previous study, Fairlie and Flett's study found perfectionistic concerns to show positive correlations with all three burnout components (exhaustion, cynicism, and inefficacy), whereas perfectionistic strivings again showed no significant correlations. Van Yperen et al. (2011) examined employees reporting mental health issues. Employees diagnosed in a clinical interview as suffering from severe job burnout showed higher levels of perfectionistic concerns, but not higher levels of perfectionistic strivings than healthy controls. Finally, Kazemi and Ziaaddini (2014) examined employees working in executive organizations. Only perfectionistic concerns showed a positive correlation with overall burnout (combining exhaustion, cynicism, and inefficacy), not perfectionistic strivings.

Other studies found much the same pattern, except that perfectionistic strivings showed negative correlations with the inefficacy component. Li et al. (2014), for example, examined a sample of employees working in information technology and found perfectionistic strivings to be unrelated to exhaustion and cynicism, but showing a negative correlation with inefficacy. Perfectionistic concerns, on the other hand, showed positive correlations with all three burnout components. Caliskan et al. (2014) examined a sample of white-collar employees working in various small- and medium-sized enterprises. Perfectionistic strivings again showed nonsignificant correlations with exhaustion and cynicism, but a negative correlation with inefficacy. In contrast, perfectionistic concerns showed positive correlations with exhaustion and cynicism, but not with inefficacy.

Finally, some studies found perfectionistic strivings to show positive correlations with burnout. However, these were restricted to the exhaustion and cynicism component and never showed for the inefficacy component (e.g., Hrabluik et al., 2012; Taris et al., 2010; Tashman et al., 2010). Moreover, the studies did not control for the overlap between perfectionistic strivings and perfectionistic concerns when examining the perfectionism–burnout relationships. Because research in other areas found that perfectionistic concerns not only suppress the positive associations of perfectionistic strivings, but also inflate their negative associations (R. W. Hill et al., 2010; Stoeber, Kobori, & Brown, in press; Stoeber & Otto, 2006), it is conceivable that the overlap with perfectionistic concerns was responsible for the positive correlations which perfectionistic strivings showed with exhaustion and cynicism and that the relationships would have been nonsignificant had the overlap been controlled for.

Unfortunately, only two studies investigating perfectionism in employees and burnout have controlled for the overlap between the two perfectionism factors. The first study (Stoeber & Rennert, 2008) examined a sample of teachers working at secondary schools. When correlations were regarded, perfectionistic strivings showed no significant correlations with any of the burnout components. However, when multiple regressions were regarded controlling for the overlap with perfectionistic concerns, perfectionistic strivings showed negative regression weights with all three components. The second study (Childs & Stoeber, 2010), mentioned previously, found perfectionistic strivings to show nonsignificant correlations with the three burnout components but significant negative regression coefficients with both cynicism and inefficacy when the overlap with perfectionistic concerns was controlled for. By contrast, perfectionistic concerns showed significant positive correlations and positive regression coefficients with all three burnout components in both studies.

In sum, the findings indicate that only perfectionistic concerns consistently show positive relationships with burnout, not perfectionistic strivings. On the contrary, when the overlap with perfectionistic concerns is controlled for, perfectionistic strivings may show *negative* relationships with burnout. Consequently, when it comes to burnout, perfectionism in employees seems to be a "double-edged sword" (cf. Stoeber, in press). On the one hand, the concerns dimension of perfectionism represents a risk of employees burning out at the job. On the other hand, the strivings dimension of perfectionism seems to counteract this risk and protect employees from burning out. The findings, however, also suggest that perfectionistic concerns are a stronger risk factor than perfectionistic strivings are a protective factor. Consequently, if we have a look at the combined effects of perfectionistic strivings and perfectionistic concerns, "overall perfectionism" is a personality disposition putting employees at increased risk of job burnout.

Summary, An Intriguing Question, and Future Research

Summary

Despite the limitations of the studies reviewed in this chapter, it is safe to conclude that perfectionism is related to all three key variables in people's working life: work engagement, workaholism, and burnout. However, when we differentiate perfectionistic strivings and perfectionistic concerns—the two superordinate factors of perfectionism (Stoeber & Otto, 2006)—we find differential relationships with two of the three variables: work engagement and burnout. Whereas both perfectionistic strivings and perfectionistic concerns appear to be positively related to workaholism, only perfectionistic strivings consistently show positive relationships with work engagement, and only perfectionistic concerns consistently show positive relationships with burnout. What is more, when the overlap with perfectionistic concerns is controlled for, perfectionistic strivings may show negative relationships with burnout.

An Intriguing Question

Because workaholism is closely related to burnout—Clark et al.'s (in press) meta-analysis found an estimated population correlation of $\rho = 0.40$ between workaholism and overall burnout aggregating findings from 18 studies comprising more than 10,000 employees—the differential pattern of relationships that perfectionistic strivings and perfectionistic concerns show raises an intriguing question: Why do perfectionistic strivings in employees predict higher levels of workaholism, but not higher levels of burnout?

There are (yet) no studies on perfectionism in employees to answer this question, but there is other research that suggests potential reasons. One reason may be work engagement. Work engagement is said to be "the antipode of job burnout" (Bakker, Schaufeli, Leiter, & Taris, 2008, p. 188). Perhaps it is also an "antidote" to job burnout. Work engagement shows only small-sized positive correlations with workaholism (Clark et al., in press, found an estimated population correlation of only $\rho = 0.05$), but shows large-sized negative correlations with burnout: In a meta-analysis summarizing findings from 54 studies with almost 30,000 employees (Crawford, LePine, & Rich, 2010), the estimated population correlation of work engagement and burnout was $\rho = -0.45$. With only perfectionistic strivings showing sizeable positive correlations with work engagement (but not perfectionistic concerns), it is conceivable that—for employees who are higher in perfectionistic strivings than perfectionistic concerns—the contributing effect that workaholism has on burnout is compensated, or even overcompensated, by the negative effect that work engagement has on burnout.

Another reason may be self-determined motivation. Research in sport psychology suggests that individual differences in autonomous versus controlled motivation may mediate the perfectionism–burnout relationship. Investigating athlete burnout, Jowett, Hill, Hall, and Curran (2013) found perfectionistic strivings to show positive correlations with autonomous motivation (comprising intrinsic motivation, integrated regulation, and identified regulation) and controlled motivation (comprising introjected regulation and external regulation), whereas perfectionistic concerns showed a positive correlation only with controlled motivation. Furthermore, Jowett et al. found autonomous motivation to show a negative correlation with burnout, whereas controlled motivation showed a positive correlation. When all variables were subjected to a mediation analysis, autonomous and controlled motivation mediated the relationship between perfectionistic strivings, perfectionistic concerns, and burnout: Perfectionistic strivings showed a positive path to autonomous motivation which showed a negative path to burnout. In contrast, perfectionistic concerns showed a positive path to controlled motivation which showed a positive path to burnout. (When the overlap with perfectionistic concerns was controlled for, the path from perfectionistic strivings to controlled motivation was nonsignificant.) Following Stoeber et al.'s (2013) findings that perfectionistic strivings in employees showed positive correlations with all aspects of autonomous motivation (intrinsic motivation, integrated regulation, identified regulation), whereas perfectionistic concerns showed positive correlations with all aspects of controlled motivation (introjected regulation, external regulation), the mediation model that Jowett et al. (2013) suggested for burnout in athletes may also hold for burnout in employees (see Fig. 12.1, Panel A).

Finally, differences in the use of adaptive versus maladaptive coping styles[7] could be a reason why perfectionistic concerns may lead to burnout, but not perfectionistic strivings. Theory and research on burnout have identified job stress to be a key factor for employees' developing symptoms of burnout (e.g., Maslach et al., 2001). People, however, differ in the ways they cope with stress with some people showing coping styles that are adaptive (because they reduce stress), whereas others show coping styles that are maladaptive (because they fail to reduce stress or even may increase stress) (cf. Lazarus & Folkman, 1984). Studies investigating

[7] With Compas (1987), we understand coping styles to represent individuals' preferred ways of coping in response to stress either across different situations or over time within a given situation.

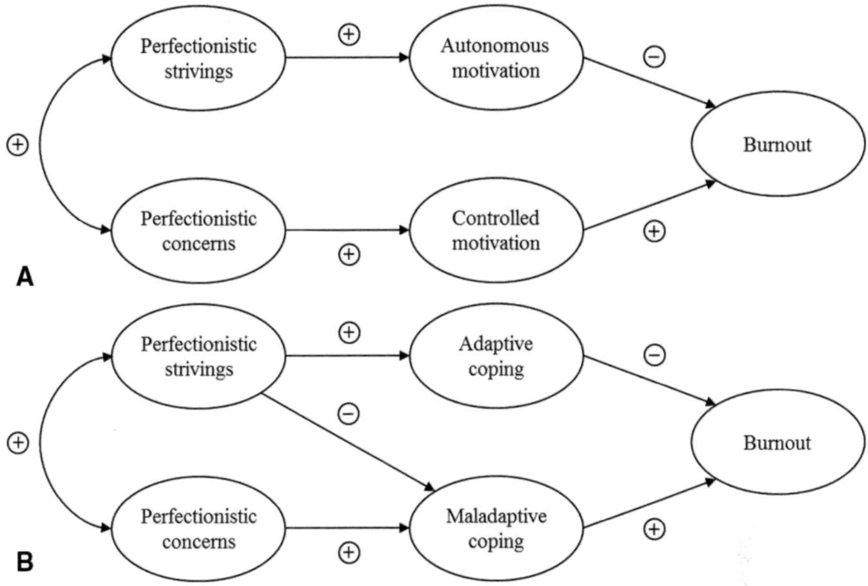

Fig. 12.1 Why perfectionistic concerns may lead to burnout, but not perfectionistic strivings: the role of autonomous versus controlled motivation (Panel A) and adaptive versus maladaptive coping (Panel B)

perfectionism and coping have established that perfectionistic concerns show positive correlations with maladaptive coping styles such as avoidant coping and denial, whereas perfectionistic strivings show positive correlations with adaptive coping styles such as problem-focused coping and planning (e.g., Dunkley, Blankstein, Halsall, Williams, & Winkworth, 2000; Gnilka, Ashby, & Noble, 2012; Stoeber & Janssen, 2011). In addition, Stoeber and Rennert (2008) found perfectionistic strivings in school teachers to show negative correlations with maladaptive coping. Taken together with other findings indicating that coping mediates the perfectionism–burnout relationship in employees (Chang, 2012; Li et al., 2014), the findings suggest that perfectionistic concerns may predict increased burnout by means of maladaptive coping, whereas perfectionistic strivings may predict decreased burnout by means of adaptive coping and an inverse relationship with maladaptive coping (see Fig. 12.1, Panel B).

Future Research

Whereas the model depicted in Panel B of Fig. 12.1 has found empirical support concerning perfectionism, coping, and burnout in athletes (see A. P. Hill, Hall, & Appleton, 2010), future research still needs to find support for the model in employees. The same goes for the mediation model of perfectionism, autonomous versus controlled motivation, and burnout shown in Panel A as well as the "antidote" effect that work engagement may have on the perfectionistic strivings–burnout relationship we suggested above.

Furthermore, future research needs to employ longitudinal designs to establish the temporal, and perhaps causal, links of the relationships suggested by the research detailed in the present chapter. To our knowledge, there is so far only one study that investigated longitudinal effects of perfectionism on burnout in employees. Childs and Stoeber (2012) examined two samples of employees—a sample of administrative and managerial staff working for the National Health Service and a sample of school teachers—and found that, across samples, perfectionistic concerns not only showed positive correlations with burnout, but also predicted increases in burnout over time.

Whereas Childs and Stoeber's findings represent a first step in the right direction, further longitudinal studies on perfectionism and burnout in employees are needed. In addition, further studies on perfectionism, work engagement, and workaholism in employees are needed. In this, future studies should continue the search for mediators and moderators of the relationships that perfectionism in employees shows with work engagement, workaholism, and burnout. Moreover, future studies need to differentiate between perfectionistic strivings and perfectionistic concerns and be aware that perfectionistic strivings may show different relationships when the overlap with perfectionistic concerns is controlled for. If so, we are certain that future research will confirm perfectionism to be a key personality characteristic that can explain why some employees are engaged in and passionate about their work, why some employees become addicted to work and develop excessive and compulsive working habits, and why some employees burn out and become disengaged, cynical, and unproductive.

Finally, and perhaps most importantly, future studies need to investigate how to help perfectionistic employees to keep their perfectionistic concerns in check so that they do not negatively impact their work–life balance, health, and well-being. There are two excellent self-help books available (Antony & Swinson, 2009; Shafran, Egan, & Wade, 2010) that may help employees to better understand their perfectionism and cope with the perfectionistic concerns and that could be recommended to employees whose perfectionism is negatively affecting their work and private life. Unguided self-help has been shown to reduce perfectionism. However, guided self-help and face-to-face counseling have been shown to be more effective and to have longer-lasting positive effects (Egan et al., in press; Pleva & Wade, 2007). Consequently, employers may want to consider offering group sessions of guided self-help involving trained psychologists to employees who are suffering from perfectionism. We hope that the present chapter will inspire such future research to help advance our knowledge about how perfectionism in employees contributes to work engagement, workaholism, and job burnout and how they affect employees' health and well-being.

References

Antony, M. M., & Swinson, R. P. (2009). *When perfect isn't good enough: Strategies for coping with perfectionism* (2nd ed.). Oakland: New Harbinger.

Attridge, M. (2009). Measuring and managing employee work engagement: A review of the research and business literature. *Journal of Workplace Behavioral Health, 24,* 383–398.

Bakker, A. B., & Bal, M. P. (2010). Weekly work engagement and performance: A study among starting teachers. *Journal of Occupational and Organizational Psychology, 83,* 189–206.

Bakker, A. B., Schaufeli, W. B., Leiter, M. P., & Taris, T. W. (2008). Work engagement: An emerging concept in occupational health psychology. *Work & Stress, 22,* 187–200.

Baron, R. M., & Kenny, D. A. (1986). The moderator-mediator variable distinction in social psychological research: Conceptual, strategic, and statistical considerations. *Journal of Personality and Social Psychology, 51,* 1173–1182.

Bieling, P. J., Israeli, A. L., & Antony, M. M. (2004). Is perfectionism good, bad, or both? Examining models of the perfectionism construct. *Personality and Individual Differences, 36,* 1373–1385.

Burke, R. J. (2000). Workaholism in organizations: Psychological and physical well-being consequences. *Stress Medicine, 16,* 11–16.

Caliskan, S. C., Arikan, S. C., & Saatci, E. Y. (2014). SMEs context of Turkey from the relational perspective of members' perfectionism, work family conflict and burnout. *International Journal of Business and Social Science, 5,* 129–139.

Chang, Y. (2012). The relationship between maladaptive perfectionism with burnout: Testing mediating effect of emotion-focused coping. *Personality and Individual Differences, 53,* 635–639.

Childs, J. H., & Stoeber, J. (2010). Self-oriented, other-oriented, and socially prescribed perfectionism in employees: Relationships with burnout and engagement. *Journal of Workplace Behavioral Health, 25,* 269–281.

Childs, J. H., & Stoeber, J. (2012). Do you want me to be perfect? Two longitudinal studies on socially prescribed perfectionism, stress and burnout in the workplace. *Work & Stress, 26,* 347–364.

Christian, M. S., Garza, A. S., & Slaughter, J. E. (2011). Work engagement: A quantitative review and test of its relations with task and contextual performance. *Personnel Psychology, 64,* 89–136.

Clark, M. A., Lelchook, A. M., & Taylor, M. L. (2010). Beyond the big five: How narcissism, perfectionism, and dispositional affect relate to workaholism. *Personality and Individual Differences, 48,* 786–791.

Clark, M. A., Michel, J. S., Zhdanova, L., Pui, S. Y., & Baltes, B. B. (in press). All work and no play? A meta-analytic examination of the correlates and outcomes of workaholism. *Journal of Management.*

Cohen, J. (1992). A power primer. *Psychological Bulletin, 112,* 155–159.

Cohen, J., Cohen, P., West, S. G., & Aiken, L. S. (2003). *Applied multiple regression/correlation analysis for the behavioral sciences* (3rd ed.). Mahwah: Lawrence Erlbaum Associates.

Compas, B. E. (1987). Coping with stress during childhood and adolescence. *Psychological Bulletin, 101,* 393–403.

Craiovan, P. M. (2014). Correlations between perfectionism, stress, psychopathological symptoms and burnout in the medical field. *Procedia-Social and Behavioral Sciences, 127,* 529–533.

Crawford, E. R., LePine, J. A., & Rich, B. L. (2010). Linking job demands and resources to employee engagement and burnout: A theoretical extension and meta-analytic test. *Journal of Applied Psychology, 95,* 834–848.

Deci, E. L., & Ryan, R. M. (1985). *Intrinsic motivation and self-determination in human behavior.* New York: Plenum.

DiBartolo, P. M., Frost, R. O., Chang, P., LaSota, M., & Grills, A. E. (2004). Shedding light on the relationship between personal standards and psychopathology: The case for contingent self-worth. *Journal of Rational-Emotive & Cognitive-Behavior Therapy, 22,* 241–254.

Diener, E., Suh, E. M., Lucas, R. E., & Smith, H. L. (1999). Subjective well-being: Three decades of progress. *Psychological Bulletin, 125,* 276–302.

Dunkley, D. M., Blankstein, K. R., Halsall, J., Williams, M., & Winkworth, G. (2000). The relation between perfectionism and distress: Hassles, coping, and perceived social support as mediators and moderators. *Journal of Counseling Psychology, 47,* 437–453.

Egan, S. J., van Noort, E., Chee, A., Kane, R. T., Hoiles, K. J., Shafran, R., & Wade, T. D. (in press). A randomised controlled trial of face to face versus pure online self-help cognitive behavioural treatment for perfectionism. *Behaviour Research and Therapy.*

Enns, M. W., & Cox, B. J. (2002). The nature and assessment of perfectionism: A critical analysis. In G. L. Flett & P. L. Hewitt (Eds.), *Perfectionism: Theory, research, and treatment* (pp. 33–62). Washington, DC: American Psychological Association.

Fairlie, P., & Flett, G. L. (2003, August). Perfectionism at work: Impacts on burnout, job satisfaction, and depression. Poster presented at the 111th Annual Convention of the American Psychological Association, Toronto, Ontario, Canada.

Flaxman, P. E., Ménard, J., Bond, F. W., & Kinman, G. (2012). Academics' experiences of a respite from work: Effects of self-critical perfectionism and perseverative cognition on postrespite well-being. *Journal of Applied Psychology, 97,* 854–865.

Frost, R. O., Marten, P., Lahart, C., & Rosenblate, R. (1990). The dimensions of perfectionism. *Cognitive Therapy and Research, 14,* 449–468.

Frost, R. O., Heimberg, R. G., Holt, C. S., Mattia, J. I., & Neubauer, A. L. (1993). A comparison of two measures of perfectionism. *Personality and Individual Differences, 14,* 119–126.

Gaudreau, P. (2012). A methodological note on the interactive and main effects of dualistic personality dimensions: An example using the 2 × 2 model of perfectionism. *Personality and Individual Differences, 52,* 26–31.

Gnilka, P. B., Ashby, J. S., & Noble, C. M. (2012). Multidimensional perfectionism and anxiety: Differences among individuals with perfectionism and tests of a coping-mediation model. *Journal of Counseling & Development, 90,* 427–436.

Hewitt, P. L., & Flett, G. L. (1991). Perfectionism in the self and social contexts: Conceptualization, assessment, and association with psychopathology. *Journal of Personality and Social Psychology, 60,* 456–470.

Hill, R. W., Huelsman, T. J., Furr, R. M., Kibler, J., Vicente, B. B., & Kennedy, C. (2004). A new measure of perfectionism: The perfectionism inventory. *Journal of Personality Assessment, 82,* 80–91.

Hill, A. P., Hall, H. K., & Appleton, P. R. (2010). Perfectionism and athlete burnout in junior elite athletes: The mediating influence of coping tendencies. *Anxiety, Stress, & Coping, 23,* 415–430.

Hill, R. W., Huelsman, T. J., & Araujo, G. (2010). Perfectionistic concerns suppress associations between perfectionistic strivings and positive life outcomes. *Personality and Individual Differences, 48,* 584–589.

Hrabluik, C., Latham, G. P., & McCarthy, J. M. (2012). Does goal setting have a dark side? The relationship between perfectionism and maximum versus typical employee performance. *International Public Management Journal, 15,* 5–38.

John, O. P., & Srivastava, S. (1999). The big five trait taxonomy: History, measurement, and theoretical perspectives. In L. A. Pervin & O. P. John (Eds.), *Handbook of personality: Theory and research* (2nd ed., pp. 102–138). New York: Guilford.

Jowett, G. E., Hill, A. P., Hall, H. K., & Curran, T. (2013). Perfectionism and junior athlete burnout: The mediating role of autonomous and controlled motivation. *Sport, Exercise, and Performance Psychology, 2,* 48–61.

Karasek, R. A. Jr. (1979). Job demands, job decision latitude, and mental strain: Implications for job redesign. *Administrative Science Quarterly, 24,* 285–308.

Kazemi, A., & Ziaaddini, M. (2014). Relationship between perfectionism, psychological hardiness, and job burnout of employees in executive organizations. *International Journal of Academic Research in Business and Social Sciences, 4,* 160–170.

Lazarus, R. S., & Folkman, S. (1984). *Stress, appraisal, and coping.* New York: Springer.

Li, X., Hou, Z.-J., Chi, H.-Y., Liu, J., & Hager, M. J. (2014). The mediating role of coping in the relationship between subtypes of perfectionism and job burnout: A test of the 2 × 2 model of perfectionism with employees in China. *Personality and Individual Differences, 58,* 65–70.

Maslach, C., Schaufeli, W. B., & Leiter, M. P. (2001). Job burnout. *Annual Review of Psychology, 52,* 397–422.

Matuska, K. M. (2010). Workaholism, life balance, and well-being: A comparative analysis. *Journal of Occupational Science, 17,* 104–111.

Mazzetti, G., Schaufeli, W. B., & Guglielmi, D. (2014). Are workaholics born or made? Relations of workaholism with person characteristics and overwork climate. *International Journal of Stress Management, 21,* 227–254.

Mitchelson, J. K. (2009). Seeking the perfect balance: Perfectionism and work-family conflict. *Journal of Occupational and Organizational Psychology, 82,* 349–367.

Mitchelson, J. K., & Burns, L. R. (1998). Career mothers and perfectionism: Stress at work and at home. *Personality and Individual Differences, 25,* 477–485.

Ng, T. W. H., Sorensen, K. L., & Feldman, D. C. (2007). Dimensions, antecedents, and consequences of workaholism: A conceptual integration and extension. *Journal of Organizational Behavior, 28,* 111–136.

Oates, W. E. (1971). *Confessions of a workaholic: The facts about work addiction.* New York: World Publishing.

Ozbilir, T., Day, A., & Catano, V. M. (in press). Perfectionism at work: An investigation of adaptive and maladaptive perfectionism in the workplace among Canadian and Turkish employees. *Applied Psychology*.

Philp, M., Egan, S., & Kane, R. (2012). Perfectionism, over commitment to work, and burnout in employees seeking workplace counselling. *Australian Journal of Psychology, 64,* 68–74.

Pleva, J., & Wade, T. D. (2007). Guided self-help versus pure self-help for perfectionism: A randomised controlled trial. *Behaviour Research and Therapy, 45,* 849–861.

Robinson, B. E. (2000). Workaholism: Bridging the gap between workplace, sociocultural, and family research. *Journal of Employment Counseling, 37,* 31–47.

Ryan, R. M., & Deci, E. L. (2000). Self-determination theory and the facilitation of intrinsic motivation, social development, and well-being. *American Psychologist, 55,* 68–78.

Schaufeli, W., & Salanova, M. (2011). Work engagement: On how to better catch a slippery concept. *European Journal of Work and Organizational Psychology, 20,* 39–46.

Schaufeli, W. B., Salanova, M., González-Romá, V., & Bakker, A. B. (2002). The measurement of engagement and burnout: A confirmative analytic approach. *Journal of Happiness Studies, 3,* 71–92.

Schaufeli, W. B., Taris, T. W., & van Rhenen, W. (2008). Workaholism, burnout, and work engagement: Three of a kind or three different kinds of employee well-being? *Applied Psychology, 57,* 173–203.

Schwenke, T. J., Ashby, J. S., & Gnilka, P. B. (2014). Sign language interpreters and burnout: The effects of perfectionism, perceived stress, and coping resources. *Interpreting, 16,* 209–232.

Shafran, R., Egan, S., & Wade, T. (2010). *Overcoming perfectionism: A self-help guide using cognitive behavioral techniques*. London: Robinson.

Sherry, S. B., Hewitt, P. L., Sherry, D. L., Flett, G. L., & Graham, A. R. (2010). Perfectionism dimensions and research productivity in psychology professors: Implications for understanding the (mal)adaptiveness of perfectionism. *Canadian Journal of Behavioural Science, 42,* 273–283.

Shih, S.-S. (2012). An examination of academic burnout versus work engagement among Taiwanese adolescents. *Journal of Educational Research, 105,* 286–298.

Shirom, A. (2002). The MBI-General Survey. In C. Maslach, S. E. Jackson, & M. P. Leiter (Eds.), *Maslach burnout inventory manual* (3rd ed., pp. 19–26). Palo Alto: Consulting Psychologists Press.

Shirom, A., & Melamed, S. (2005). Does burnout affect physical health? A review of the evidence. In A.-S. G. Antoniou & C. L. Cooper (Eds.), *Research companion to organizational health psychology* (pp. 599–622). Cheltenham: Edward Elgar.

Slaney, R. B., & Ashby, J. S. (1996). Perfectionists: Study of a criterion group. *Journal of Counseling and Development, 74,* 393–398.
Slaney, R. B., Rice, K. G., Mobley, M., Trippi, J., & Ashby, J. S. (2001). The revised Almost Perfect Scale. *Measurement and Evaluation in Counseling and Development, 34,* 130–145.
Snir, R., & Harpaz, I. (2006). The workaholism phenomenon: A cross-national perspective. *Career Development International, 11,* 374–393.
Spence, J. T., & Robbins, A. S. (1992). Workaholism: Definition, measurement, and preliminary results. *Journal of Personality Assessment, 58,* 160–178.
Stöber, J. (1998). The frost multidimensional perfectionism scale revisited: More perfect with four (instead of six) dimensions. *Personality and Individual Differences, 24,* 481–491.
Stoeber, J. (in press). Perfectionism in sport and dance: A double-edged sword. *International Journal of Sport Psychology.*
Stoeber, J., & Childs, J. H. (2010). The assessment of self-oriented and socially prescribed perfectionism: Subscales make a difference. *Journal of Personality Assessment, 92,* 577–585.
Stoeber, J., & Eysenck, M. W. (2008). Perfectionism and efficiency: Accuracy, response bias, and invested time in proof-reading performance. *Journal of Research in Personality, 42,* 1673–1678.
Stoeber, J., & Janssen, D. P. (2011). Perfectionism and coping with daily failures: Positive reframing helps achieve satisfaction at the end of the day. *Anxiety, Stress, & Coping, 24,* 477–497.
Stoeber, J., & Otto, K. (2006). Positive conceptions of perfectionism: Approaches, evidence, challenges. *Personality and Social Psychology Review, 10,* 295–319.
Stoeber, J., & Rennert, D. (2008). Perfectionism in school teachers: Relations with stress appraisals, coping styles, and burnout. *Anxiety, Stress, & Coping, 21,* 37–53.
Stoeber, J., & Stoeber, F. S. (2009). Domains of perfectionism: Prevalence and relationships with perfectionism, gender, age, and satisfaction with life. *Personality and Individual Differences, 46,* 530–535.
Stoeber, J., Otto, K., Pescheck, E., Becker, C., & Stoll, O. (2007). Perfectionism and competitive anxiety in athletes: Differentiating striving for perfection and negative reactions to imperfection. *Personality and Individual Differences, 42,* 959–969.
Stoeber, J., Davis, C. R., & Townley, J. (2013). Perfectionism and workaholism in employees: The role of work motivation. *Personality and Individual Differences, 55,* 733–738.
Stoeber, J., Kobori, O., & Brown, A. (in press). Examining mutual suppression effects in the assessment of perfectionism cognitions: Evidence supporting multidimensional assessment. Assessment.
Taris, T. W. (2006). Is there a relationship between burnout and objective performance? A critical review of 16 studies. *Work & Stress, 20,* 316–334.
Taris, T. W., van Beek, I., & Schaufeli, W. (2010). Why do perfectionists have a higher burnout risk than others? The mediational effect of workaholism. *Romanian Journal of Applied Psychology, 12,* 1–7.
Tashman, L. S., Tenenbaum, G., & Eklund, R. (2010). The effect of perceived stress on the relationship between perfectionism and burnout in coaches. *Anxiety, Stress, & Coping, 23,* 195–202.
Tremblay, M. A., Blanchard, C. M., Taylor, S., Pelletier, L. G., & Villeneuve, M. (2009). Work extrinsic and intrinsic motivation scale: Its value for organizational psychology research. *Canadian Journal of Behavioural Science, 41,* 213–226.
Tziner, A., & Tanami, M. (2013). Examining the links between attachment, perfectionism, and job motivation potential with job engagement and workaholism. *Journal of Work and Organizational Psychology, 29,* 65–74.
van Beek, I., Taris, T. W., & Schaufeli, W. B. (2011). Workaholic and work engaged employees: Dead ringers or worlds apart? *Journal of Occupational Health Psychology, 16,* 468–482.
Van Yperen, N. W., Verbraak, M., & Spoor, E. (2011). Perfectionism and clinical disorders among employees. *Personality and Individual Differences, 50,* 1126–1130.
Wittenberg, K. J., & Norcross, J. C. (2001). Practitioner perfectionism: Relationship to ambiguity tolerance and work satisfaction. *Journal of Clinical Psychology, 57,* 1543–1550.

Wojdylo, K., Baumann, N., Buczny, J., Owens, G., & Kuhl, J. (2013). Work craving: A conceptualization and measurement. *Basic and Applied Social Psychology, 35,* 547–568.
Zhang, Y., Gan, Y., & Cham, H. (2007). Perfectionism, academic burnout and engagement among Chinese college students: A structural equation modeling analysis. *Personality and Individual Differences, 43,* 1529–1540.

Chapter 13
Perfectionism, Health, and Well-Being: Epilogue and Future Directions

Danielle S. Molnar and Fuschia M. Sirois

As the contributions in the present volume attest, we have gained a much deeper understanding of the role of perfectionism in health and well-being over the past 25 years. Advances in the theoretical conceptualizations of perfectionism, the way we measure perfectionism, and a growing appreciation of the substantial role of personality and individual difference factors in health and well-being and across different contexts have collectively converged to contribute to the development of a promising body of literature focused on understanding when, where, and why perfectionism may create risk or resilience for health and well-being. Indeed, each of the contributions in this edited volume address these important issues from novel and unique perspectives, often highlighting the commonalties of the complexities and controversies that abound. In this final chapter, we have selected four key themes emerging from these works that we believe deserve closer attention because they have the potential to pave the way for future research for the next generation of researchers in the field. Specifically, we will discuss (1) issues in the conceptualization and measurement of perfectionism, (2) the pervasiveness of perfectionism, (3) the adaptive versus maladaptive perfectionism debate, and (4) issues in measuring health and well-being in relation to perfectionism. These themes afford us new insights into links among perfectionism, health, and well-being that can guide scholars to new and exciting questions to further propel the field forward.

D. S. Molnar (✉)
Research Institute on Addictions, University at Buffalo, The State University of New York, Buffalo, NY, USA
e-mail: dmolnar@ria.buffalo.edu

Department of Psychology, Brock University, St. Catharines, ON, Canada

F. M. Sirois
Department of Psychology, University of Sheffield, 309 Western Bank, S10 2TP Sheffield, UK
e-mail: f.sirois@sheffield.ac.uk

Centre for Research on Aging, Sherbrooke, QC, Canada

F. M. Sirois, D. S. Molnar (eds.), *Perfectionism, Health, and Well-Being*,
DOI 10.1007/978-3-319-18582-8_13

Theme 1: Issues in the Conceptualization and Measurement of Perfectionism

Issue 1. Different levels of Analysis

With respect to the application of perfectionism to the study of health and well-being, there are some key conceptual and measurement issues that continue to be a challenge for scholars in the field. First, we need to be cognizant that there are different lenses through which we can explore perfectionism. Indeed, researchers and clinicians alike can treat perfectionism as a global personality disposition following from the trait approach (e.g., the Multidimensional Perfectionism Scale, MPS-F; Frost, Marten, Lahart, & Rosenblate, 1990; the Multidimensional Perfectionism Scale, MPS-HF; Hewitt & Flett, 1991; Almost Perfect Scale—Revised, APS-R; Slaney, Rice, Mobley, Trippi, & Ashby, 2001), focus on the frequency in which individuals' experience automatic perfectionistic thoughts, from a cognitive perspective (e.g., Perfectionistic Cognitions Inventory (PCI); Flett, Hewitt, Blankstein, & Gray, 1998; The Multidimensional Perfectionism Cognitions Inventory—English (MPCI-E); Kobori, 2006; Stoeber, Kobori, & Tanno, 2010), or concentrate on perfectionistic behavior in the form of perfectionistic self-presentation, which reflects the tendency for some perfectionists to engage in active perfectionistic self-promotion while hiding any perceived flaws from others (Perfectionistic Self-Presentation Scale (PSPS); Hewitt et al., 2003). This is an issue of paramount importance as conceptualizing perfectionism as a trait, cognition, or behavior will have direct implications in terms of intervention and treatment.

Generally speaking, perfectionism researchers tend to exhibit a strong bias toward assessing perfectionism as a deeply ingrained personality trait that colors all facets of the self. This approach harkens back to classic theorist views of perfectionism (e.g., see Adler, 1956; Horney, 1950; Pacht, 1984) and is also consonant with highly influential contemporary models of perfectionism such as the models of multidimensional perfectionism put forth by Frost and associates (1990) and Hewitt and Flett (1991). Furthermore, highlighting the trait elements of perfectionism also permits researchers to situate their findings relating perfectionism to health-related outcomes within the broader literature of personality and health (e.g., Friedman, 2000; Smith, 2006). Clearly, this approach has merit when considering perfectionism's role in the arenas of health and well-being, as contemporary researchers have confirmed early scholar's assertions that perfectionism is a critical factor for a host of outcomes such as health problems (Flett, Hewitt, & Molnar, Chap. 2; Kempke, Van Houdenhove, Claes, & Luyten, Chap. 5, this volume; Molnar, Reker, Culp, Sadava, & DeCourville, 2006; Sirois & Molnar, 2014), distress (Dunkley, Solomon-Krakus, & Moroz, Chap. 7, this volume), psychopathology (Burgess & DiBartolo, Chap. 8; Flett, Hewitt, & Nepon, Chap. 6, this volume), and even early mortality (Fry & Debats, 2009).

In light of these findings, research should undoubtedly continue to be directed at further elucidating models of trait perfectionism and how they influence indicators of health and well-being. Yet, it is also crucial to broaden our focus to understanding how perfectionistic cognitions and perfectionistic self-presentation are related to health functioning, psychopathology, and well-being, as these conceptualizations of perfectionism remain to be relatively understudied. Flett et al. (see Chap. 6, this volume), for example, make a strong case for focusing more attention on the cognitive aspects of perfectionism, by introducing and providing evidence to support their Cognitive Theory of Perfectionism, which posits that automatic perfectionist thoughts can impair physical functioning and well-being by prolonging and exacerbating the stress and emotional distress of perfectionists. The notion that perfectionistic self-presentation merits further consideration is discussed by Molnar, Sirois, and Methot-Jones (see Chap. 4, this volume) in their examination of the role of perfectionism in coping with chronic illness. As these authors note when elucidating their Stress and Coping Cyclical Amplification Model of Perfectionism in Illness, perfectionistic self-presentation can specifically undermine coping efforts and disease management by interfering with support-seeking behaviors. In other words, by hiding behind a mask of stoicism, perfectionists suffering from chronic illness may exacerbate their health problems and protract their stress because potential support providers, such as physicians, friends, and significant others may never know the stress, pain, and physical limitations that they are actually struggling with.

Issue 2. Unidimensional Versus Multidimensional?

A second issue concerns whether to conceptualize trait perfectionism as a unidimensional construct or as a multidimensional construct. At present, the majority of leading researchers in the field have moved beyond relying solely on unidimensional measures of perfectionism (e.g., Burns, 1980) to models underscoring the importance of unique features of perfectionism, including both intra- and interpersonal aspects, such as a compulsive striving for unreasonably high standards, strong concerns over making mistakes, nagging doubts about actions, high levels of self-criticism, perceiving large discrepancies between one's goals and one's progress toward those goals, high standards for others, being orderly, neat and tidy, and making self-worth conditional on acceptance from others (e.g., Frost et al., 1990; Hewitt & Flett, 1991; Hill, Huelsman, Furr, Kibler, & Vicente, 2004; Slaney et al., 2001), often employing one of the three most influential multidimensional models of perfectionism in their studies (i.e., the MPS-F, Frost et al., 1990; the MPS-HF, Hewitt & Flett, 1990, 1991; and the APS-R, Slaney et al., 2001).

The adoption of multidimensional conceptualizations of perfectionism is clearly a critical development in the field, as these models allow researchers to not only emphasize the complexity of this personality construct, but to highlight the importance of distinguishing different dimensions of perfectionism for health and well-being, which allow for more targeted clinical interventions and treatments. For instance, it appears that socially prescribed perfectionism (MPS-HF, Hewitt & Flett, 1990; 1991) concern over mistakes (MPS-F, Frost et al., 1990) and discrepancy

(APS-R, Slaney et al., 2001) are the most relevant dimensions of trait perfectionism for various forms of psychopathology, such as depression, suicidal ideation, and anxiety (Burgess & DiBartolo, see Chap. 8, this volume, Frost et al., 1990; Flett, Hewitt, & Heisel, 2014; Hewitt & Flett, 1991; Rice, Leever, Christopher, & Porter, 2006; Shafran & Mansell, 2001). Further, self-oriented perfectionism is uniquely predictive of early mortality (Fry & Debats, 2009). However, these distinctions do not appear to be as pertinent for other aspects of health and well-being, such as in the context of coping with chronic illness (see Molnar et al., Chap. 4, this volume; Sirois & Molnar, 2014) or in the area of eating disorders (see Wade et al., Chap. 9, this volume). This has prompted some experts in the field to advocate for returning to unidimensional models of perfectionism which emphasize self-focused aspects of perfectionism that they contend may be most relevant in clinical settings (e.g., Clinical Perfectionism; Shafran, Cooper, & Fairburn, 2002). Continued research on the role of perfectionism in these two specific domains of health and well-being is clearly needed to help provide greater insight into this issue.

Issue 3. The Two-Factor Model

A third and related issue pertains to scholars' ostensible reliance on the two-factor model of perfectionism in health and well-being. Since Frost, Heimberg, Holt, Mattia, and Neubauer's (1993) original factor analysis demonstrating that two underlying factors could be extracted from the Multidimensional Perfectionism Scales (MPS-F; Frost et al., 1990; MPS-HF; Hewitt & Flett, 1991), mounting evidence indicates that two basic forms of perfectionism, often referred to as "Perfectionistic Strivings" and "Perfectionistic Concerns," or as "Personal Standards" and "Self-Critical Perfectionism" can be extrapolated from virtually any trait measure of perfectionism (e.g., Dunkley, Blankstein, Masheb, & Grilo, 2006; Rice & Dellwo, 2002; Stoeber & Otto, 2006) using a variety of data analytic strategies (e.g., factor analysis, cluster analysis) and in a variety of samples such as students (Enns, Cox, Sareen, & Freeman, 2001; Frost, Heimberg, Holt, Mattia, & Neubauer, 1993; Rice & Dellwo, 2002), athletes (Haase et al., 1999; 2002), individuals from the general community (Molnar et al., 2006), and individuals experiencing psychopathology (Terry-Short, Owens, Slade, & Dewey, 1995). Although many researchers continue to be drawn to the parsimony afforded by the two-factor model of perfectionism and the convincing evidence showing that these factors are differentially associated with indicators of physical health, psychopathology, and well-being (Stoeber & Otto, 2006), not everyone has fully embraced it (Flett & Hewitt, 2006).

Indeed, the literature has become quite convoluted as researchers apply different labels to refer to these two high-order factors of perfectionism (e.g., "normal" versus "neurotic" perfectionists, Hamachek, 1978; "positive" versus "negative" perfectionism, Terry-Short et al., 1995; "passive" versus "active" perfectionism, Adkins & Parker, 1996; "adaptive" versus "maladaptive" perfectionism, Rice, Ashby, & Slaney, 1998; "personal standards" versus "maladaptive evaluation concerns" perfectionism, Frost et al., 1993; "healthy" versus "dysfunctional" perfectionism, Parker & Stumpf, 1995; "healthy" versus "unhealthy" perfectionism, Stumpf & Parker, 2000; "personal standards" versus "self-critical" perfectionism, Dunkley, Zuroff, & Blankstein, 2003; and "positive achievement striving" versus "maladaptive evaluative concerns" perfectionism, DiBartolo, Li, & Frost, 2008) and use different operational definitions of perfectionism to assess each form. Most germane to health and well-being is the fact that most researchers have largely ignored how these basic and underlying perfectionism factors are related to actual physical health. This is problematic given that some directly refer to these factors of perfectionism as "healthy" versus "unhealthy" without directly assessing health and well-being (e.g., Sapieja, Dunn, & Holt, 2011; Stumpf & Parker, 2000) and in light of evidence documenting that some indicators of "healthy" perfectionism (e.g., self-oriented perfectionism from the MPS-HF; Hewitt & Flett, 1991) are associated with poorer health and early mortality (Fry & Debats, 2009; Hadjistavropoulos, Dash, Hadjistavropoulos, & Sullivan, 2007; Saboonchi & Lundh, 2003).

Finally, it could be argued that this more condensed model also equates to the loss of precision and richness of description that was originally offered by the more nuanced assessments of multidimensional perfectionism. It seems likely that the essence of socially prescribed perfectionism, for example, which uniquely emphasizes interpersonal aspects of perfectionism and an overarching sense of helplessness (Flett et al., 2014; Hewitt & Flett, 1991) gets lost when collapsing it with other indicators of "Perfectionistic Concerns" that highlight intrapersonal elements of perfectionism. Consequently, this potential loss of precision or fidelity could result in a loss of targeted clinical interventions that could possibly undermine treatment efforts.

Perhaps, one way to handle this issue is to create a hybrid model of perfectionism, as has been done in the subjective well-being literature (e.g., see Busseri, Sadava, & DeCourville, 2007). That is, a second-order perfectionism factor could be created including each of the dimensions of perfectionism, which would decompose the variance in perfectionism into both common and dimension-specific sources. This type of model would help researchers clarify the relationship between perfectionism and indicators of health and well-being by allowing them to test simultaneously how both the common variance and the dimension-specific sources of variance in perfectionism are related to health and well-being. For instance, it could be that the dimension-specific sources of variance demonstrate more consistent and robust relationships with indices of health and well-being compared to the common variance, which would underscore the unique facets of perfectionism. Alternatively, it could be that it is only the common variance among dimensions of perfectionism that is substantively related to health and well-being. These questions can be addressed by assessing the relations between both common and dimension-specific sources of variance in perfectionism and indices of health and well-being. When we consider that the constructs of health and well-being can themselves be assessed at both broad and more specific levels, the potential for even more nuanced and complex relations among perfectionism dimensions, health, and well-being becomes apparent.

A second way to address these issues is to employ person-centered approaches, which allow researchers to detect different configurations of perfectionism as they occur within individuals, without setting the dimensions in opposition to one another. Consequently, these procedures allow researchers to consider the dimensions simultaneously without losing the shared variance and the original essence of the constructs. Put differently, when employing the person-centered approach, the goal is to discover patterns of thinking, feeling, and behaving within people. So, it is not the individual components of perfectionism that are of paramount interest, as the person-centered approach places priority on integrated configurations of perfectionism dimensions within people (Magnusson, 2003). As noted in Rice et al. (Chap. 11, this volume), person-centered analyses have not only helped to shed light on the prevalence and associated features of different types of perfectionism in students across a variety of academic settings, but also have addressed the issue of the relative adaptiveness of having high standards for performance. Furthermore, some of our work demonstrates that there are indeed unique profiles of perfectionism within individuals who are coping with chronic illness (assessed by MPS-HF; Hewitt & Flett, 1991). Moreover, the relative healthiness of self-oriented perfectionism varies as a function of the other dimensions of perfectionism included, such that self-oriented perfectionism does not appear to be associated with poorer health or well-being unless it was combined with high levels of other-oriented and socially prescribed perfectionism (Molnar, Flett, Sirois, & Hewitt, forthcoming).

Issue 4. Suppression

Suppression effects are becoming an increasingly salient issue in our field. Indeed, the potentially adaptive effects of Perfectionistic Strivings (or its components) often are only uncovered once the joint variance between Perfectionistic Strivings and Perfectionistic Concerns has been statistically accounted for in the analyses (see Hill, Huelsman, & Araujo, 2010; Stoeber, Kobori, & Brown, 2014a). Some researchers suggest that it is important to test multiple dimensions of perfectionism simultaneously so that researchers can statistically control for the joint variance among the dimensions of perfectionism so as to "purify" the dimension of interest (Aldea & Rice, 2006; Stoeber, Schneider, Hussain, & Matthews, 2014b). These suppression effects have been replicated numerous times suggesting that they are not simply a statistical artefact that can be brushed under the proverbial carpet. Suppression effects clearly should be carefully attended to in the field of perfectionism. The questions are how best to model these suppression effects and how best to interpret them?

With regard to modeling these suppression effects, most researchers simply include both Perfectionistic Strivings and Perfectionistic Concerns in their regression equations simultaneously. There is nothing ostensibly wrong with this approach from a statistical point of view. However, when employing analytic techniques such as ordinary least squares regression or structural equation modeling, this general approach may limit the amount of information that can be gleaned from such analyses because it does not permit researchers to directly model the often substantial joint variance between Perfectionistic Strivings and Perfectionistic Concerns. However, employing a hybrid model or a person-centered approach to the study of perfectionism in health and well-being may potentially provide researchers with alternate methods of handling suppression. As outlined above, the hybrid approach would allow researchers to directly and simultaneously model both the common variance and unique variance of Perfectionistic Strivings and Concerns, providing greater information and a more nuanced analysis. A person-centered approach would also appear to be quite appropriate for gaining a better understanding of these suppression effects. Indeed, when explaining how to interpret suppression effects in the context of perfectionistic cognitions, Stoeber et al. (2014a) asserted that "-if we have two individuals who report the same frequency of perfectionistic concerns cognitions, but different frequencies of perfectionistic strivings cognitions-the individual reporting a higher frequency of strivings cognitions should feel better (more positive affect, less negative affect, fewer depressive symptoms) than the individual reporting a lower frequency of strivings cognitions (p.657)." These hypothesized within person configurations of perfectionistic cognitions (and analogously, within person configurations of trait perfectionism) along with the hypothesized differences between these different groups of individuals can be directly and empirically tested with a person-centered approach, such as Latent Profile Analysis.

Yet, even when employing these sophisticated statistical techniques we are still left with the nagging question as to what Perfectionistic Strivings really represent when its joint variance with Perfectionistic Concerns has been accounted for in the analyses, especially when we consider that the shared variance among the different dimensions of perfectionism is often quite sizeable (i.e., correlations typically ranging from 0.40 to 0.70; Enns et al., 2001; Stoeber & Otto, 2006; Stoeber et al., 2014a). One plausible interpretation put forth by Stoeber et al. (2014a) is that "including perfectionistic concerns in the equation therefore clears out the "negativity" in perfectionistic strivings' predictive validity that is due to its covariance with perfectionistic concerns, thereby making room for the positive effects of perfectionistic strivings to show (p.657)." In other words, Perfectionistic Strivings itself may be uniquely adaptive or at least not as maladaptive relative to Perfectionistic Concerns. This explanation is quite viable. However, when we hold Perfectionistic Concerns constant in our analyses, thus accounting for the overlapping variance between Perfectionistic Strivings and Perfectionistic Concerns, are we still assessing Perfectionistic Strivings per se or is the variant we are left with more akin to conscientiousness rather than perfectionism? This is a question that deserves further consideration, given the consistent positive associations between Perfectionistic Strivings and conscientiousness and the general lack of association between Perfectionistic Concerns and conscientiousness (Hewitt & Flett, 2007; Hill, McIntire, & Bacharach, 1997; Stoeber, Otto, & Dalbert, 2009). Indeed, most people would argue that striving for excellence or having high standards is adaptive, but according to historical accounts and present models of perfectionism (e.g., Ellis, 2002; Horney, 1950; Frost et al., 1990; Hewitt & Flett, 1991) Perfectionistic Strivings does not simply reflect striving for excellence, but a compulsive need to be absolutely perfect. Therefore, researchers are urged to direct greater attention to disentangling the effects of conscientiousness and Perfectionistic Strivings in future studies, especially when examining perfectionism in the context of health and well-being, where both constructs are highly relevant.

Theme 2: The Pervasiveness of Perfectionism

One theme that becomes abundantly clear throughout the present volume is that the effects of perfectionism do not appear to be circumscribed to particular facets of health and well-being, but cut across multiple indicators and across multiple life domains. Indeed, the chapters that comprise this volume provide compelling evidence indicating that perfectionism not only contributes to the etiology and maintenance of a host of psychopathologies, such as anxiety (see Burgess & DiBartolo, Chap. 8, this volume), eating disorders (see Wade, O'Shea, & Shafran, Chap. 9, this volume), and depression (see Flett et al., Chap. 6, this volume), but is also highly relevant in the realm of physical health, as perfectionism has been implicated in physical health problems (see Flett et al., Chap. 2, this volume), coping with chronic illness (see Kempke et al., Chap. 5; Molnar et al., Chap. 4, this volume), and in the practice of health behaviors (see Sirois, Chap. 3, this volume). Researchers also recognize that perfectionism may exert many of its effects on health and well-being via its involvement in the generation, enhancement, and protraction of stress responses often via poor coping abilities (see Dunkley et al., Chap. 7, this volume).

Finally, convincing evidence from the last section of this volume indicates that the health-related effects of perfectionism also generalize across a broad spectrum of social contexts. Sherry, Mackinnon, and Gautreau (see Chap. 10, this volume), for example, present their expanded social disconnection model (SDM) of perfectionism, which highlights the interpersonal ramifications of perfectionism for health and well-being. Their expanded SDM provides a comprehensive understanding of how different perfectionism dimensions create vulnerabilities for poor interpersonal relationships; which, in turn, lead to a host of negative outcomes concerning health and well-being. Rice, Richardson, and Ray (see Chap. 11, this volume), on the other hand, review new evidence linking perfectionism to academic outcomes and to well-being in students across various academic settings. They thoughtfully conclude that perfectionism is highly relevant in this domain and that a multivalenced model of perfectionism is most appropriate when examining perfectionism in the context of academic settings, as their review indicates that Perfectionistic Strivings tends to be linked with positive academic indicators such as self-reported GPA, mastery goal orientations, and self-determination, whereas Perfectionistic Concerns tend to be related to poorer academic outcomes, such as perceiving courses as being more difficult, test anxiety, and experiencing higher levels of negativity before exams.

In a similar vein, Stoeber and Damian (see Chap. 12, this volume) provide an insightful analysis of the role of perfectionism with respect to three fundamental aspects of individuals' professional lives that are concomitant with employees' health and well-being: work engagement, workaholism, and job burnout. In their chapter, they provide clear evidence linking both Perfectionistic Strivings and Perfectionistic Concerns to workaholism. Yet, Stoeber and Damian highlight the complexity of studying perfectionism in the context of work, by demonstrating that Perfectionistic Strivings and Perfectionistic Concerns can be differentiated when studying work engagement and job burnout, such that Perfectionistic Strivings appear to be generally associated with positive outcomes in employees, such as greater work engagement and less burnout, whereas Perfectionistic Concerns tend to contribute to poorer outcomes for employees, such as less work engagement and greater burnout. They close by offering two conceptual models grounded by theory and the extant literature in an effort to guide future researchers explicate why Perfectionistic Strivings and Perfectionistic Concerns are differentially related to burnout.

From the purview of this edited volume, there is little doubt that perfectionism's associations with health and well-being are far-reaching. However, in light of the importance of person by situation interactions (e.g., Funder, 2008; Swan & Selye, 2005) and some evidence indicating that perfectionism may be more relevant for some life domains (e.g., work, academic, and social relationships; Sherry et al., Chap. 10, this volume; Rice et al., Chapter, 11, this volume; Slaney & Ashby, 1996; Stoeber & Damian, Chap. 12, this volume; Stoeber & Stoeber, 2009) relative to others, needed at this point is more programmatic research aimed at assessing how different life contexts can shape and contour relations among perfectionism, health, and well-being. For example, despite some promising new findings (see Kempke et al., Chap. 5, Molnar et al., Chap. 4, this volume), very little research has explored how perfectionism may contribute to health functioning and engagement in health-related behaviors in the context of chronic illness.

Moreover, the majority of studies have almost exclusively concentrated on aspects of perfectionism in the patient who is experiencing the illness, rather than exploring the psychosocial context in which the patient lives, including family members and/or other significant individuals in the person's life. Consequently, research has failed to systematically study how perfectionism in caregivers contributes to the patient's health and well-being and conversely how perfectionism in patients affects the health and well-being of caregivers (for a noteworthy exception, see Hewitt, Flett, & Mikail, 1995). This omission in the literature is rather perplexing given the convincing findings illustrating dyadic effects of perfectionism (Mackinnon et al., 2012; Sherry et al., Chap. 10, this volume) and work demonstrating that family members imposed standards on the patients can communicate to them that they must be "perfect" patients (Anderson & Wolpert, 2004).

Finally, although an extensive literature supports that perfectionism is prevalent in children and represents a public health issue for this population (Flett & Hewitt, 2014), the role of perfectionism in children's health functioning and problems remains a pressing issue in the field. Analogous to findings in adults, perfectionism has been associated with a host of adjustment difficulties and stress in children and adolescents (Flett & Hewitt, 2012). The high levels of stress inherent in perfectionism likely contribute to health problems in children and adolescents, as they do in adults, but this is an open question. Likewise, we continue to lack a clear understanding of the mechanisms that may link perfectionism to health in children.

From a developmental psychopathology framework, the impact of perfectionism on health in children may occur through several pathways. For instance, perfectionism can affect children's health via dysregulation of the hypothalamic–pituitary–adrenal axis (HPA) and overactivation of inflammatory processes. A second potential pathway is through a higher constellation of maternal, paternal, and environmental risk characteristics (including parental perfectionism), and the effects of these risk characteristics on parenting quality that lead to both higher levels of child perfectionism and poorer health in these children. Finally, the developmental psychopathology framework also suggests that not all children who are high in perfectionism will exhibit poor health, highlighting the importance of potential moderators.

Theme 3: Adaptive Versus Maladaptive Perfectionism

It is not uncommon for individuals who have achieved remarkable success to directly attribute their success to their perfectionism. For example, Tiger Woods, Justin Timberlake, Barbara Streisand, Anna Wintour, and Martha Stewart (just to name a few) have all publically referred to themselves as perfectionists and have suggested that perfectionism is an important ingredient for their success, which dovetails with research indicating that individuals are often hesitant to relinquish their perfectionism because they attribute their successes to it and believe that it is fundamental to their identity (Slaney & Ashby, 1996; Slaney, Chadha, Mobley, & Kennedy, 2000). The notion that perfectionism can actually have some adaptive value is appealing to many given how deeply woven perfectionism is in our society. Yet, there is also a growing awareness of the costs of perfectionism, particularly in the areas of health and well-being, suggesting that our love affair with perfectionistic ambitions based on the underlying assumption that striving for perfection leads to a "perfect" life lacks foundational support.

Several chapters in the present volume touch on this popular issue to varying degrees, with some authors directly championing the notion that perfectionism has some adaptive value for health and well-being (e.g., Rice et al., Chap. 11, Stoeber et al., Chap. 12, this volume) and others contending that perfectionism is by its very nature maladaptive and unhealthy (e.g., Flett et al., Chaps. 2 and 6). Indeed, full discussions on this topic can be found in several papers (e.g., see Flett & Hewitt, 2006; Greenspon, 2000; Stoeber & Otto, 2006). Yet, the chapters that comprise this volume clearly demonstrate the need to move beyond asking whether perfectionism is simply adaptive or maladaptive, especially with regard to Perfectionistic Strivings, because the findings that emerge reveal that the answers to this question are far more complicated than this question affords.

Although the research presented in this volume provides overwhelming evidence indicating that Perfectionistic Concerns is a risk factor for poorer health and well-being (see Burgess & DiBartolo, Chap. 8; Flett et al., Chap. 6; Molnar et al., Chapter, 4; Sirois, Chap. 3) and that this association is largely explained by stress processes (Dunkley et al., Chap. 7, this volume) and social disconnection (Sherry et al., Chap. 10, this volume), the findings concerning Perfectionistic Strivings suggest that it is neither healthy nor unhealthy in the absolute sense. Rather, the relative healthiness or unhealthiness of Perfectionistic Strivings depends on several factors, such as the population under study, whether the overlapping variance between Perfectionistic Strivings and Perfectionistic Concerns has been accounted for in the analyses, the context under study, and whether particular indirect pathways (e.g., stress, social disconnection, health-related behaviors) that link Perfectionistic Strivings with indices of health and well-being are included in the study or not. Thus, it is time to begin asking more complex questions that will provide much more substantive information, such as under what circumstances, and for whom, does Perfectionistic Strivings have the most harmful or beneficial consequences?

Perhaps, Perfectionistic Strivings are less detrimental for health and well-being in relatively young and healthy samples or in contexts, such as academic and work settings, where perfectionism is highly valued and consistently awarded (see Rice et al., Chap. 11; Stoeber & Damian, Chap. 12, this volume). Yet, emerging evidence indicates that Perfectionistic Strivings may be a vulnerability factor for poor health and well-being in the context of chronic illness, when individuals can no longer relentlessly strive toward their unrealistically high standards. Indeed, Sirois, Molnar, and Methot-Jones (forthcoming) provide compelling evidence to support this notion. Our meta-analysis of 65 studies on perfectionism and health demonstrates that the association between Perfectionistic Strivings and health problems varies as a function of sample type with Perfectionistic Strivings contributing to poorer health in chronically ill samples and to a lesser degree in community samples. However, we also found that Perfectionistic Strivings is not significantly related to health in university students. Our results further demonstrate the need to attend to measurement issues when assessing the relative adaptiveness of perfectionism for health; we found that Perfectionistic Strivings was associated with greater health problems when assessed with the relevant subscales from the MPS-HF and the MPS-F, but was associated with fewer health problems when assessed with the Standards subscale from the APS-R.

Finally, our study also provides evidence that highlights the importance of evaluating sex-related differences when examining the role of perfectionism in health (Sirois et al., forthcoming). Specifically, we found that Perfectionistic Strivings was only linked with poorer health outcomes in women. Perhaps, these sex-related differences represent discrepancies in stress, such that women tend to experience higher levels of stress than men, likely due to the multiple social roles that women fulfill (Matud, 2004). Taken together, these results directly speak to the complexity inherent in the study of perfectionism in health and well-being and to the importance of considering key contextual variables as moderators when examining associations between Perfectionistic Strivings and health. Indeed, recognizing this complexity is critical for perfectionism research to continue to make meaningful progress, as greater awareness of these complications increases the scope of applications of perfectionism in the fields of health and well-being.

Theme 4: Issues in Measuring Health and Well-Being in Relation to Perfectionism

Understanding the ways in which perfectionism may be differentially related to health and well-being depends not only on the ways in which perfectionism is conceptualized and measured, but also on the ways in which health and well-being are assessed. As noted by Sirois and Molnar (see Chap. 1, this volume), there is considerable overlap between health and well-being, with physical health outcomes playing a key role in outcomes related to psychological well-being. In this regard, research that aims to address how and why perfectionism is linked to health or well-being should consider assessing both outcomes simultaneously rather than separately. This would also provide opportunities for more sophisticated analyses of the potentially dynamic and reciprocal process linking perfectionism to these related outcomes.

Another key consideration in assessing the significance of perfectionism for health and well-being centers on the specificity versus breadth issue. Increasing understanding about the ways that perfectionism may create risk or resilience for health and well-being will require assessing the links to a range of health-related outcomes. However, the level at which these outcomes are assessed is equally important. For example, researchers are beginning to investigate perfectionism in the context of specific chronic conditions such as chronic fatigue syndrome (e.g., Kempke et al., Chap. 5 this volume; Sirois & Molnar, 2014), fibromyalgia (Molnar, Sadava, Flett, & Colautti, 2012), and inflammatory bowel disease (IBD; Flett, Baricza, Gupta, Hewitt, & Endler, 2011). As tempting as it may be to cull together the evidence from these and other studies on a limited set of chronic health conditions to draw broad conclusions about the implications of perfectionism for chronic illness, it is important to acknowledge the potential differences between different chronic health conditions which may attenuate or amplify the effects of perfectionism. As noted by Molnar et al. (Chap. 4, this volume), certain chronic conditions such as IBD may amplify the social disconnection experienced by perfectionists and thus exacerbate stress and troubling physical symptoms. Expanding the scope of chronic illnesses examined with respect to perfectionism is clearly needed as is more applied work with different clinical samples to further understand which processes are unique to or generalizable across multiple populations.

The issue of specificity is also important when considering other important health-related outcomes such as health behaviors. Much of the work on health behaviors and perfectionism has tended to lump both health-promoting and health compromising behaviors together when examining the links to perfectionism dimensions (see Sirois, Chap. 3 this volume). This can obscure potential differential relations with Perfectionistic Strivings and Perfectionistic Concerns and result in inaccurate conclusions about the role of perfectionism in health behaviors. The other extreme, only examining single health behaviors, can also be problematic as this approach may yield equivocal results that are hard to reconcile across different studies because of the specific health behaviors examined. Using an established and empirically informed framework for conceptually organizing health behaviors, such as that proposed by Vickers, Conway, and Hervig (1990) may be one way to address these issues.

A final issue centers on the point that much of the research on perfectionism, health, and well-being has relied solely on self-report assessments of health outcomes. While this may be convenient and necessary in some instances, advances in our understanding of the health outcomes associated with perfectionism depend upon employing more sophisticated and objective methods of assessment. As noted by Dunkley et al. (Chap. 7, this volume), research assessing stress and markers of HPA axis activity using biological measures such as cortisol can help clarify the nature of the relationships between Perfectionistic Strivings and Perfectionistic Concerns to the physical effects of stress that may go beyond self-reported perceptions of stress. Accordingly, to gain a genuine appreciation of the complexity inherent in the study of perfectionism in the context of health and well-being, it will be critical for us to conduct integrative multi-method studies from multidisciplinary teams with expertise in areas such as biology, psychology, and sociology that reflect biopsychosocial models of health and well-being.

Concluding Remarks and Additional Ideas for Future Research

As noted throughout this volume, perfectionism appears to be endemic to Western society, with evidence indicating that perfectionistic tendencies are prevalent both in adults (Stoeber & Stoeber, 2009) and in children (Chan 2009; Rice, Ashby, & Gilman, 2011). The pervasiveness and promotion of perfectionism is truly alarming given that perfectionism is associated with significant costs to individual's health and well-being such as early mortality (Fry & Debats, 2009), psychopathology (Burgess & DiBartolo, Chap. 8, this volume; Flett et al., Chap. 6, this volume; Shafran & Mansel, 2001), greater stress (Dunkley et al., Chap. 7, this volume), less engagement in health-promoting behaviors (Sirois, Chap. 3, this volume), and poorer physical health (Molnar et al., Chap. 4, Kempke et al., Chap. 5, this volume) that cut across an extensive array of social contexts such as interpersonal relationships (Sherry et al., Chap. 10, this volume), academic pursuits (Rice et al. Chapter 11, this volume), and work (Stoeber et al., Chap. 12, this volume). Undoubtedly, a greater appreciation of the role of perfectionism in health and well-being has never been so essential. However, scholars in the field are now well-armed to tackle these important issues.

The next era of research examining perfectionism in health and well-being will likely be influenced by many of the themes emphasized by the contributors of the present volume including broadening our scope of inquiry to incorporate multiple levels of perfectionism, such as perfectionistic traits, cognitions, and self-presentational behavior; expanding our methodological and analytical repertoires to include hybrid models of perfectionism, person-centered approaches, daily diary studies, dyadic studies, and social network analyses, and both long- and short-term prospective longitudinal studies of perfectionism, health and well-being; placing greater emphasis on conceptual models to guide our work; being more cognizant of how different social contexts can help shape perfectionism's association with health and well-being; and moving beyond the simplistic debate of whether perfectionism is adaptive or maladaptive to more interesting questions that concern the specific mechanisms and processes that may render certain perfectionists particularly vulnerable to poor health and well-being, but leave other perfectionists less vulnerable to these same consequences.

Importantly, the chapters that comprise this volume indicate that it is time to move beyond studying simple bivariate correlations between perfectionism and health and between perfectionism and well-being. Rather, researchers should examine the underlying mechanisms that explicate the relations between perfectionism and indices of health and well-being. This will not only have important theoretical implications on which more concise models of perfectionism and health can be built, but will provide insight into developing more specific interventions to help perfectionists avoid the possible negative health implications of perfectionism.

Unfortunately, though, apart from a few noteworthy exceptions, investigations directed at increasing our understanding of perfectionism in health and well-being have largely been atheoretical. Consequently, we believe that the paramount contribution of this book is the wealth of new theoretically based models provided by leading researchers in the field that not only help to clarify the specific processes that link perfectionism to health and/or well-being, but also consider the importance of key factors that likely influence the processes under study. These rich theoretical insights will surely be invaluable to both new and seasoned researchers alike, as they provide fertile ground to expand our knowledge base on the role of perfectionism in health and well-being.

References

Adkins, K. K., & Parker, W. (1996). Perfectionism and suicidal preoccupation. *Journal of Personality and Social Psychology, 64,* 529–543.

Adler, A. (1956). The neurotic disposition. In H. L. Ansbacher & R. R. Ansbacher (Eds.), *The individual psychology of Alfred Adler* (pp. 239–262). New York: Harper.

Aldea, M. A., & Rice, K. G. (2006). The role of emotional dysregulation in perfectionism and psychological distress. *Journal of Counseling Psychology, 53*(4), 498–510.

Anderson, B. J., & Wolpert, H. A. (2004). A developmental perspective on the challenges of diabetes education and care during the young adult period. *Patient Education and Counseling, 53,* 347–352.

Burgess, A., & DiBartolo, P. M. (in press). Anxiety and perfectionism: Relationships, mechanisms, and conditions. In F. M. Sirois & D. S. Molnar (Eds.), *Perfectionism, health, and well-being* (pp. TBA). New York: Springer.

Burns, D. D. (1980). The perfectionist's script for self-defeat. *Psychology Today, 14,* 34–52.

Busseri, M., Sadava, S. W., & DeCourville, N. (2007). A hybrid model for research on subjective well-being: Examining common and component-specific sources of variance in life satisfaction, positive affect, and negative affect. *Social Indicators Research, 83,* 413–445.

Chan, D. W. (2009). Dimensionality and typology of perfectionism: The use of the Frost mutidimensional perfectionism scale with Chinese gifted students in Hong Kong. *Gifted Child Quarterly, 53,* 174–187. doi:10.1177/0016986209334963.

DiBartolo, P., Li, C., & Frost, R. O. (2008). How do the dimensions of perfectionism relate to mental health? *Cognitive Therapy and Research, 32,* 401–417. doi:10.1007/s10608-007-9157-7.

Dunkley, D. M., Zuroff, D. C., & Blankstein, K. R. (2003). Self-critical perfectionism and daily affect: Dispositional and situational influences on stress and coping. *Journal of Personality and Social Psychology, 84,* 234–252.

Dunkley, D. M., Blankstein, K. R., Masheb, R. M., & Grilo, C. M. (2006). Personal standards and evaluative concerns dimensions of "clinical" perfectionism: A reply to Shafran et al. (2002, 2003) and Hewitt et al. (2003). *Behaviour Research and Therapy, 44,* 63–84.

Dunkley, D. M., Solomon-Krakus, S., & Moroz, M. (in press). Personal standards and self-critical perfectionism and distress: Stress, coping, and perceived social support as mediators and moderators. In F. M. Sirois & D. S. Molnar (Eds.), *Perfectionism, health, and well-being* (pp. TBA). New York: Springer.

Ellis, A. (2002). The role of irrational beliefs in perfectionism. In G. L. Flett & P. L. Hewitt (Eds.), *Perfectionism: Theory, research, and treatment* (pp. 217–229). Washington, DC: American Psychological Association.

Enns, M. W., Cox, B. J., Sareen, J., & Freeman, P. (2001). Adaptive and maladaptive perfectionism in medical students: A longitudinal investigation. *Medical Education, 35,* 1034–1042.

Flett, G. L., & Hewitt, P. L. (2006). Positive versus negative perfectionism in psychopathology: A comment on Slade and Owens's dual process model. *Behavior Modification, 30*(4), 472–495.

Flett, G. L., & Hewitt, P. L. (2012). Perfectionism and cognitive factors in distress and dysfunction in children and adolescents: Introduction to the special issue. *Journal of Rational-Emotive and Cognitive-Behavior Therapy, 30,* 53–61.

Flett, G. L., & Hewitt, P. L. (2014). A proposed framework for preventing perfectionism and promoting resilience and mental health among vulnerable children and adolescents. *Psychology in the Schools, 51,* 899–912.

Flett, G. L., Hewitt, P. L., Blankstein, K. R., & Gray, L. (1998). Psychological distress and the frequency of perfectionistic thinking. *Journal of Personality & Social Psychology, 75*(5), 1363–1381.

Flett, G. L., Baricza, C., Gupta, A., Hewitt, P. L., & Endler, N. S. (2011). Perfectionism, psychosocial impact and coping with irritable bowel disease: A study of patients with crohn's disease and ulcerative colitis. *Journal of Health Psychology, 16*(4), 561–571.

Flett, G. L., Hewitt, P. L., & Heisel, M. J. (2014). The destructiveness of perfectionism revisited: Implications for the assessment of suiced risk and the prevention of suicide. *Review of General Psychology, 18,* 156–172.

Flett, G. L., Hewitt, P. L., & Nepon, T. (in press). Perfectionism, worry, and rumination in health and mental health: A review and a conceptual framework for a cognitive theory of perfectionism. In F. M. Sirois & D. S. Molnar (Eds.), *Perfectionism, health, and well-being* (pp. TBA). New York: Springer.

Flett, G. L., Hewitt, P. L., & Molnar, D. S. (in press). Perfectionism in health and illness from a person-focused, historical perspective. In F. M. Sirois & D. S. Molnar (Eds.), *Perfectionism, health, and well-being* (pp. TBA). New York: Springer.

Friedman, H. S. (2000). Long-term relations of personality and health: Dynamisms, mechanisms, tropisms. *Journal of Personality, 68*(6), 1089–1107.

Frost, R. O., Marten, P. A., Lahart, C., & Rosenblate, R. (1990). The dimensions of perfectionism. *Cognitive Therapy and Research, 14,* 449–468.

Frost, R. O., Heimberg, R. G., Holt, C. S., Mattia, J. I., & Neubauer, A. L. (1993). A comparison of two measures of perfectionism. *Personality and Individual Differences, 14*(1), 119–126.

Fry, P. S., & Debats, D. L. (2009). Perfectionism and the five-factor personality traits as predictors of mortality in older adults. *Journal of Health Psychology, 14*(4), 513–524.

Funder, D. C. (2008). Persons, situations, and person-situation interactions. In O. P. John, R. W. Robins, & L. A. Pervin (Eds.), *Handbook of personality: Theory and research* (pp. 568–580). New York: Guilford.

Greenspon, T. S. (2000). "Healthy perfectionism" is an oxymoron! Reflections on the psychology of perfectionism and the sociology of science. *Journal of Secondary Gifted Education, 22,* 176–181.

Haase, A. M., Prapavessis, H., & Owens, R. G. (1999). Perfectionism and eating attitudes in competitive rowers: Moderating effects of body mass, weight classification and gender. *Psychology and Health, 14,* 643–657.

Haase, A. M., Prapavessis, H., & Owens, R. G. (2002). Perfectionism, social physique anxiety and disordered eating: A comparison of male and female elite athletes. *Psychology of Sport and Exercise, 3,* 209–222.

Hadjistavropoulos, H., Dash, H., Hadjistavropoulos, T., & Sullivan, T. (2007). Recurrent pain among university students: Contributions of self-efficacy and perfectionism to the pain experience. *Personality and Individual Differences, 42,* 1081–1091.

Hamachek, D. E. (1978). Psychodynamics of normal and neurotic perfectionism. *Psychology: A Journal of Human Behavior, 15,* 27–33.

Hewitt, P. L., & Flett, G. L. (1991). Perfectionism in the self and social contexts: Conceptualization, assessment, and association with psychopathology. *Journal of Personality and Social Psychology, 60,* 456–470.

Hewitt, P. L., & Flett, G. L. (1990). Perfectionism and depression: A multidimensional analysis. *Journal of Social Behavior and Personality, 5,* 423–438.

Hewitt, P. L., & Flett, G. L. (2007). When does conscientiousness become perfectionism? *Current Psychiatry, 6,* 49–60.

Hewitt, P. L., Flett, G. L., & Mikail, S. F. (1995). Perfectionism and relationship adjustment in pain patients and their spouses. *Journal of Family Psychology, 9*(3), 335–347.

Hewitt, P. L., Flett, G. L., Sherry, S. B., Habke, M., Parkin, M., Lam, R. W., McMurtry, B., Ediger, E., Fairlie, P., & Stein, M. (2003). The interpersonal expression of perfection: Perfectionistic self-presentation and psychological distress. *Journal of Personality and Social Psychology, 84,* 1303–1325.

Hill, R. W., McIntire, K., & Bacharach, V. R. (1997). Perfectionism and the Big Five factors. *Journal of Social Behavior & Personality, 12,* 257–270.

Hill, R. W., Huelsman, T. J., & Araujo, G. (2010). Perfectionistic concerns suppress associations between perfectionistic strivings and positive life outcomes. *Personality and Individual Differences, 48,* 584–589.

Hill, R. W., Huelsman, T. J., Furr, M., Kibler, J., & Vicente, B. B. K. C. (2004). A new measure of perfectionism: The perfectionism inventory. *Journal of Personality Assessment, 82*(1), 80–91.

Horney, K. (1950). *Neurosis and human growth.* New York: Norton.

Kempke, S., Van Houdenhove, B., Claes, S., & Luyten, P. (in press). The role of perfectionism in chronic fatigue syndrome. In F. M. Sirois & D. S. Molnar (Eds.), *Perfectionism, health, and well-being* (pp. TBA). New York: Springer.

Kobori, O. (2006). *A cognitive model of perfectionism: The relationship of perfectionism personality to psychological adaptation and maladaptation.* Unpublished doctoral dissertation, University of Tokyo, Tokyo.

Mackinnon, S. P., Sherry, S. B., Antony, M. M., Stewart, S. H., Sherry, D. L., & Hartling, N. (2012). Caught in a bad romance: Perfectionism, conflict, and depression in romantic relationships. *Journal of Family Psychology, 26,* 215–225.

Magnusson, D. (2003). The person-centered approach: Concepts, measurement models, and research strategy. *New Directions in Child and Adolescent Development, 101,* 3–23.

Matud, M. P. (2004). Gender differences in stress and coping styles. *Personality and Individual Differences, 37,* 1401–1415. doi:10.1016/j.paid.2004.01.010.

Molnar, D. S., & Sirois, F. M. (in press). Perfectionism in the context of chronic illness. In F. M. Sirois & D. S. Molnar (Eds.), *Perfectionism, health, and well-being* (pp. TBA). New York: Springer.

Molnar, D. S., Reker, D. L., Culp, N. A., Sadava, S. W., & DeCourville, N. H. (2006). A mediated model of perfectionism, affect, and physical health. *Journal of Research in Personality, 40*(5), 482–500.

Molnar, D. S., Sadava, S. W., Flett, G. L., & Colautti, J. (2012). Perfectionism and health-related quality of life in women with fibromyalgia. *Journal of Psychosomatic Research, 73,* 295–300.

Molnar, D. S., Flett, G. L., Sirois, F. M., & Hewitt, P. L. (forthcoming). A person-centered approach to multidimensional perfectionism in chronic illness: Perfectionism profiles in physical functioning, psychological health, and social resources.

Pacht, A. R. (1984). Reflections on perfectionism. *American Psychologist, 39,* 386–390.

Parker, W. D., & Stumpf, H. (1995). An examination of the multidimensional perfectionism scale with a sample of academically talented children. *Journal of Psychoeducational Assessment, 13,* 372–383.

Rice, K. G., & Dellwo, J. P. (2002). Perfectionism and self-development: Implications for self-esteem, depression, and college adjustment. *Journal of Counseling & Development, 80,* 188–196.

Rice, K. G., Ashby, J. A., & Slaney, R. B. (1998). Self-esteem as a moderator between perfectionism and depression: A structural equations analysis. *Journal of Counseling Psychology, 45,* 304–314.

Rice, K. G., Leever, B. A., Christopher, J., & Porter, J. D. (2006). Perfectionism, stress, and social (dis)connection: A short-term study of hopeless, depression, and academic adjustment among honors students. *Journal of Counseling Psychology, 53,* 524–534.

Rice, K. G., Ashby, J. S., & Gilman, R. (2011). Classifying adolescent perfectionists. *Psychological Assessment, 23*(3), 563–577.

Rice, K. G., Richardson, C. M., & Ray, M. E. (in press). Perfectionism in academic settings. In F. M. Sirois & D. S. Molnar (Eds.), *Perfectionism, health, and well-being* (pp. TBA). New York: Springer.

Saboonchi, F., & Lundh, L.-G. (2003). Perfectionism, anger, somatic health, and positive affect. *Personality and Individual Differences, 35,* 1585–1599. doi:10.1016/S0191-8869(02)00382-3.

Sapieja, K. M., Dunn, J. G. H., & Holt, N. L. (2011). Perfectionism and perceptions of parenting styles in male youth soccer. *Journal of Sport & Exercise Psychology, 33,* 20–39.

Shafran, R., & Mansell, W. (2001). Perfectionism and psychopathology: A review of research and treatment. *Clinical Psychology Review, 21,* 879–906.

Shafran, R., Cooper, Z., & Fairburn, C. G. (2002). Clinical perfectionism: A cognitive-behavioural analysis. *Behaviour Research and Therapy, 40*(7), 773–791.

Sherry, S. B., Mackinnon, S. P., & Gautreau, C. M. (in press). Perfectionists don't play nicely with others: Expanding the social disconnection model. In F. M. Sirois & D. S. Molnar (Eds.), *Perfectionism, health, and well-being* (pp. TBA). New York: Springer.

Sirois, F. M. (in press). Perfectionism and health behaviors: A self-regulation resource perspective. In F. M. Sirois & D. S. Molnar (Eds.), *Perfectionism, health, and well-being* (pp. TBA). New York: Springer.

Sirois, F. M., & Molnar, D. S. (2014). Perfectionism and maladaptive coping styles in patients with chronic fatigue syndrome, irritable bowel syndrome and fibromyalgia/arthritis and in healthy controls. *Psychotherapy and Psychosomatics, 83*(6), 384–385.

Sirois, F. M., Molnar, D. S., & Methot-Jones, T. (forthcoming). Does striving for perfection guarantee perfect health?: A meta-analysis of perfectionism, stress, and health.

Slaney, R. B., & Ashby, J. (1996). Perfectionists: Study of a criterion group. *Journal of Counseling and Development, 74,* 393–398.

Slaney, R. B., Chadha, N., Mobley, M., & Kennedy, S. (2000). Perfectionism in Asian Indians: Exploring the meaning of the construct in India. *The Counseling Psychologist, 28,* 10–31.

Slaney, R. B., Rice, K. G., Mobley, M., Trippi, J., & Ashby, J. S. (2001). The revised almost perfect scale. *Measurement and Evaluation in Counseling and Development, 34*(3), 130–145.

Smith, T. W. (2006). Personality as risk and resilience in physical health. *Current Directions in Psychological Science, 15,* 227–231.

Stoeber, J., & Damian, L. E. (in press). Perfectionism in employees: Work engagement, workaholism, and burnout. In F. M. Sirois & D. S. Molnar (Eds.), *Perfectionism, health, and well-being* (pp. TBA). New York: Springer.

Stoeber, J., & Otto, K. (2006). Positive conceptions of perfectionism: Approaches, evidence, challenges. *Personality and Social Psychology Review, 10,* 295–319.

Stoeber, J., & Stoeber, F. S. (2009). Domains of perfectionism: Prevalence and relationships with perfectionism, gender, age, and satisfaction with life. *Personality and Individual Differences, 46,* 530–535.

Stoeber, J., Otto, K., & Dalbert, C. (2009). Perfectionism and the big five: Conscientiousness predicts longitudinal increases in self-oriented perfectionism. *Personality and Individual Differences, 47,* 363–368.

Stoeber, J., Kobori, O., & Tanno, Y. (2010). The multidimensional perfectionism cognitions inventory-English (MPCI-E): Reliability, validity, and relationships with positive and negative affect. *Journal of Personality Assessment, 92,* 16–25.

Stoeber, J., Kobori, O., & Brown, A. (2014a). Examining mutual suppression effects in the assessment of perfectionism cognitions: Evidence supporting multidimensional assessment. *Assessment, 21,* 647–660.

Stoeber, J., Schneider, N., Hussain, R., & Matthews, K. (2014b). Perfectionism and negative affect after repeated failure: Anxiety, depression, and anger. *Journal of Individual Differences, 35*(2), 87–94.

Stumpf, H., & Parker, W. D. (2000). A hierarchical structural analysis of perfectionism and its relation to other personality characteristics. *Personality and Individual Differences, 28,* 837–852.

Swann, W. B. Jr., & Seyle, C. (2005). Personality's comeback and its emerging symbiosis with social psychology. *Personality and Social Psychology, 31,* 155–165.

Terry-Short, L. A., Owens, R. G., Slade, P. D., & Dewey, M. E. (1995). Positive and negative perfectionism. *Personality and Individual Differences, 18*(5), 663–668.

Vickers, R. R., Conway, T. L., & Hervig, L. K. (1990). Demonstration of replicable dimensions of health behaviors. *Preventive Medicine, 19,* 377–401.

Wade, T. D., O'Shea, A. O., & Shafran, R. (in press). Perfectionism and eating disorders. In F. M. Sirois & D. S. Molnar (Eds.), *Perfectionism, health, and well-being* (pp. TBA). New York: Springer.

Index

F. M. Sirois, D. S. Molnar (eds.), *Perfectionism, Health, and Well-Being*,
DOI 10.1007/978-3-319-18582-8

MIX
Papier aus verantwortungsvollen Quellen
Paper from responsible sources
FSC® C105338
FSC
www.fsc.org

If you have any concerns about our products,
you can contact us on
ProductSafety@springernature.com

In case Publisher is established outside the EU,
the EU authorized representative is:
Springer Nature Customer Service Center GmbH
Europaplatz 3, 69115 Heidelberg, Germany

Printed by Libri Plureos GmbH
in Hamburg, Germany